Edwin R. Gerler Jr.
Editor

Handbook
of School Violence

Pre-publication
REVIEWS,
COMMENTARIES,
EVALUATIONS . . .

"The *Handbook of School Violence* offers an eclectic collection of chapters about school violence. It provides quality chapters that cover a wide range of topics. Of particular note are chapters about the importance of positive 'connectedness' and 'identification with academics' as ways of thinking about positively developing our youth and preventing them from violent behavior.

This book is important as it evidences the arrival of solid academic research on the topic of school violence. That the research is offered by young, new academics bodes well for future efforts on the topic of school violence both in the research arena and the arena where it counts the most: the schools that will benefit from such researchers as they work to establish and maintain safe learning environments for all students."

Joanne McDaniel, MPA
Director, Center for the Prevention
of School Violence, Raleigh, NC

"The *Handbook of School Violence* is an important addition to the growing literature of school violence. Gerler has assembled an array of topics on school violence that have not yet been published in one book. The topics span the causes of school violence and progress nicely to prevention and intervention topics. The special focus on crisis intervention is very important to all students in pupil personnel programs including social work, psychology, nursing, and counseling. These kinds of crisis skills are essential for every PPS school professional. Professionals in the field who want to learn more about school violence issues and interventions also would benefit from this book. I commend the contributors to and editor of this handbook. Many children and schools will benefit from their efforts."

Ron Avi Astor, PhD
Associate Professor,
University of Southern California
Schools of Social Work and Education

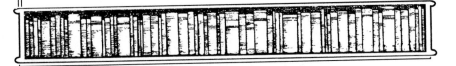

More pre-publication
REVIEWS, COMMENTARIES, EVALUATIONS . . .

"**G**erler has assembled an impressive, cross-disciplinary team of authors that discuss central issues in the conceptualization of root causes of school violence and best practices in its prevention and response. Readers will be challenged to think about school violence in new and innovative ways, while also having access to pragmatic strategies that can be used by any school to enhance its comprehensive school safety plan. It is a must-read for researchers and practitioners."

Michael Furlong, PhD
Professor, University of California,
Santa Barbara Center for School-Based
Youth Development

THRP

The Haworth Reference Press
An Imprint of The Haworth Press, Inc.
New York • London • Oxford

Handbook
of School Violence

THE HAWORTH PRESS
School Violence
Edwin R. Gerler Jr.
Senior Editor

Handbook of School Violence edited by Edwin R. Gerler Jr.

Additional titles of related interest

Bullying Behavior: Current Issues, Research, and Interventions edited by Robert A. Geffner, Marti T. Loring, and Corinna Young

Threats in Schools: A Practical Guide for Managing Violence by Joseph T. McCann

Bullying, Peer Harassment, and Victimization in the Schools: The Next Generation of Prevention edited by Maurice J. Elias and Joseph E. Zins

Issues in School Violence Research edited by Michael J. Furlong, Gale M. Morrison, Dewey G. Cornell, and Russell Skiba

Kids and Violence: The Invisible School Experience edited by Catherine N. Dulmus and Karen M. Sowers

Handbook
of School Violence

Edwin R. Gerler Jr.
Editor

The Haworth Reference Press
An Imprint of The Haworth Press, Inc.
New York • London • Oxford

Published by

The Haworth Reference Press, an imprint of The Haworth Press, Inc., 10 Alice Street, Binghamton, NY 13904-1580.

Cover design by Marylouise E. Doyle.

Library of Congress Cataloging-in-Publication Data

Handbook of school violence / Edwin R. Gerler, Jr., editor.
    p. cm.
   Includes bibliographical references and index.
   ISBN 0-7890-1623-0 (hard : alk. paper)—ISBN 0-7890-1624-9 (soft : alk. paper)
   1. School violence—United States—Prevention—Handbooks, manuals, etc. 2. Conflict management—United States—Handbooks, manuals, etc. 3. School crisis management—United States—Handbooks, manuals, etc. I. Gerler, Edwin R.
   LB3013.32.H36 2004
   371.7'82—dc21

                                                     2003012287

CONTENTS

ABOUT THE EDITOR

Edwin R. Gerler Jr., EdD, is Professor in the College of Education at North Carolina State University, where he is also the past Associate Dean for Research and External Affairs. He has been a teacher, counselor, and consultant in schools throughout the United States. His major interest is in the application of computer and Internet technology to education and human services.

Dr. Gerler has written extensively, served as Editor in Chief of two national counseling journals, and coproduced a film on elementary school counseling. He is the founding co-editor of the online publication *Meridian: A Middle School Computer Technologies Journal* (http://www.ncsu.edu/meridian/). He is also the founding editor of the *Journal of School Violence* (http://genesislight.com/JSV.html).

Dr. Gerler's books include *Counseling the Young Learner, Elementary School Counseling in a Changing World,* and *The Challenge of Counseling in Middle Schools.* His most recent textbook (with Stanley Baker) is *School Counseling for the 21st Century, Fourth Edition.* More information about this textbook is available at <http://vig.prenhall.com/catalog/academic/product/0,4096,0130494852-DES.00.html>.

His most recent book, *How the Naked Ape Got to the Land of Nod,* reflects his interest in using psychology, theology, and humor to examine human difficulties creatively. More information about his latest book is available at <http://www.genesislight.com>.

CONTRIBUTORS

Stephen E. Brock currently serves as an assistant professor at California State University, Sacramento. He previously worked for 18 years as a school psychologist. He has lectured nationally and published extensively in the area of school crisis response. He co-authored the book *Preparing for Crises in the Schools* and is the lead editor of the National Association of School Psychologists' (NASP) publication *Best Practices in School Crisis Prevention and Intervention.* Brock serves as a contributing editor to NASP's newsletter, *Communiqué,* and is on the editorial board of *The California School Psychologist.*

Dewey G. Cornell is the Curry Memorial Professor of Education in the Curry School of Education at the University of Virginia. He is the director of the Virginia Youth Violence Project, whose mission is to identify effective methods and policies for youth violence prevention, especially in school settings. Cornell is also a forensic clinical psychologist and a faculty associate of the Institute of Law, Psychiatry, and Public Policy. Since 1984, Dr. Cornell has conducted research on juvenile homicide, psychological assessment of violent youth, and school safety, authoring more than 90 professional publications in psychology and education. One of his current projects concerns the development and implementation of guidelines for schools to use in responding to student threats of violence.

Maura Dillon graduated from the University of California in 1989 with a bachelor's degree in community studies, and then moved to Vermont to work as a social activist on issues such as domestic violence, biotechnology, and independent media. In 1992 she moved to Berlin, Germany, where she studied political philosophy at the Free University. She then moved to Durham, North Carolina, where she enrolled as a PhD student at Duke University. After four years of academic immersion, she sought a more practical application of her ideas and chose to pursue a master's in counseling at North Carolina State University. Although she believes her own mediation and negotiation skills date back to becoming the oldest child of four in her family at age two and a half, she received her first formal mediation training at the Dispute Settlement Center in Durham. She currently resides in Pittsboro, North Carolina, where she works for child and family services at the OPC Area Program and makes functional pottery.

Shane R. Jimerson is a professor of counseling, clinical, and school psychology and child and adolescent development at the University of California, Santa Barbara. He is a co-editor of the NASP *Best Practices in School Crisis Prevention and Intervention* book and the author and co-author of more than 60 journal articles, chapters, and books. He is the co-author of a five-book series titled *Mourning Child Grief Support Group Curriculum* (published by Taylor and Francis, 2001). His scholarship and contributions have been recognized by multiple awards, including the Best Research Article Award from the Society for the Study of School Psychology/*Journal of School Psychology* (1998, 2000), the Outstanding Research Article of the Year from the National Association of School Psychologists/*School Psychology Review* (2001), and the 2002 Early Career Scholar Award from the American Educational Research Association: Division E Human Development. He is the editor of *The California School Psychologist* journal and serves on the editorial boards of the *Journal of School Psychology, School Psychology Quarterly,* and *Journal of Early Childhood Research and Practice.* Jimerson serves as the co-chair of the International Crisis Response Network of the International School Psychology Association, and is also an active member of the school crisis prevention and response committees of the California Association of School Psychologists and the National Association of School Psychologists.

Cheryl Kaiser-Ulrey was a doctoral student at Florida State University's APA-approved PhD program in counseling psychology and school psychology. She began her internship in fall 2002 and graduated in the summer of 2003.

Laura Kallus received her master's degree in anthropology with a concentration in development at George Washington University. She completed life history interviews with Latino gang members and disseminated the preliminary results in a publication of the American

Anthropology Association, Committee on Refugees and Immigrants. She has had extensive experience working with and advocating for gang members. She is currently the vice president of research and evaluation for a consulting firm in Miami, Florida, a firm that evaluates more than 45 youth crime prevention programs throughout Miami Dade County.

Michael J. Karcher is an assistant professor of education and human development at the University of Texas at San Antonio. He received a PhD from the University of Texas at Austin in counseling psychology and an EdD from Harvard University in human development and psychology. For his research agenda on developmental interventions, he has developed measures of adolescent connectedness for preadolescents, adolescents, and late adolescents, for which he has published several empirical and validation studies. These measures have been translated into Spanish, Chinese, and French, which are used in both of his school-based, developmental intervention research programs, as well as in his research linking connectedness to both positive youth development and risk-taking behaviors, such as smoking and alcohol use. His research and teaching interests focus on school-based developmental interventions that promote adolescents' connectedness and social cognitive development, specifically developmental mentoring and pair counseling. His mentoring research reflects his own model of structured, cross-age mentoring in schools as well as his examination of best practices of adult-youth mentoring in schools. He is currently working with David L. DuBois on a handbook of youth mentoring, and, in collaboration with Communities in Schools, is conducting research on mentoring with Hispanic students in 40 schools in Austin and San Antonio. He has published his theoretical and empirical work on pair counseling, a developmental play therapy for children in dyads (or pairs), in the *International Journal of Play Therapy*, other journals, and book chapters. His expertise in school-based counseling and interventions informs his work on the editorial boards for two school counseling journals: *Professional School Counseling* and *Psychology in the Schools*.

Helen Lupton-Smith is an adjunct professor at North Carolina State University. She has a PhD in counselor education. Much of her research efforts and publications have focused on peer mediation. While obtaining her doctorate, she worked part-time with the Wake County

Public School System in Raleigh, North Carolina, assisting with the implementation of peer mediation programs and conflict resolution curricula in various pilot elementary, middle, and high schools. Her research, which evolved from that experience, focused on training high school students to be peer mediators and peer mediation trainers of elementary school students. The developmental benefits of the high school students involved in that experience were assessed.

David C. May is an associate professor and school safety fellow in the Department of Correctional and Juvenile Justice Services at Eastern Kentucky University. He received his PhD in sociology with emphasis in criminology from Mississippi State University in 1997. He has published numerous articles in the areas of causes of juvenile delinquency and adolescent fear of crime and a book that examines the relationship between adolescent fear of crime and weapon-related delinquency. He is presently co-authoring another book examining the antecedents of gun ownership and possession among adolescent male delinquents. His free time is spent with his wife, Natalie, and three small children, James, William, and Grace. He was activated for military duty in support of Operation Enduring Freedom and returned to his academic endeavors in 2003.

Robert L. McGlenn is a clinical and school psychologist who, in addition to maintaining a private practice since 1977, has experience in a variety of mental health areas. He has worked as a school psychologist at both the elementary and secondary school levels, trained and supervised doctoral-level interns at area psychiatric hospitals and community-based clinics, and consulted with a residential treatment center for severely disturbed adolescents. McGlenn designed and directed the implementation of the crisis response plan to the Santana and Granite Hills High School shootings in March 2001. He presently serves as the coordinator of the Santana Recovery Project, which provides services and treatment to those traumatized by the event. Since the incident, he has spoken to numerous groups concerning school safety, treatment, and violence prevention, and has worked for the National School Safety Center as a trainer for the Community Oriented Policing Services program (COPS).

Jason W. Osborne is an assistant professor of educational psychology at North Carolina State University. His research interests focus on how the structure and nature of the self influences particular outcomes, such as academic and related nonacademic outcomes. He received his PhD in educational psychology from the University of Buffalo, where he also received significant training in self theory and social psychology.

Stephen A. Rollin is a professor in the combined program in counseling psychology and school psychology, as well as associate dean for graduate studies and research in Florida State University's College of Education. He is also the principal investigator on an Office of Juvenile Justice and Delinquency Prevention (OJJDP) sponsored grant on school violence prevention that is part of the Hamilton Fish Institute at George Washington University. He is director of the Center for Policy Studies at Florida State. Rollin received his EdD in counseling and guidance in 1970 from the University of Massachusetts. He is a licensed psychologist in the State of Florida, and is a member of the following professional organizations: American Psychological Association, Division of Counseling Psychology, Division of International Psychology; American Educational Research Association; and the American Society for Clinical Hypnosis.

Stacey Scheckner is currently a predoctoral intern working with adolescents at Sharp Mesa Vista Hospital in San Diego, California. She has worked on an individual and group basis with a variety of adolescent problems, such as eating disorders, self-mutilation, depression, suicidal ideation, past abuse, violent tendencies, and family problems. She is specifically dedicated to at-risk youth and aspires to having her own practice, helping children/adolescents and families. Her previous research efforts include Project KICK (Kids in Corporation with Kids), a drug/alcohol-based program that also teaches social skills, conflict resolution, communication skills, and self-esteem building. Scheckner's other endeavors include an elementary truancy prevention program with other doctoral students and professors at Florida State University. She is currently preparing an article that describes her dissertation work, detailing the implementation and empirical validation of a computer-mediated school violence prevention program at the elementary school level. She has also worked in a variety of settings, including hospitals, private practice, and university counseling center. Scheckner graduated with her PhD in counseling psychology and school psychology from Florida State University in August of 2003.

Richard Wagner is a professor in the Department of Psychology at Florida State University with a special interest in cognitive and behavioral science. His major area of research interest is the acquisition of complex cognitive knowledge and skills, which he has pursued in two domains. In the domain of reading, his research has focused on the role of reading-related phonological processing abilities in normal and abnormal development of reading skills and in the prediction, prevention, and remediation of dyslexia. In the domain of human intelligence, his research has focused on the role of practical knowledge and intelligence in intellectual performance manifested outside the classroom setting.

Preface

When I was like eleven, I was hanging out. I used to go to a middle school. It was for bad people, only bad people go there. It's a school just for bad people that had gotten kicked out of school. And I had got kicked out of my school cause they found me with a gun . . . I took it out on this dude. We had got in a fight, a Spanish dude. We started fighting and then I got mad and I took out the gun. I got locked up and they put me in that school. And then I started hanging out with wrong people. Started breaking into houses and stuff, started smoking weed and drinking Old English.

This is the voice of a gang member featured in Chapter 7 of the *Handbook of School Violence*. The book brings together many voices: the voices of violent youngsters and of the helpers who provide needed care; the voices of students who feel no connection with their families or with their work at school; the voices of those who strive to prevent these students from acting on their feelings of alienation; the voices of scholars—new and old—who create theory and research, laying the foundation for school violence prevention and intervention.

FEATURES OF THE HANDBOOK

The *Handbook of School Violence* addresses the causes of school violence, the prevention of school violence, and interventions in cases of school violence. The handbook features:

- an Internet site—<http://genesislight.com/hsv%20files>—that brings scholars and practitioners together to invent online and print products for school violence prevention and intervention;
- writing from new scholars, blended with the work of some veteran authors, to provide a foundation for creative thinking about school violence prevention and intervention;

- a new look at how "connectedness" with family, school, and academic success influences school violence;
- means to prevent school violence using (1) threat assessment techniques, (2) peer mediation programs, (3) empathy with youngsters involved in gangs, and (4) approaches for reducing weapons in schools;
- a focus on crisis intervention and support services that is rooted in field-based experience with school violence, particularly in the aftermath of the Santana High School shootings on March 5, 2001, in San Diego, California;
- an overview of how various domains of human functioning contribute to understanding the causes of school violence and to developing strategies for school violence prevention and intervention.

THE HANDBOOK AND THE INTERNET

This handbook is the foundation for a future series of books from The Haworth Press to present new thinking and scholarship on school violence. International discussions via the Internet will bring together ideas for other books in the series. In addition, the handbook is a companion work to the *Journal of School Violence,* a new professional journal launched in 2002 by The Haworth Press. Although they are print documents, both the handbook and the journal are living products in the sense that they will evolve hour by hour, day by day on the Internet and will be enriched by the varied, future possibilities offered by the Web. The Web sites for these products are as follows:

> *Handbook of School Violence:* <http://genesislight.com/hsv %20files/index.html>
> *Journal of School Violence:* <http://genesislight.com/JSV.html>

Those of us who are exploring the opportunities and the challenges of the Internet for confronting school violence see the Web as an amazing new tool. The print version of the *Handbook of School Violence,* for example, will be enriched as scholars and practitioners across the world and across cultures use the handbook's Internet site to offer immediate critique and new thinking to what exists in the book. The Internet also offers a visual companion to the words that are often insufficient in depicting the grief brought by school violence. Some of the Internet sites that have contributed to my thinking as I developed this handbook include the following:

Bullying Online
<http://www.bullying.co.uk/>
This site is part of the United Kingdom's National Grid for Learning and is linked to government departments, from health department Web sites, as well as from Web sites of more than 60 local governing councils and 12 U.K. police forces. The site incorporates approximately 30 different sections, including several on different types of school bullying policy and on other issues, such as mobile phone abuse and how to deal with racism.

Center for the Prevention of School Violence
<http://www.ncsu.edu/cpsv/>
Established in 1993, the center serves as a primary resource for dealing with the problem of school violence. The center, a public agency not motivated by profit, focuses on ensuring that schools are safe and secure so that every student is able to attend a school that is free of fear and conducive to learning.

Center for the Study and Prevention of Violence
<http://www.colorado.edu/cspv/>
Located at the University of Colorado, this site provides extensive resources for understanding the many facets of school violence.

Connect
<http://www.gold.ac.uk/connect/>
This initiative brings together practitioners and researchers throughout Europe to provide substantial and authoritative reports on school violence and to examine intervention strategies that appear most promising in terms of prior work and wide European applicability.

European Observatory of Violence in Schools
<http://www.obsviolence.pratique.fr/indexgb.html>
The observatory was founded in Bordeaux in September 1998 (jointly funded by Bordeaux University, the European Commission,

and the French Ministry of Education), as a research center for the study of violence in schools and urban violence in Europe.

Hamilton Fish Institute
<http://www.hamfish.org/>
The institute, with assistance from the U.S. Congress, was founded in 1997 to serve as a national resource to test the effectiveness of school violence prevention methods and to develop more effective strategies. The institute's goal is to determine what works and what can be replicated to reduce violence in America's schools and communities.

Harvard Youth Violence Prevention Center
<http://www.hsph.harvard.edu/hicrc/prevention.html>
An interdisciplinary center based in the Department of Health Policy and Management at the Harvard School of Public Health, the Harvard Youth Violence Prevention Center's (HYVPC) focus is on research partnerships and violence prevention within communities. HYVPC's area partners include: (1) the Education Development Center in Newton, MA, (2) the New England Medical Center, (3) seven Boston-based community agencies, and (4) representatives from a variety of government organizations, including the Boston Public Health Commission, the Boston Police Department, and the Boston mayor's office. Areas of particular focus include violence prevention, community improvement, and youth development.

Institute on Violence and Destructive Behavior
<http://darkwing.uoregon.edu/~ivdb/>
The Institute helps schools and social service agencies understand violence and destructive behavior to ensure the safety of young people and to facilitate the academic achievement and healthy social development of children and youth.

Keys to Safer Schools
<http://keystosaferschools.com/CriticalTraining.htm>
Keys to Safer Schools is dedicated to helping parents, schools, and other youth-oriented organizations to have a safer place to learn, work, and play in today's climate of rising youth violence. Keys to Safer Schools is an organization based in Bryant, Arkansas, with a

global presence through their extensive Web site, training, and network of associates.

National Association of Students Against Violence Everywhere
<http://nationalsave.org/>
SAVE's mission is to decrease the potential for violence in schools and communities by involving students in meaningful crime prevention, conflict management, and community service activities.

Nature and Prevention of Bullying
<http://www.gold.ac.uk/tmr/>
Sponsored by the research training initiative of the European Commission, this project studies the causes and prevention of bullying and social exclusion in schools.

October Center for the Study and Prevention of Youth Violence
<http://www.octobercenter.vcu.edu/index.html>
The October Center for the Study and Prevention of Youth Violence is a partnership between Virginia Commonwealth University and the Greater Richmond Community. The center is dedicated to the promotion of culturally sensitive strategies that effectively interrupt the cycle of violence, contribute to healing, and create safe environments where youth and families can grow and thrive, free of violence. The October Center was established by the Centers for Disease Control and Prevention as one of ten National Academic Centers of Excellence on Youth Violence Prevention.

Virginia Youth Violence Project
<http://youthviolence.edschool.virginia.edu/>
The mission of this project is to identify effective methods and policies for youth violence prevention, especially in school settings. The project conducts and disseminates research on the understanding and reduction of violent behavior, and provides education, consultation, and training for educators, psychologists, and other colleagues in the social, legal, and human services professions.

Youth Violence Prevention Center
<http://www.sph.umich.edu/yvpc/index.shtml>
Located at the University of Michigan's School of Public Health, the Youth Violence Prevention Center (YVPC) develops, implements,

and monitors comprehensive strategies that help prevent youth violence and promote healthy development through collaboration among community, university, and health department partners. The focus of the center is on interdisciplinary, ecologically and culturally relevant, community-based approaches to violence prevention. Its work is carried out by three distinct cores: training, implementation, and evaluation. The specific aims of the center are to: (1) build the scientific infrastructure to support the development of community-wide youth violence prevention interventions; (2) promote interdisciplinary strategies that foster collaboration; (3) work with community members to address youth violence prevention; (4) institutionalize violence prevention in health provider practice and training; and (5) develop an evaluation plan and surveillance system to monitor progress. The Youth Violence Prevention Center is based in Flint, Michigan, and is a community organization. Elementary through high school students participate in the center through the Youth Against Violence group. The YVPC is funded by the Centers for Disease Control and Prevention.

SOME THOUGHTS ABOUT THE CONTRIBUTORS TO THE HANDBOOK

The individuals who contributed chapters to this handbook include a variety of new scholars, joining a few of us who have been around a long time and who have a history of writing about topics related to school violence. Why did I choose these new scholars to contribute to this book? As is true with many creative endeavors, this book evolved from a series of fortunate accidents. As editor of the *Journal of School Violence,* I have had Internet contact with experts throughout the world, many of them veteran thinkers and writers on violence in schools and elsewhere. These experts have built a growing body of literature that invites new and creative thought from people whose scholarly careers are just beginning to take shape and who have lengthy futures ahead for creative thinking and conducting studies on school violence. These new scholars are confronted with special challenges as they think about integrating the study of school violence into their careers, challenges that sharpen their work and make them particularly valuable contributors to this handbook. These new scholars must find ways for their research efforts to add value and make a difference to the citizens and donors who support their institutions.

In spite of—or perhaps because of—new challenges, emerging scholars bring to the study of school violence a kind of uncharted energy. One of them wrote to me: "I feel really good about the chapter—I think it may be the best thing I've ever written, at least it is what I am most proud of." Another wrote: "I really owe you a note of thanks for suggesting this chapter. In wrestling with this chapter I have been forced to think through my theories and ideas at a much higher level than I have to this point, and I think that this process is taking me to a whole new level in my research and thinking." Still another wrote: "I am interested in doing a follow-up/long-term study on my topic—do you have any suggestions for such a project? I envision something that includes photos as I have many from the last five years. I have the connections to develop a big project."

As someone who is at the "beginning of the end" of his academic career, I enjoy collaborating with scientists, artists, and pioneers whose ideas are newly forming and are apparently unfettered. Those of us who have been around for a while know our limits too well and need to be energized by explorers who have learned, as yet, only a few limits to creative ventures.

CONCLUDING COMMENTS

School violence exists along a lengthy continuum, at one end marked by minor incidents involving everyday fighting, name-calling, bullying, and minor property destruction and at the other end marked by extortion, rape, homicide, and mass murder. The continuing evolution of terrorism makes the prospects of mass violence in our schools horrific on a new scale. Likewise, the use of the Internet as a tool to incite violence is still in its infancy. The *Handbook of School Violence* is a first step in the creation of new print and online products that will offer innovative and practical ideas for addressing the problem of school violence in its various manifestations.

PART I:
CAUSES OF SCHOOL VIOLENCE

Psychologist Harry Stack Sullivan (1947) wrote: "In most general terms, we are all much more simply human than otherwise, be we happy and successful, contented and detached, miserable and mentally disordered, or whatever" (p. 7). He believed that troubled humans often delude themselves into thinking that they are alienated—alone in the world—that they have problems and concerns unlike those of others. This construct, known as the "delusion of uniqueness," seems to be at the root of school violence—where young people, often alienated from their peers, feeling unconnected with the school community and the world around them, resort to planning and implementing violent acts that win the attention and notoriety of their immediate worlds (and beyond, through constant and thorough media coverage).

This may seem to some an overly simple view of what causes school violence, and, in fact, it is only a small part of the picture. Psychologist Arnold Lazarus (1981) has argued persuasively that the foundation of troubled behavior, including abusive and violent acts, may be found in several domains of human functioning, which he identified using a convenient acronym, BASIC ID:

B—Behavior
A—Affect
S—Sensation
I—Imagery
C—Cognition
I—Interpersonal Relations
D—Diet and Physical Functioning

1

The following is a cursory examination of how each domain helps in understanding the causes of school violence.

Behavior

Certain elements in the school and social environments of young people foster and maintain acts of violence. Extraordinary misbehavior, for example, often elicits significant attention from peers, from teachers and school administrators, and—in especially noteworthy cases—from the media. On the other hand, behaviors that pertain to the central mission of schooling, in particular, behaviors that contribute to academic achievement, are less impressive, less visible, and are often ignored by peers—or worse, ridiculed. Violent and destructive behaviors are also more likely to be featured in movies and video games than are the routine and persistent behaviors required for achievement. Violent and destructive behaviors, therefore, are in a much stronger position to be emulated.

Affect

Many schools have large enrollments and unmanageable class sizes, which make it difficult for educators to attend to how children feel about themselves and the world surrounding them. Teachers and other professionals in the schools are often unable to create the classroom conditions that renowned theorist Carl Rogers (1961) deemed crucial for emotional growth and development, namely, genuineness, empathy, and positive regard. Some children who also lack emotional support at home and elsewhere outside of school therefore feel further diminished and devalued at school—and are prone to lash out in violent and abusive ways.

Sensation

We become aware of the world through our senses. For children, learning about the world is often unplanned and informal. This learning involves a seemingly endless barrage of new and varied sensory stimuli. In a world where our senses are constantly stimulated by technological marvels, students often characterize school as a place that lacks stimuli promoting learning, exploring, and discovering. Although the more stoic among us may view such characterizations as self-serving excuses for irresponsibility, students who simply exist at school—who see the classroom as boring and unstimulating—may resist the environment in angry and abusive ways. Students may also attempt to escape this environment with alcohol, drugs, and other substances that destroy the capacity for learning and increase the propensity for violence.

Imagery

How students experience the world through mental images is open to speculation and is in need of research. How students translate their mental images into overt behavior and action is also an area open to exploration. The portrayal of violence in the media and elsewhere undoubtedly structures the imagery that children experience regularly in their lives. We know from firsthand testing that some children translate this troubling imagery into unspeakable acts of violence that seemingly defy explanation. Other children are able to impede this imagery or channel it into more positive directions. We need to hear about the violent mental images our children nourish, and then we need to discover ways to block the growth of these images into violent acts.

Cognition

Psychologist Albert Ellis (1971) has noted that violent and abusive behavior is often the product of irrational thinking. When, for example, I become upset or angry, the emotion is, according to Ellis, a product of "catastrophizing" (blowing out of proportion) something that I have encountered in my daily routine. Those of us who are older remember saying as children, "Sticks and stones may break my bones but names will never hurt me." Or we said, "I'm rubber. You're glue. What you say to me bounces off me and sticks to you." These simple sayings helped us inhibit overblown retaliation for relatively harmless verbal attacks. Physical violence at school is sometimes the product of irrational, overblown retaliation for verbal abuse. The more rational students can be about the difficult challenges they face at school and elsewhere, the less likely they will become involved in acts of violence.

Interpersonal Relations

Students often lack the motivation to interact compassionately toward their peers, challenging one another when appropriate, but supporting one another when necessary. Students often find it difficult to tolerate ethnic, cultural, and religious differences. Many find it hard to treat these differences as sources of curiosity and exploration rather than barriers to friendship and excuses for violence among student groups. Youngsters often lack a sense of community at school. They feel alienated and—in extreme cases—the desire to strike out violently.

Diet and Physical Functioning

How students care for themselves physically is likely to contribute to how they feel about the world and how they react to the circumstances they face. Students whose diets are problematic, whose physical well-being is far less than adequate, may feel insecure and unworthy—alienated in an affluent society where attractive, able-bodied youngsters are sought after and admired. In extreme cases, young people who face ridicule because of their physical presence may retaliate in abusive and violent ways.

An Overview of Part I

Part I of the *Handbook of School Violence* cannot cover all the possible causes for violence in schools. Instead, it focuses on the ways that connectedness and identification with academics influence school violence. In his thought-provoking chapter, "Connectedness and School Violence: A Framework for Developmental Interventions," Michael Karcher notes:

> All adolescents need to achieve a minimum amount of connectedness across their social ecology, but not all are able to establish sufficient connectedness within the family, school, and other conventional contexts and relationships. Youths at risk for

engaging in violence often establish an imbalance, having more unconventional than conventional forms of connectedness.

Jason Osborne's chapter, "Identification with Academics and Violence in Schools," builds on the theme of connectedness, focusing on the concept of bonding to school. Osborne addresses two interesting scenarios:

> In the first case, students who removed academics as a source of self-esteem are likely to replace academics with peer relationships, which might facilitate undesirable behavior. In the second case, students who were academically disidentified would experience significant levels of frustration at being forced to continue attending school, which might lead to violent behaviors.

As more books appear in this series, scholars will examine other causes of school violence. In addition, as the *Handbook of School Violence* Internet site evolves, practitioners, graduate students, and other scholars will be able to go online to critique and build on what is presented here on the causes of school violence. Individuals may follow the evolution of the handbook's Internet site at the following address: <http://genesislight.com/ hsv%20files/>.

REFERENCES

Ellis, A. (1971). *Reason and emotion in psychotherapy.* New York: Lyle Stuart.
Lazarus, A. A. (1981). *The practice of multimodal therapy.* New York: McGraw-Hill.
Rogers, C. R. (1961). *On becoming a person.* Boston: Houghton Mifflin.
Sullivan, H. S. (1947). *Conceptions of modern psychiatry.* Washington, DC: William Alanson White Psychiatric Foundation.

Chapter 1

Connectedness and School Violence: A Framework for Developmental Interventions

Michael J. Karcher

Adolescent connectedness significantly impacts violence in schools. The main goals of this chapter are to define the mechanisms by which promoting connectedness can prevent youth violence and to present a framework for constructing developmental intervention programs to prevent violence in schools. Developmental interventions provide myriad opportunities for school counselors and prevention programs to prevent violence in schools. Central to developmental interventions is the tenet that by helping youths establish a balance of connectedness to school, family, and friends, they will become less likely to engage in violent behavior (Hawkins, Farrington, and Catalano, 1998; Mulvey and Cauffman, 2001). Three principles from a framework for implementing developmental interventions are presented to highlight how connectedness-promoting interventions can fill a very important void in comprehensive violence-prevention programming in the schools. To illustrate these principles, two developmental interventions are profiled at the end of the chapter.

The model of connectedness presented in this chapter is derived from ecological and developmental theory. The model holds that each social world of the adolescent—school, friends, family, and neighborhood—can be characterized along a continuum of conventionality. Highly conventional worlds include those contexts, relationships, and activities that are structured, sanctioned, and supervised by adults in society. These contexts of connectedness are antithetical to problem behaviors and risk taking (Donovan, Jessor, and Costa, 1988). Conventional connectedness usually includes the social worlds of school, teachers, reading, religion, and family, all of which are structured by adults and directed toward the future. Positive orientations toward and active involvement in all of these serve to buffer against violence (Honora and Rolle, 2002; O'Donnell, Hawkins, and Abbott, 1995). Connectedness to peers, friends, and the neighborhood may be conventional if the nature of these relationships and activities reflects attitudes and conventions prescribed by adults. However, the neighborhood and time spent with peers, friends, and romantic partners, given their unsupervised nature, often elicit activities that can lead to problem behaviors. The unconventional worlds of connectedness are those social ecologies in which youths themselves typically dictate the norms, activities, and structure that govern what youths do. Youths' neighborhoods and friendships are the most common examples of contexts in which unconventional connectedness develops. All adolescents need to achieve a minimum amount of connectedness across their social ecology, but not all are able to establish sufficient connectedness within the family, school, and other conventional contexts and relationships. Youths at risk for engaging in violence often establish an imbalance, having more unconventional than conventional forms of connectedness.

Connectedness also varies developmentally and ecologically in ways that bear directly on violence in schools. This chapter provides definitions of connectedness, highlights its variations across contexts during adolescence, and illustrates the different effects of conventional and unconventional connectedness on violent and delinquent behavior in order to identify important parameters and practices for promoting connectedness in schools. These principles may be used to create interpersonally focused, developmental interventions to prevent and reduce violence in schools.

CONNECTEDNESS

A Critical Target for Violence Prevention in Schools

Promoting connectedness to school serves to counterbalance the increasing importance of connectedness to peers and friends in adolescence. This counterbalance is important because connectedness to friends and peers who engage in unconventional, problem behaviors is one of the best predictors of violent behavior (Olin, 2001). Youths who engage with peers and friends in unconventional, illicit behaviors, and who denounce school and other conventional contexts and relationships are most prone to violence. In contrast, youths who are actively involved in, enjoy, and feel good at school are less likely to engage in violent behavior (Cernovich and Giordana, 1992; Farrington, 1991; O'Donnell, Hawkins, and Abbott, 1995). For this reason, promoting active engagement in school and positive feelings about school (namely, connectedness to school) should be at least one of the primary targets of school-based violence prevention programs. Promoting connectedness to friends who engage in conventional, prosocial behaviors should be another.

Connectedness has several precursors, including attachment to caregivers, relatedness to others, and feelings of belongingness within social groups. Connectedness is a function of attachment, interpersonal social support, and group-level experiences of belonging because connectedness—active involvement and caring for others—is a reciprocation of the support and positive affect that other people, in specific places, have provided youths, and that have supported the youths' self-esteem and skill development. These processes reveal opportunities and parameters for structuring programs and experiences in schools that can assuage violent behaviors.

Active Involvement and Persistent Caring in One's Social Ecology

The concept of connectedness has sometimes been restricted to participation or involvement in interpersonal relationships (Gilligan, 1991; Jordan et al., 1991), but this definition is needlessly restrictive and inconsistent with the public's broader use of the term. More broadly, connectedness includes the acts of giving back to, being involved with, and being affectively invested in other people, places, and activities. "Connectedness occurs when a person is actively involved with another person, object, group or environment, and that involvement promotes a sense of comfort, well-being, and anxiety-reduction" (Hagerty et al., 1993, p. 293). For example, youths can be connected to school and reading just as they may care for, enjoy, and be actively involved with a teacher, peer, friend, or parent.

The ecology of adolescent connectedness includes all of the significant micro-, macro-, and mesosystems that adolescents experience in their day-to-day lives (Bronfenbrenner, 1979). Microsystems include youths' important relationships in the home with parents and siblings, in the school with teachers and peers, and in the neighborhood with friends. The macrosystems of connectedness are the larger institutions in youths' lives, such as the neighborhood, family, school, religion, and cultural group membership. The mesosystems are those processes of connection that link micro- and macrosystems. For example, one main mesosystem in schools is reading, an activity that links youths to school, teachers, and friends. Adolescent connectedness generalizes from dyadic relationships (or microsystems) toward the activities and contexts associated with these contexts. Connectedness reflects an extension and reciprocation of basic attachment and bonding processes to the adolescents' widening social ecology. As with indicators of attachment, connectedness reflects proximity seeking and positive affect for people, places, and activities in the adolescent's life.

The Reciprocation of Experiences of Belonging, Relatedness, and Attachment

Connectedness has, as its source, those positive relationships and experiences with others in which one experiences esteem and competence. Early in life, positive attachments with caregivers provide children with their initial sources of support, esteem, and praise (Ainsworth, 1989; Kohut, 1977). Later, other forms of social support enter the lives of youths, such as interpersonal relatedness (e.g., with siblings, teachers, peers, and friends) and experiences of group belonging. Therefore, attachment and social support can be viewed as the initial sources of relatedness and belonging, which youths reciprocate through connectedness.

Attachment

The presence of connectedness early in life takes the form of a strong caregiver-child bond. It reflects the behavioral reciprocation of affective experiences (Chodorow, 1978; Stem, 1985) by the child to the caregiver through proximity seeking and positive affect. Like the toddler, the adolescent becomes connected in those worlds that provide the adolescent the basic interpersonal ingredients of self-development—empathy, praise, and attention within relationships in which they receive clear, consistent structure (Kohut, 1977; Kohut and Elson, 1987). It is well known that toddlers who have healthy, secure attachments with caregivers demonstrate positive affect and proximity seeking toward caregivers (Ainsworth, 1989). Similarly, adolescents report the most positive affect and demonstrate proximity seeking toward those people—whether parents, siblings, peers, friends, or teachers—who have provided them empathy, praise, and attention in a clear and consistent manner. It is out of these relationship contexts that skills, talents, and interests (self-developments) develop, because youth make the greatest efforts to demonstrate interpersonal competence with those supportive people (Kohut, 1977).

Youths report and demonstrate greater connectedness in the worlds in which they have felt praised (and thus competent), empathized with (and thus understood), and attended to as special (and thus important)—whether in school, home, neighborhood, or religious contexts. This is key to intervention and may explain why these qualities have been found in the most effective prevention programs (Schorr, 1988; Catalano et al., 2002). It is arguable that no amount of skills training or heightened knowledge will effectively curb violent behavior among youths if such interventions are devoid of positive interpersonal relationships in which youths can feel competent, understood, and important.

Social Support

It appears that youths' past and present levels of social support will affect their receptivity to interpersonal interventions. Evidence suggests that early attachment experiences predict individuals' openness to receiving help and willingness to accept social support during adolescence. Mallinckrodt (1991) found that the quality of late adolescents' relationships with their families and with important nonfamily members were significant predictors of the quality of their therapeutic working alliance. He argued that "the ability to meaningfully connect with others is presumed to be a good indicator of their capacity to form productive working alliances" (p. 402). Therefore, adolescents' ability to benefit from social support appears to be constrained by the quality of their past experiences with other people, such that those who have received the least social support may be the hardest to reach. In fact, aggressive youths who tend to overestimate their social relatedness (and report excessively high self-esteem) can be the most difficult to reach through interventions (Prasad-Gaur, Hughes, and Cavell, 2001).

Relatedness

In a similar way, security in the caregiver-child relationship determines to some degree the interpersonal relatedness youths experience in later relationships with peers, friends, and teachers. Relatedness is the felt sense of closeness and being valued by another individual. Hagerty et al. (1993) suggest that relatedness is a "functional, behavioral system rooted in early attachment behaviors and patterns," such that "affiliation or exploration are activated only after the attachment behavioral system" (p. 292). Breaks in relatedness, such as through forced separations or empathic lapses, undermine connectedness by lessening youths' willingness to invest time and energy in relationships with others (Richters and Martinez, 1993). For example, Midgley, Feldlauffer, and Eccles (1989) reported that students who moved from elementary classrooms where they experienced high teacher support to middle school classrooms in which they perceived less teacher support showed decreases in their interest in learning. In short, where relatedness is undermined, connectedness will lapse as well. Youths whose teachers do not provide consistent sources of empathy, praise, and attention and clear, consistent structure will become less involved in school and will become less inclined to seek out these ingredients of self-development in school and school-based relationships (van Aken and Asendorpf, 1997).

Belonging

When relatedness is experienced collectively from multiple people in a defined context, the result is the experience of belonging. Belonging becomes of paramount importance to adolescents. The need to belong is defined, not as the need to be the passive recipient of supportive relationships, but as the need for "frequent [positive and pleasing] interaction plus persistent caring" (Baumeister and Leary, 1995, p. 292). Hagerty and colleagues (1993) describe connectedness to others, as well as to organizations and their activities, as a reciprocation of experienced belonging and relatedness that has, directly or indirectly, as its source primary attachment relationships. How accepted and valued a youth feels by particular groups shapes how connected—involved and concerned—that youth will be with people and activities in those groups or organizations. One confirms or acknowledges the experience of belonging and being related by becoming connected through increased interaction and caring for other people and places (see Figure 1.1).

Defined from an ecological point of view, adolescent connectedness reflects a youth's volitional involvement in relationships, contexts, and activities which he or she finds positive, worthwhile, and important. It is the reciprocation of one's positive experiences of relatedness and belonging with others in particular places. Connectedness is a function of both the social support presented to individuals as well as their openness to receiving that social support and to feeling secure in those relationships and contexts.

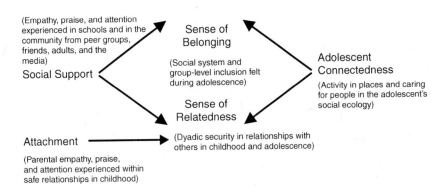

FIGURE 1.1. A hypothesized model of the sequence of attachment, social support, relatedness, and belonging in the development of adolescent connectedness

Because connectedness reflects the presence of such profoundly important experiences, it has been linked to physical health as well as to clinical disorders and risk-taking behaviors (Bonny et al., 2000; Hendry and Reid, 2000; Resnick, Harris, and Blum, 1993). Indeed, a great deal of research on delinquency and violent behavior shows that connectedness and alienation are intimately linked with problem behaviors among youths (Hawkins, Catalano, and Miller, 1992; Hirschi, 1969; Jessor and Jessor, 1977), and therefore are important targets of effective violence-prevention programs (Allen, Kuperminc, et al., 1994; Hawkins, Von Cleve, and Catalano, 1991; Jason and Kobayashi, 1995; Jessor, 1992). Given these findings, promoting connectedness seems like a logical and worthwhile goal. However, the protective functions of connectedness appear to vary across the relationships and contexts in adolescents' lives, such that not all forms of connectedness decrease one's risk for violent behavior.

Conventionality in Adolescent Connectedness

Jessor and Jessor's (1977) theory of problem behavior argues that the concept of conventionality plays a significant role in delinquency, risk taking, and substance use, all of which contribute to or co-occur with violence. Depending on the individual youth and the specific set of peers, connectedness to peers can reflect either the conventions of the adult world or the unsupervised activities and norms of the adolescent world. Associating with conventional peers is one of the best protective factors against violent behavior (Hawkins, Farrington, and Catalano, 1998; Hawkins, Von Cleve, and Catalano, 1991; Olin, 2001). Although connectedness to friends could be called conventional, because most families want their children to have friends, connectedness to friends serves a different function than does connectedness to school or family.

Connectedness to friends has both positive and negative effects on violent behavior. On the one hand, any connectedness is better than none in terms of promoting social development, avoiding experiences of alienation, and preventing aggression (Collins, 2002; Nakkula and Selman, 1991). On the other hand, when connectedness to friends is high with little conventional connectedness to school or family, youths' risk for engaging in violence increases.

Adolescents who ... strongly identify with parents and teachers show more positive school adjustment and motivation, whereas emulation of friends is negatively related to these variables. (Lynch and Cicchetti, 1997, pp. 83-84)

Spending unsupervised time in the neighborhood, with friends, and in other youth-governed contexts increases the risk that youths will engage in unconventional behaviors (Dishion, McCord, and Poulin, 1999; Patterson, Dishion, and Yoerger, 2000; Jessor, 1992). Taken to the extreme, unconventional connectedness leads to unconventional activities that are unlawful and potentially damaging to self and others (Jessor and Jessor, 1977). Behaviors such as stealing, drinking, delinquency, and violence, are most common when strong connectedness to friends is not balanced by equally strong connectedness to school or to family (Hirschi, 1969; Olin, 2001), because conventional connectedness serves as a control against nonnormative, antisocial, illicit and aggressive behaviors (Hirschi, 1969).

There appears to be an interaction between forms of conventional and unconventional connectedness, such that when connectedness is not achieved in one context it will be overemphasized in others (Ainsworth, 1989). Baumeister and Leary (1995) argue that because the need to belong is pervasive, a "compensatory function" exists that allows the absence of belonging in one ecology (e.g., family) to be countered by belonging in another (e.g., friends). They argue that "relationships should substitute for each other, to some extent, as would be indicated by effective replacement of lost relationships partners and by a capacity for social relatedness in one sphere to overcome potential ill effects of social deprivation in another" (Baumeister and Leary, 1995, p. 500). Although the absence of conventional connectedness with one parent can be compensated for by connectedness with the other, unconventional connectedness, such as with friends, cannot take the place of absent parental connectedness (van Aken and Asendorpf, 1997). The intervention opportunity presented by this compensatory function is the possibility for conventional experiences and relationships, such as in after-school programs, to compensate for prior deprivations of conventional connectedness that resulted from poor parental bonding, peer rejection, or school failure and underachievement.

Yet often it appears that aggressive and alienated youths engender further disconnection from their conventional peers and teachers. In a study of rural, middle school adolescents, Karcher (2002) reported three findings that present challenges to successful intervention. First, parenting practices predicted violent behavior, and parenting interventions are often beyond the scope of many school violence programs (Cooper, Lutenbacher, and Faccia, 2000). Second, parenting practices contributed to connectedness to teachers, specifically poor parenting practices predicted lower levels of connectedness to teachers and school. Third, controlling for the effects of parenting practices on teacher connectedness, violent behavior had a negative effect on teacher connectedness. Youths who engaged in violent behavior became less connected to their teachers. This reveals the cycle of violence in which disconnection (i.e., from parents) leads to violence, which further decreases connectedness (e.g., to teachers). Therefore, teachers must actively work to break this cycle, knowing that violent teens may be predisposed to establish weak bonds with them (Prasad-Gaur, Hughes, and Cavell, 2001).

Further analysis of data from this study of 139 rural, Caucasian middle school students (Karcher, 2002) reveals the interaction effect of conventional/unconventional connectedness and violent behavior. Correlations between connectedness and the frequency of violent behaviors were examined using a survey of the number of times a youth has engaged in particular types of adolescent violence (Kingery, 1998) and an ecological measure of adolescent connectedness that uses a five-point anchored scale (Karcher, 2001). Friend, parent, and school connectedness correlated negatively with the frequency of several of the more severe forms of violence, such as menacing language, impulsive violence, and inventive violence, but not with common forms of violence. For example, both connectedness to friends ($r = -.18$) and to parents ($r = -.20$) were negatively correlated with severe menacing behavior, such that more connectedness predicted less violence. An interaction between connectedness to parents and to friends also existed, such that only those youths who reported low connectedness to both friends and parents reported engaging in severe menacing behavior, $F(3, 132) = 7.06$, $p < 001$. The interaction in Figure 1.2 was computed by charting one standard deviation above and below the mean frequency of engaging in acts of severe menacing behavior for both types of connectedness. The interaction was computed such that

the rate of severe menacing = $4.108 - 1.501(b_{\text{parents}}) - .874$
$(b_{\text{friends}}) + .352 (b_{\text{parents}} \times b_{\text{friends}})$.

The interaction reveals that severe menacing violent behavior is most likely when no connectedness to friends exists to compensate for absent connectedness to parents. This provides one more reason why promoting connectedness among disconnected youths should be a primary goal of comprehensive violence prevention programs in schools.

DEVELOPMENTAL TRENDS IN CONNECTEDNESS TO FRIENDS, SCHOOL, AND FAMILY

Unfortunately, in terms of violence prevention, it is normative for unconventional connectedness, such as to peers and friends, to increase during adolescence and for conventional connectedness to decline.

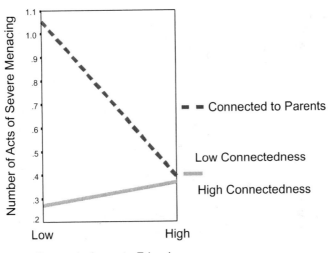

FIGURE 1.2. The interaction between connectedness to friends and to parents in explaining youths' engagement in acts of severe menacing violent behavior. Only youths with low connectedness to friends and low connectedness to parents reported, on average, having engaged in one or more such violent acts.

Lynch and Cicchetti (1997) illustrated that between elementary and middle school, a shift occurs in children's connection to family and teachers (it wanes) as the strength of their connection to friends and peers increases. This explanation supports psychoanalytic (Blos, 1962) descriptions of adolescence as a time of separation from the family and of extending early attachments to the peer group.

Lynch and Cicchetti's explanation is ecological, but somewhat incomplete. They argue that context changes cause these changes in connectedness:

> In school, children are exposed to a new community of unfamiliar peers and adults, and they are presented with a new set of context specific challenges. In particular, integration into the peer group, acceptable performance in the classroom, and appropriate motivational orientation for achievement are all part of this stage-salient developmental task. (Lynch and Cicchetti, 1997, p. 81)

This explanation is partly true, but it does not fully explain why youth disengage from teachers but not from peers.

The Role of Perspective Taking in Connectedness Development

Another explanation for these developmental patterns can be found in changes in the primary sources of self-esteem and cognitive development between preadolescence and adolescence. Theorists of self-development, from Mead (1934) to Harter (1999), suggest that it is from close interpersonal relationships that empathy, praise, and attention are drawn that provide the basis for self-esteem and self-development (Kohut, 1977; Kohut and Wolf, 1978). Youths' primary sources of esteem, however, begin to shift during preadolescence. For the preadolescent, primary sources of social support are parents and teachers, but for older adolescents, friends and peers become increasingly important sources of social support. Several reasons account for this, one of which is the task of self-development and another is the growth of perspective-taking abilities during this time.

Erik Erikson (1968) described the processes of identity development in considerable detail and expanded his earlier description of the stages (Erikson, 1959) of what can be called self-developments. These stages reflect developmentally specific self-developments. Kohut and Wolf (1978) argue that self-developments (skills, talents, and self-esteem) result from empathy, praise, and attention in the context of clear, consistent structure provided by competent adults. Erikson's (1968) developmental model illustrates that each stage of development (e.g., the establishment of trust in the parent-child relationship) contributes to later identity developments (e.g., autonomy and initiative). For Erikson, self-developments are the manifestation of youths' cognitive differentiation and integration of their own skills, roles, and self-awareness in the larger social contexts and social groups in their lives. That is, self-developments result from seeing oneself in relationship to others in increasingly complex ways.

Unfortunately, not all of the self-developments in Erikson's developmental model are couched within the connectedness developments that implicitly precede and inform them. The importance of connectedness appears to be relegated to the developmental periods before childhood and at the end of adolescence. After trust (or mistrust) is established in the infant and toddler eras, the next three developmental achievements are related to autonomy, separateness, and distinctiveness as manifested through (1) initiative, (2) industry, and (3) identity achievements (see Figure 1.3). The next developmental achievement in Erikson's model, intimacy, appears only after the development of identity in late adolescence. Not presented in Erikson's taxonomy is the role of connectedness developments in each successive self-development.

Joan Erikson (1988) wrote about the weaving tension of developmental growth as a process of moving back and forth between connectedness and self-developments. What links growth in connectedness and self-development is the phenomenon of social cognitive development (Kegan, Noam, and Rogers, 1982). Each of Erik Erikson's "I" developments (initiative, industry, and identity) reflects an increasingly differentiated social perspective taken on the self in the context of others. Therefore, each "I" self-development grows out of a developmentally distinct form of connectedness, and each subsequent form of connectedness reflects youths' abilities to take the perspective of others and use it for self-understanding.

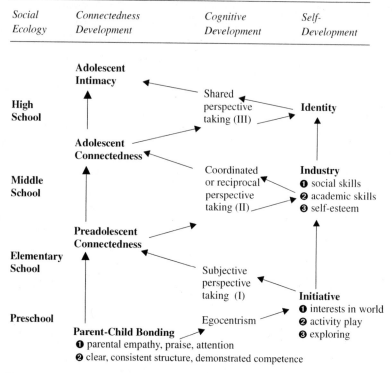

Social Ecology	*Connectedness Development*	*Cognitive Development*	*Self-Development*

Adolescent Intimacy

High School

Shared perspective taking (III)

Identity

Adolescent Connectedness

Middle School

Coordinated or reciprocal perspective taking (II)

Industry
❶ social skills
❷ academic skills
❸ self-esteem

Preadolescent Connectedness

Elementary School

Subjective perspective taking (I)

Initiative
❶ interests in world
❷ activity play
❸ exploring

Preschool

Egocentrism

Parent-Child Bonding
❶ parental empathy, praise, attention
❷ clear, consistent structure, demonstrated competence

FIGURE 1.3. A topographical model illustrating the weaving tension of developmental growth between involvement with others (connectedness) and development of the self as a function of cognitive developments in perspective-taking abilities. The achievement of connectedness in each new social ecology is dependent on the successful implementation of burgeoning perspective-taking skills and social skills in relationships in social contexts. Each of the self-developments described by Erikson results from the successful establishment of connectedness and the subsequent use of perspective-taking skills to construct a more differentiated and integrated self-understanding.

Understanding the connection between self-developments, connectedness developments, and perspective-taking abilities is important for the prevention of violence in two ways. First, violence, both physical and verbal, reflects the dominance of one's own needs and wants over another's. Violence is, therefore, evidence of limited perspective taking (Selman et al., 1992). This may be due either to an unwillingness or an inability to consider and respect others' points of view. For example, it is commonly agreed that increases in empathy result in decreases in aggression and violence (Chandler, 1973; van Manen and Emmelkamp, 2001), and that gains in empathy require mature social perspective taking (Eisenberg, 1992; Eisenberg et al., 1996). Second, neither the promotion of skills nor of connectedness will be possible without understanding the constraints that cognitive development places on successful intervention, because attachment-based working models are understood by the individual differently at each successive level of cognitive development (Fischer and Ayoub, 1996). Interventionists should understand the manner in which perspective taking develops and contributes to both connectedness and self-developments.

Four levels of perspective taking develop between childhood and late adolescence (Selman, 1980), and each differently shapes the way in which connectedness and self-developments occur. The *egocentric point of view* (level 0) is revealed through behavioral indicators of one's transitory needs, wants, and feelings. Impulsive violence is one indicator of egocentric (level 0) perspective taking in action (Selman et al., 1992). *Subjective perspective taking* (level I) reflects a spoken point of view that can be explained and justified but does not realistically consider others' needs. *Reciprocal perspective taking* (level II) reflects the ability to coordinate others' wants, needs, and feelings (i.e., points of view) with one's own in terms of making decisions, planning, and feeling empathic. This is a critical development in terms of violence prevention, because it allows for empathy and cooperation (Tice and Baumeister, 1993). Finally, *shared perspective taking* (level III) allows a youth to step back and see himself or herself in important relationships from a third-person point of view. This perspective helps the youth see the impact of his or her actions on enduring relationships. It also helps youth to understand better that sometimes what an individual wants must become subordinate to the relationship's perspective if the relationship is to survive and thrive, or if one is to avoid being the target of reciprocated violence and hostility from others in the future.

Adolescent Connectedness

Each advance in perspective taking evokes new self-understanding and developments, both of which allow for new forms of connectedness to develop between youths and those people and places in their lives. In addition to the shift in emphasis in childhood from connectedness to adults to an emphasis on connectedness to peers and to friends in adolescence, the emergence of abstract (level III) perspective taking elicits heightened attention by youths to connectedness to groups, youth values, and abstract ideas. Adolescent connectedness reflects not only affection for and activity with significant people (parents, siblings, teachers, and peers) in the important social systems (school, family, neighborhood) that youths participate in regularly, but also reflects attention to the larger, principle-based ecologies (religion, culture, and future) that inform identity development. Preadolescent connectedness is less differentiated. It is more dyad specific, interpersonal, and reflects affection for and activity with those individuals (parents, siblings, teachers, friends, and peers) in the important social worlds (school, family, and neighborhood) where youths negotiate their immediate needs in the contexts of others. Preadolescent connectedness reveals youths' interest in pleasing and getting along with individual peers or adults, whereas mature adolescent connectedness reflects a desire to develop group-based identities and to maintain satisfying relationships. Successful intervention requires understanding the constraints cognitive development places on the manifestations of connectedness, as well as understanding the self-developments to which connectedness leads.

The Interactive Nature of Connectedness, Perspective Taking, and Self-Developments

It appears from attachment studies that safe exploration and self-differentiation depends on the establishment of a secure bond with caregivers (Ainsworth, 1989; Bretherton, 1999). It is out of this secure place that the child's egocentrism is overcome through the discovery of his or her own interests and joy in exploring and playing. The child who experiences a positive parent-child bond uses this social support as a springboard for developing the initiative to explore his or her own interests, play activities, and the larger world beyond the parent-child relationship (Tolman, Diekmann, and McCartney, 1989). The child's autonomy and initiative, the first of Erikson's self-developments, helps the child to develop, define, and articulate his or her own perspective—to be able to articulate what he or she likes, enjoys, and wants (see Figure 1.3).

The child's initiative and subjective perspective taking help him or her to elicit further empathy, praise, and attention from parents and teachers. Through the same connectedness → perspective taking → self-development sequence, preadolescent connectedness results from parents and teachers valuing, praising, and encouraging the child's initiative. The preadolescent uses this connectedness to teachers and parents as a secure base from which to develop academic and social skills. One primary mechanism by which these skills develop is as a function of taking the perspective of their teachers and parents. When the child's perspective-taking developments allow him or her to understand what teachers and parents want—i.e., what activities result in positive reinforcement, praise, and attention—the child becomes more likely to practice those skills and activities. Acting industriously in ways that garner praise and approval from adults becomes the youth's main goal, because the goals and beliefs of adults are seen as correct forms of behavior to emulate so that one can receive their social support (Kohut, 1977).

By middle school, adolescent connectedness is derived from youths linking their own industriousness to that of their peers. Socially competent middle school students are consistently praised by parents and teachers for developing positive attitudes, as well as for demonstrating social and academic skills. At the same time, the ability to coordinate two social perspectives also allows youths to consider their peers' points of view. Youths begin to experience relatedness with other youths who share similar interests, skills, and attitudes. Often youths' unique interests are validated by their peers and friends in ways that parents cannot. Youths experience this form of relatedness in dyads, cliques, and friendships (Sullivan, 1953). Youths sharing similar perspectives become increasingly significant sources of relatedness and begin to compete with adults as primary sources of empathy, praise, and attention.

By early high school, youths' third-person or shared perspective-taking abilities help them to see that these cliques and dyads reflect interests, values, and activities that are shared by members of groups—such as teams, clubs, and gangs. Youths, like adults, become drawn to those groups whose members share their own points of view. As occurred during middle school through dyads and friendships, high school youths come to receive praise and attention from peer and social groups that they feel they cannot access from most adults. This praise and attention leads youths to become more involved in and to highly value these peer groups. This connectedness to peer groups becomes the centerpiece of most youths' evolving identity.

The identity youths create will reflect the balance of the conventional and unconventional connectedness in their lives. Youths' identities are born out of relationships in which they feel valued. Youths who identify with others who value school and who work hard tend to maintain their connectedness to school, parents, teachers, and conventionally oriented peers during adolescence, but youths who identify only with friends who discourage their connectedness to school, teachers, and parents are at a greater risk for engaging in violence and risk taking.

DISCONNECTION AND VIOLENCE

Some changes in connectedness are a normal part of development. The normative and predictable changes in connectedness between childhood and adolescence described previously provide targets for interventions designed to prevent violence by promoting connectedness. It is important to keep in mind, however, that disconnection also can result from unsatisfactory relationships with adults and poor performance in conventional contexts or activities (Allen, Hauser, et al., 1994). Adolescents will tend to report lower than normal connectedness in those contexts and relationships in which they have experienced misunderstanding, criticism, and rejection. For example, school disconnection is typically a function of past experiences of underachievement in school and subsequent experiences of misunderstanding, criticism, and rejection. Similarly, family neglect, peer rejection, religious intolerance, and racial/ethnic misunderstandings experienced by youths may result in lower connectedness in the forms of less involvement, less positive affect, and less caring about their performance in those social worlds.

Hirschi (1969) argued that youths who are not able to get their affective needs for closeness and social bonding met within the conventional worlds of the school or the family are left to get those needs met from other youths. Not feeling liked and supported by adults in their schools or families, such youths discount the importance of those social ecologies. Finding a cohort of peers who also share their anticonventional outlook leads alienated youth to engage in unconventional and sometimes unlawful activities. These activities and their unconventional connectedness to friends become their primary sources of self-esteem and markers of self-development, and serve as primary triggers for youth violence (Olin, 2001).

Sometimes youths' disconnection from school and heightened connectedness to friends is a function of the parenting styles they experience at home (Karcher, 2002). The important role of parental connectedness in the development of adolescents' connectedness to friends reveals the indirect effect of poor parenting on youth violence. Parental contributions to youths' self-esteem and self-development are mediated (or manifest) through youths' connectedness to friends, because parents influence the kind of friends their children seek out (Brown et al., 1993). Youths who experience harsh and inconsistent parenting tend to feel disconnected from their families and associate with delinquent peers.

INTERVENTIONS: WHAT TO DO?

Although connectedness contributes to self-developments, specifically identity development, skills development, and self-esteem, the question of how to prevent violence is not as simple as promoting connectedness to school and family for all youth. Prevention programs that overemphasize promoting connectedness for youths who require skill-building interventions can be futile or problematic. However, it is difficult to teach academic skills to aggressive and delinquent youths who have not already established a positive connection with program or school staff. Barkley (1990) noticed this problem when first implementing his behavioral approach for the treatment of attention deficit hyperactivity disorder (ADHD). He found that unless the connection between the parent and child was reestablished through activities that provided the child empathy, praise, and attention, the child often would refuse to participate in any system of behavior modification.

Indeed, the tension regarding whether schools should intervene to affect attitudes and behavioral patterns (i.e., promote conventional connectedness) or teach interpersonal skills, such as cooperation and negotiation, remains unanswered. With regard to the targets of intervention, Harter (1999) casts the question in terms of self-esteem and asks,

> should one identify the self-evaluations themselves as the target, for example, by attempting to enhance global self-worth directly, or should one focus primarily on improving actual skills in particular domains? The goals of these different educational programs reflect two competing orientations toward change. As Caslyn and Kenny (1997) have noted, "self-enhancement" theorists believe that efforts should focus on enhancing self-concept and self-esteem directly. In contrast, "skills" theorists argue that attitudes about the self are consequences of successful achievement and thus pedagogical efforts should be directed toward enhancing specific academic skills. In recent years, the pendulum has clearly shifted toward the skills learning orientation in which interventions target specific domains. (p. 311)

In the end, Harter suggests that specific skills and experiences be the focus of intervention with enhanced self-esteem a distal outcome or goal of the program. The rationale for this argument is that improved skills, such as in negotiation or academics, will result in improvements in self-esteem. However, absent from this debate is the importance of youths' connectedness to teachers and program staff. Self-evaluations often reflect how we think we are seen by others (Mead, 1934), which requires the ability to understand others' perspectives (Selman, 1980). Therefore, improved skills in contexts and relationships devoid of connectedness are not likely to affect self-esteem because meaningful experiences of empathy, praise, and attention are lacking.

The model of adolescent connectedness presented in this chapter suggests that a weaving back and forth exists between self-developments (both in self-esteem and in skills) and connectedness developments during adolescence. Following each growth in connectedness are particular sets of self-developments, part of which reflect youths' estimations of how they are viewed by others and their desire to attain the skills that will be appreciated by those in their lives whom they value. Therefore, the target of a developmental intervention designed to prevent violence will depend on the adolescent's relative achievements of connectedness, perspective taking, and self-development.

DEVELOPMENTAL INTERVENTIONS FOR THE PREVENTION OF YOUTH VIOLENCE

From the model in Figure 1.3, three principles of youth development can be hypothesized to provide guidelines for intervention and the prevention of youth violence.

Central Principles

1. *Connectedness and self-developments are mutually dependent.* (a) Age-appropriate forms of connectedness are a result of perspective-taking skill development, prior self-developments, and earlier experiences of connectedness. To promote connectedness, interventions should build on prior self-developments and help children take a perspective on both their own and others' interests, experiences, and talents. (b) Growth in self-developments is a function of perspective-taking skill developments, prior connectedness, and prior achievements in self-development. To facilitate self-developments, interventions must target the use of perspective-taking skills within significant relationships. For example, once preadolescent connectedness is established, self-developments emerge through the process of perspective taking. By identifying their own skills (both social and academic), youth come to better understand their subjective perspective and uniqueness, which informs self-esteem, but also allows them to understand how they are similar and dissimilar to others. Coordinated or reciprocal perspective taking (level II) is a prerequisite for comparing and contrasting one's own attitudes, interests, skills, and experiences with those of others. This reflection on self-developments leads youths to participate in activities with like-minded peers, which facilitates belonging and results in group-based adolescent connectedness.

2. *Successful intervention requires developmental assessments and goal setting.* Successful intervention will depend, in part, on the ac-

curacy of adults' assessments of youths' relative strengths and deficits in the areas of connectedness, perspective taking, and self-development. Interventions should target areas of deficits, either connectedness, perspective taking, or self-development, by promoting the precursors of each development. Although a good assessment of strengths and weaknesses in these three areas is critical to establishing targets for intervention, it is not as important that youth achieve some criterion level of each through the intervention, but rather that they participate in and enjoy the process. Connectedness, perspective taking, social and academic skills, and self-esteem can be measured, quantified, and subjected to specific evaluative criteria. However, the model in Figure 1.3 is intended to convey these as interrelated experiences more than as specific, independent achievements. The goal of each intervention should be to help youths experience, practice, and engage in the process of being connected, taking others' perspectives, esteeming oneself, and learning skills.

3. *Development occurs within ongoing relationships.* Developmental interventions should occur within authentic, ongoing relationships between youth and their peers. These peer interactions should be structured with activities that promote specific developments in connectedness, perspective taking, or domains of the self (e.g., skills or self-esteem). Adults should work to ensure that the unconventional activities, attitudes, and behaviors do not develop as a result of the intervention (Dishion, McCord, and Poulin, 1999).

The main mechanisms of growth in all three areas are the two related experiences of (1) empathy, praise, and attention, and (2) clear, consistent structure from competent others. Kohut (1977) suggests that empathy, praise, and attention evoke self-esteem and establish connectedness with significant others. When those significant others act in a clear, consistent, and competent fashion, this leads youths to idealize and want to model the behaviors of others (whether adults or peers). Youths want to act in ways that will continue to evoke empathy, praise, and attention from others, and so they seek out specific skills and talents. When talents and skills are achieved, youths see that others are pleased by these self-developments, and connectedness results in the form of the youths liking and wanting to be around those significant others. These esteeming, praising, and attending processes must be included along with skill learning opportunities in interventions that are designed to strengthen conventional connectedness.

Age- and Context-Specific Developmental Interventions

The model in Figure 1.3 and the three principles just discussed reveal age-specific opportunities for violence prevention. At each age, specific forms of connectedness, perspective taking, and self-developments are required. Deficits in any area increase youths' risk for engaging in or being the target of violent behavior. Youths are more likely to engage in violent behavior when they lack empathy, feel alienated and disconnected, or suffer the consequences of deficits in skill development (van Manen and Emmelkamp, 2001). Successful intervention requires accurate assessment of the presence of each skill and deficit and the targeted use of structured, peer-based interventions, preferably in the conventional context of school.

Developmental interventions in preschool and early elementary school could promote initiative in the form of motivating children to explore their environment, engage in parallel peer play, and pursue the activities that interest them. However, children might not be ready for this self-development in cases in which early caretaking experiences did not facilitate strong caregiver-child bonding. In the absence of a secure attachment to primary caregivers, promoting adult-child bonding should be the target of intervention. Interventions and relationship contexts could be structured so that caregivers can provide (1) empathy, praise, and attention, and (2) clear, consistent structure. These adults would need sufficient training and supervision to ensure they feel competent in providing such experiences. Once caregiver bonding is strengthened through interventions such as parent training or quality day care, children could be provided environments that engage the child's interest, activity, and exploration and thereby promote the child's initiative and motivation.

As illustrated in the framework in Figure 1.3, the goals of developmental interventions in elementary school should be to solidify the child's initiative and motivation, facilitate the child's awareness of his or her own unique perspective, and use both of these experiences to encourage preadolescent connectedness. Preadolescent connectedness is important because it supports the development of social (e.g., negotiation) skills, academic skills, and self-esteem in late elementary school and middle school. Preadolescent connectedness is demonstrated through the child's active engagement and positive attitudes toward school, the family, and dyadic relationships with teachers, peers, friends, parents, and siblings.

Developmental interventions in late elementary and middle school should encourage engagement in peer relationships and contexts that (1) facilitate the acquisition of social and academic skills, and (2) provide opportunities for self-reflection, social comparison, and cooperation. Intervention examples include peer counseling and developmental mentoring. Both of these developmental interventions, described in greater detail in the next section, promote social skills, connectedness, and perspective taking, as well as negotiation skills in the context of structured and supervised peer relationships. Positive experiences by children in interventions such as these, which promote preadolescent connectedness and perspective taking, should effect self-developments in social skills, academic skills, and self-esteem that prevent violence.

For youths in early middle school who have firmly established social skills, academic skills, and self-esteem, but who demonstrate negative school attitudes or weakening bonds to conventional contexts and people (e.g., family and school), the goal of developmental interventions should be to promote adolescent connectedness to teachers, peers, parents, and conventional activities (such as reading), to promote the student's vision of himself or herself in the future, and to facilitate participation in prosocial, conventional group activities (e.g., sports, band, clubs, volunteerism) that can promote conventional forms of connectedness. Interventions should provide opportunities to coordinate skills around shared goals within teams and groups (e.g., sports, clubs) in order to promote the application of self-developments (e.g., social skills, school achievement, and self-esteem) within conventional relationships and to facilitate shared, third-person perspective taking. Both of these should strengthen adolescents' connectedness and lessen youths' risk for and engagement in violence at school.

By late middle school and early high school, a central goal of developmental interventions should be to facilitate conventional identity development through deepened involvement in conventional activities and relationships. Erikson (1968) forewarned of processes by which an overemphasis on unconventional connectedness can lead to a negative identity. Both conventional and unconventional adolescent connectedness affect identity development, self-esteem, risk taking, academic success, and interpersonal happiness (Bonny et al., 2000; Bush, 2000; Grotevant and Cooper, 1998; Hendry and Reid, 2000; Resnick et al., 1997), and the effect of adolescent connectedness on identity development is mediated by perspective-taking skills (Grotevant and Cooper, 1986; Selman, 1977, 1981). As one example, seeing oneself as a member of this or that group helps solidify one's identity. Yet the precursors to identity must be in place for identity-development interventions to be effective. For example, a balance of unconventional and conventional forms of connectedness should already be established and secure in youths' lives. Interventions should provide opportunities to reflect on experiences with peer groups in contexts of conventional connectedness that confirm these as important parts of youths' self-understanding. For example, by mentoring a younger child or volunteering time in a school or community, older youths can receive positive, conventionally based empathy, praise, and attention, which helps to confirm a degree of conventionality in their developing identities. Similarly, school-based interventions and school-to-work programs can promote both connectedness and self-developments. Most effective will be those interventions that promote (1) principle-driven social involvement, (2) coordinated, supervised activities for a social cause that promote shared (third-person) conventional perspective taking, or (3) structured and collaborative team, club, or civic involvement. Each of these activities should facilitate gains in identity development (assuming the experiences are positive) and further integrate the use of level-three shared perspective taking into the everyday lives of adolescents.

Ideally, these interventions would be part of a system of intervention activities that span across adolescents' ecology and developmental periods. Many school developmental guidance programs have coordinated and sustained interventions as their ultimate goal (Gysbers and Henderson, 2000). In the prevention of violence, it seems that enduring activities that are well integrated into the school, community, or family organizations have the greatest impact (Dryfoos, 1990; Embry et al., 1996; Larson, 1994; Schorr, 1988). For this reason, the following section describes two interventions that target youths in primary and secondary school contexts and provide ongoing, developmentally appropriate opportunities for growth in perspective taking, connectedness, and self-development.

DYADIC APPROACHES TO VIOLENCE PREVENTION

Two intervention approaches that are designed to promote all three developmental intervention targets—connectedness, perspective taking, and self-development—are developmental mentoring and pair counseling. Both occur within ongoing relationships with peers, and have been found effective in reducing or preventing violent, aggressive, and delinquent behavior (Karcher and Lewis, 2002; Selman et al., 1992; Shehan et al., 1999). They are used most commonly with older children and young adolescents who demonstrate delayed development in skills, connectedness, or perspective taking, and who are, therefore, at increased risk for violent behavior (Dodge and Frame, 1982; Selman et al., 1992). In both interventions, peer relationships are structured by adults in order to facilitate connectedness to others and to school, to encourage age-appropriate perspective taking within these relationships, and to help youths learn academic and social skills.

Developmental Mentoring

In developmental mentoring, children (as mentees) are paired with high school mentors. This is a form of cross-age, peer group, structured mentoring that typically takes place after school (Karcher, Davis, and Powell, 2002). Initially, the mentee uses developmental mentoring either to establish preadolescent connectedness within the ecology of the school, or to develop social skills, academic achievement, and self-esteem. Some youths need to capitalize on their prior skill developments to achieve connectedness, whereas others need to build on their already established connectedness to develop new skills, interests, and self-understandings. Program coordinators help the adolescent mentors decide whether to focus on (1) providing mentees empathy, praise, and attention, or (2) helping the children develop skills by modeling and guiding age-appropriate academic and social skills in a playful, peer group context.

Developmental mentoring provides an opportunity for youth to participate in the program across their elementary, middle, and high school years by providing different roles in the program. Children in middle school who have grown beyond their roles as mentees can become protégés who serve as assistants to one or more mentors. Being protégés allows youths to draw on their previously developed social skills, school achievement experiences, and own positive memories in the program to help other mentor and mentee dyads. Ideally, the protégé makes repeated efforts to take other youths' points of view (both the mentors' and mentees') to assist them with their relationship. This serves to increase protégés' empathy for others by taking others' (third-person) perspectives. For teenagers, serving as mentors allows them to try and recreate their own experiences of conventional connectedness with others and to more fully develop the conventional aspects of their identities by making this time commitment to volunteering. By promoting empathy and facilitating involvement in conventional relationships, activities, and contexts, both protégés and mentors should become less likely to engage in or instigate violent behaviors.

Pair Counseling

Pair counseling is a dyadic form of play therapy designed to help children utilize social perspective-taking skills within real relationships (Selman and Schultz, 1990). It requires the counselor to accurately assess which type of perspective taking development is needed by the children, and whether each child needs help developing connectedness or developing skills. One child might negotiate through aggression and simply need help learning how to articulate his or her own perspective (level I). Another child might need help listening to and working with others' points of view (level II). This assessment of perspective taking helps determine the goals of the pair counseling.

In pair counseling, two children play under the watchful supervision of a counselor. The counselor works to promote empathy, praise, and attention within the pair; model competent negotiation skills; and provide opportunities for the children to practice these social skills. The counselor helps the children negotiate conflicts when they arise (e.g., manage their separateness) and understand how their actions affect their relationship (i.e., their connectedness).

Whether the counselor focuses on connectedness or self-developments depends on the children and the relationship. The child who knows what to do, has the skills to be successful, but typically does not use the skills, can be helped to take the perspective of the other child and to understand the impact of his or her immature behaviors on the friendship (Nakkula and Selman, 1991). Conversely, the child who understands the power of friendship and desires connectedness but who does not have the skills to get his or her own needs met within the relationship, can be taught social skills and assertiveness as alternatives to aggression and violence, and given opportunities to practice these skills in an ongoing, supervised peer relationship.

CONCLUSION

Promoting connectedness in the lives of adolescents is critical to violence prevention in many ways. Beyond the role of alienation and disconnection as precursors to violence, promoting connectedness also is key to successful violence prevention. Lasting gains in skills and self-esteem, as well as interest in conventional relationships and activities as a result of intervention, may first require interventionists to reestablish youths' connectedness to teachers, school, the family, and other conventional people and places. Once reestablished, connectedness can serve as a foundation for youths to use their burgeoning perspective-taking skills to develop new social and academic skills, and thereby to strengthen their self-esteem. Thus, connectedness is critical to violence prevention not solely through its direct effect on violence, but also through its indirect effects. One indirect effect is that promoting connectedness to adults and peers in a prevention program increases the likelihood that youths will be receptive to establishing conventional relationships and engaging in the conventional prevention activities that are believed to directly reduce youths' propensity toward violence.

REFERENCES

Ainsworth, M. D. (1989). Attachments beyond infancy. *American Psychologist, 44,* 709-716.

Allen, J. P., Hauser, S. T., Eickholt, C., Bell, K. L., and O'Connor, T. G. (1994). Autonomy and relatedness in family interactions as predictors of expressions of negative adolescent affect. *Journal of Research on Adolescence, 4*, 535-552.

Allen, J. P., Kuperminc, G., Philliber, S., and Herre, K. (1994). Programmatic prevention of adolescent problem behaviors: The role of autonomy, relatedness, and volunteer service in the Teen Outreach Program. *American Journal of Community Psychology, 22*(5), 617-638.

Barkley, R. A. (1990). Attention deficit disorders: History, definition, and diagnosis. In M. Lewis and S. Miller (Eds.), *The handbook of developmental psychopathology*. New York: Plenum.

Baumeister, R. F. and Leary, M. R. (1995). The need to belong: Desire for interpersonal attachments as a fundamental motivation. *Psychological Bulletin, 117*(3), 497-529.

Blos, P. (1962). *On adolescence: A psychoanalytic perspective*. New York: The Free Press.

Bonny, A. E., Britto, M. T., Klostermann, B. K., Hornung, R. W., and Slap, G. B. (2000). School disconnectedness: Identifying adolescents at risk. *Pediatrics, 106*(5), 1017-1021.

Bretherton, I. (1999). Updating the "internal working model" construct: Some reflections. *Attachment & Human Development, 1*(3), 343-357.

Bronfenbrenner, U. (1979). *The ecology of human development: Experiments by nature and design*. Cambridge, MA: Harvard University Press.

Brown, B. B., Mounts, N., Lamborn, S. D., and Steinberg, L. (1993). Parenting practices and peer group affiliation in adolescence. *Child Development, 64*, 467-482.

Bush, K. R. (2000). Separatedness and connectedness in the parent-adolescent relationship as predictors of adolescent self-esteem in U.S. and Chinese samples. *Marriage & Family Review, 30*(1-2), 153-178.

Catalano, R. F., Berglund, M. L., Ryan, J. A. M., Lonczak, H. S., and Hawkins, J. D. (2002). Positive youth development in the United States: Research findings on evaluations of positive youth development programs. *Prevention & Treatment, 5*, June 24, article 15. Retrieved October 9, 2002, from <http://journals.apa.org/prevention/volume2005/preoo50015a.html>.

Cernkovich, S. A. and Giordana, P. C. (1992). School bonding, race, and delinquency. *Criminology, 31*, 261-291.

Chandler, M. J. (1973). Egocentrism and anti-social behavior: The assessment and training of social perspective-taking skills. *Developmental Psychology, 9*, 326-332.

Chodorow, N. (1978). *The reproduction of mothering*. Berkeley: The University of California Press.

Collins, W. A. (2002). The development of physical aggression from early childhood to adolescence. Paper presented at the Society for Research on Adolescence ninth biennial meeting, New Orleans, April 13.

Cooper, W. O., Lutenbacher, M., and Faccia, K. (2000). Components of effective youth violence prevention programs for 7- to 14-year-olds. *Archives of Pediatric and Adolescent Medicine, 154*(November), 1134-1139.

Dishion, T. J., McCord, J., and Poulin, F. (1999). When interventions harm: Peer groups and problem behavior. *American Psychologist, 54,* 755-764.

Dodge, K. A. and Frame, C. L. (1982). Social cognitive biases and deficits in aggressive boys. *Child Development, 53,* 620-635.

Donovan, J. E., Jessor, R., and Costa, F. M. (1988). Syndrome of problem behavior in adolescence: A replication. *Journal of Consulting and Clinical Psychology, 56,* 762-765.

Dryfoos, J. G. (1990). *Adolescents at risk: Prevalence and prevention.* New York: Oxford University Press.

Eisenberg, N. (1992). *The caring child.* Cambridge: Harvard University Press.

Eisenberg, N., Fabes, R., Murphy, B., Karbon, M., Smith, M., and Maszk, P. (1996). The regulations of children's dispositional empathy-related responding to their emotionality, regulation, and social functioning. *Developmental Psychology, 32*(2), 195-209.

Embry, D. D., Flannery, D. J., Vazsonyi, A. T., Powell, K. E., and Atha, H. (1996). PeaceBuilders: A theoretically driven, school-based model for early violence prevention. *American Journal of Preventive Medicine, 12*(5), 91-100.

Erikson, E. H. (1959). *Identity and the life cycle.* New York: W. W. Norton.

Erikson, E. H. (1968). *Identity: Youth and crisis.* New York: W. W. Norton.

Erikson, J. M. (1988). *Wisdom and the senses: The way of creativity.* New York: W. W. Norton.

Farrington, D. (1991). Childhood aggression and adult violence: Early precursors and later life outcomes. In D. Pepper and K. Rubin (Eds.), *The development and treatment of childhood aggression* (pp. 5-29). Hillsdale, NJ: Erlbaum.

Fischer, K. W. and Ayoub, C. (1996). Analyzing development of working models of close relationships: Illustration with a case of vulnerability and violence. In K. W. Fischer and G. G. Noam (Eds.), *Development and vulnerability in close relationships. The Jean Piaget symposium series* (pp. 173-199). Mahwah, NJ: Lawrence Erlbaum Associates.

Gilligan, C. (1991). Women's psychological development: Implications for psychotherapy. Special Issue: Women, girls, and psychotherapy: Reframing resistance. *Women and Therapy, 11*(3-4), 5-31.

Grotevant, H. D. and Cooper, C. R. (1986). Individualization in family relationships: A perspective on individual differences in the development of identity and role-taking skill in adolescence. *Human Development, 29,* 82-100.

Grotevant, H. D. and Cooper, C. R. (1998). Individuality and connectedness in adolescent development: Review and prospects for research on identity, relationships, and context. In E. Skoe and A. von der Lippe (Eds.), *Personality development in adolescence: A cross-national and life span perspective* (pp. 3-37). London: Routledge.

Gysbers, N. C. and Henderson, P. (2000). *Developing and managing your school guidance program,* Third edition. Alexandria, VA: American Counseling Association.

Hagerty, B. M., Lynch-Sauer, J., Patusky, K., and Bouwsema, M. (1993). An emerging theory of human relatedness. *IMAGE: Journal of Nursing Scholarship, 25*(4), 291-296.

Harter, S. (1999). *The construction of the self: A developmental perspective.* New York: The Guilford Press.

Hawkins, J. D., Catalano, R. F., and Miller, J. Y. (1992). Risk and protective factors for alcohol and other drug problems in adolescence and early adulthood: Implications for substance abuse prevention. *Psychological Bulletin, 112*(1), 64-105.

Hawkins, J. D., Farrington, D., and Catalano, R. F. (1998). Reducing violence through the schools. In D. S. Elliott, B. A. Hamburg, and K. R. Williams (Eds.), *Violence in American schools* (pp. 188-216). Cambridge: Cambridge University Press.

Hawkins, J. D., Von Cleve, E., and Catalano, R. F. (1991). Reducing early childhood aggression: Results of a primary prevention program. *Journal of the American Academy of Child Adolescent Psychiatry, 30*(2), 208-217.

Hendry, L. B. and Reid, M. (2000). Social relationships and health: The meaning of social "connectedness" and how it relates to health concerns for rural Scottish adolescents. *Journal of Adolescence, 23*(6), 705-719.

Hirschi, T. (1969). *Causes of delinquency.* Berkeley: University of California Press.

Honora, D. and Rolle, A. (2002). A discussion of the incongruence between optimism and academic performance and its influence on school violence. *Journal of School Violence, 1*(1), 67-82.

Jason, L. A. and Kobayashi, R. B. (1995). Community building: Our next frontier. *Journal of Primary Prevention, 15*(3), 195-208.

Jessor, R. (1992). Risk behavior in adolescence: A psychosocial framework for understanding and action. *Developmental Review, 12*, 374-390.

Jessor, R. and Jessor, S. L. (1977). *Problem behavior and psychological development: A longitudinal study of youth.* New York: Academic Press.

Jordan, J. V., Kaplan, A. G., Miller, J. B., Stiver, I., and Surrey, J. (1991). *Women's growth in connection: Writings from the Stone Center.* New York: Guilford Press.

Karcher, M. J. (2001). Measuring adolescent connectedness: Four validation studies. Poster session presented at the annual meeting of the American Psychological Association, San Francisco, August 21.

Karcher, M. J. (2002). The cycle of violence and disconnection among rural middle school students: Teacher disconnection as a consequence of violence. *The Journal of School Violence, 1*(1), 35-51.

Karcher, M. J., Davis, C. I., and Powell, B. (2002). Developmental mentoring in the schools: Testing connectedness as a mediating variable in the promotion of academic achievement. *School Community Journal, 12*(2), 37-52.

Karcher, M. J. and Lewis, S. S. (2002). Pair counseling: The effects of a dyadic developmental play therapy on interpersonal understanding and externalizing behaviors. *International Journal of Play Therapy, 11*(1), 19-41.

Kegan, R., Noam, G. G., and Rogers, L. (1982). The psychologic of emotion: A neo-Piagetian view. *New Directions for Child Development, 16*, 105-128.

Kingery, P. M. (1998). The adolescent violence survey: A psychometric analysis. *School Psychology International, 19*(1), 43-59.

Kohut, H. (1977). *Restoration of the self.* New York: International Universities Press.

Kohut, H. and Elson, M. (1987). *The Kohut seminars on self psychology and psychotherapy with adolescents and young adults.* New York: W. W. Norton.

Kohut, H. and Wolf, E. S. (1978). The disorders of the self and their treatment: An outline. *International Journal of Psychoanalysis, 59,* 413-426.

Larson, J. (1994). Violence prevention in the schools: A review of selected programs and procedures. *School Psychology Review, 23*(2), 151-164.

Lynch, M. and Cicchetti, D. (1997). Children's relationships with adults and peers: An examination of elementary and junior high school students. *Journal of School Psychology, 35*(1), 81-99.

Mallinckrodt, B. (1991). Clients' representations of childhood emotional bonds with parents, social support, and formation of the working alliance. *Journal of Counseling Psychology, 38,* 401-409.

Mead, G. H. (1934). *Mind, self, and society: From the standpoint of a social behaviorist.* Chicago: The University of Chicago Press.

Midgley, C., Feldlauffer, H., and Eccles, J. S. (1989). Student/teacher relations and attitudes towards mathematics before and after the transition to junior high. *Child Development, 60,* 981-992.

Mulvey, E. P. and Cauffman, E. (2001). The inherent limits of predicting school violence. *American Psychologist, 56*(10), 797-802.

Nakkula, M. and Selman, R. (1991). How people "treat" each other: Pair therapy as a context for the development of interpersonal ethics. In W. M. Kurtines and J. L. Gewirtz (Eds.), *Handbook of moral behavior and development, Volume 3: Application* (pp. 179-211). Hillsdale, NJ: Lawrence Erlbaum.

O'Donnell, J., Hawkins, J. D., and Abbott, R. D. (1995). Predicting serious delinquency and substance use among aggressive boys. *Journal of Consulting and Clinical Psychology, 63,* 529-537.

Olin, S. S. (2001). Youth violence: Report from the surgeon general. *The Child, Youth, and Family Services Advocate, 24*(2), 1-7.

Patterson, G. R., Dishion, T. J., and Yoerger, K. (2000). Adolescent growth in new forms of problem behavior: Macro- and micro-peer dynamics. *Prevention Sciences, 1,* 3-13.

Prasad-Gaur, A., Hughes, J. H., and Cavell, T. (2001). Implications of aggressive children's positivity biased relatedness views for future relationships. *Child Psychiatry and Human Development, 31*(3), 215-230.

Resnick, M. D., Bearman, P. S., Blum, R. W., Bauman, K. E., Harris, K. M., Jones, J., Tabor, J., Beuhring, T., Sieving, R. E., Shew, M., Ireland, M., Bearinger, L. H., and Udry, J. R. (1997). Protecting adolescents from harm: Findings from the National Longitudinal Study on Adolescent Health. *JAMA, 278,* 823-832.

Resnick, M. D., Harris, L. J., and Blum, R. W. (1993). The impact of caring and connectedness on adolescent health and well-being. *Journal of Paediatrics & Child Health, 23,* S3-S9.

Richters, J. E. and Martinez, P. E. (1993). Violent communities, family choices, and children's chances: An algorithm for improving the odds. *Development and Psychopathology, 5,* 609-627.

Schorr, L. B. (1988). *Within our reach: Breaking the cycle of disadvantage.* New York: Doubleday.

Selman, R. L. (1977). A structural-developmental model of social cognition: Implications for intervention research. *Counseling Psychologist, 6*(4), 3-6.

Selman, R. L. (1980). *The growth of interpersonal understanding: Developmental and clinical analyses.* New York: Academic Press.

Selman, R. L. (1981). The development of interpersonal competence: The role of understanding in conduct. *Developmental Review, 1*(4), 401-422.

Selman, R. L. and Schultz, L. H. (1990). *Making a friend in youth: Developmental theory and pair therapy.* Chicago, IL: University of Chicago Press.

Selman, R. L., Schultz, L. H., Nakkula, M., Barr, D., Watts, C., and Richmond, J. (1992). Friendship and fighting: A developmental approach to the study of risk and prevention of violence. *Development and psychopathology, 4,* 529-558.

Sheehan, K., DiCara, J. A., LeBailly, S., and Christoffel, K. K. (1999). Adapting the gang model: Peer mentoring for violence prevention. *Pediatrics, 104*(1), 50-54.

Stern, D. (1985). *The interpersonal world of the infant: A view from psychoanalysis and developmental psychology.* New York: Basic Books.

Sullivan, H. S. (1953). *The interpersonal theory of psychiatry.* New York: Norton.

Tice, D. M. and Baumeister, R. F. (1993). Controlling anger: Self-induced emotion change. In D. M. Wegner and J. W. Pennebaker (Eds.), *Handbook of mental control* (pp. 393-408). Englewood Cliffs, NJ: Prentice-Hall.

Tolman, A. E., Diekmann, K. A., and McCartney, K. (1989). Social connectedness and mothering: Effects of maternal employment and maternal absence. *Journal of Personality and Social Psychology, 56*(6), 942-949.

van Aken, M. A. G. and Asendorpf, J. B. (1997). Support by parents, classmates, friends, and siblings in preadolescence: Covariation and compensation across relationships. *Journal of Social and Personal Relationships, 14*(1), 79-93.

van Manen, T. G. and Emmelkamp, P. M. G. (2001). Assessing social cognitive skills in aggressive children from a developmental perspective: The social cognitive skills test. *Clinical Psychology and Psychotherapy, 8,* 341-351.

Chapter 2

Identification with Academics and Violence in Schools

Jason W. Osborne

For our purposes here, school violence will be considered to be a special case of violent behavior perpetrated by adolescents, which occurs in or around school grounds, usually during or immediately preceding or following school hours. All indications are that behavior of this nature is at disturbingly high levels. In fact, the Centers for Disease Control and Prevention (CDC) (Tatem Kelley et al., 1997) has advocated thinking about school violence as a communicable disease. From this perspective, school violence is at pandemic proportions. Adolescents have the highest rates of crime and victimization of any age group (Snyder and Sickmund, 1999; Tatem Kelley et al., 1997). An estimated 2.7 million violent crimes occur at or near schools annually (Nolin, Davies, and Chandler, 1996). For youths ages 12 to 15, 37 percent of violent crime victimizations occur on school property (Friday, 1996). Forty percent of high school students report being involved in a physical fight, 33 percent have had property stolen or vandalized, 9 percent of students carry weapons on school property, 7 percent have been threatened or injured with a weapon at school, and 4 percent report staying home from school for

I would like to thank Brenda Major, Jennifer Crocker, Sydney Shrauger, and Ladd Wheeler who, at various times, contributed substantially to my understanding of, and passion for, the study of the self and the processes through which this mysterious entity works. Comments and correspondence should be directed to Jason W. Osborne at <jason_osborne@ncsu.edu> or at Educational Research and Leadership, NCSU, Poe Hall 608, Raleigh, NC, 27695. An earlier version of this chapter was presented at the 2002 annual meeting of the American Educational Research Association. I would like to thank Blandy Costello for her assistance in preparing this manuscript.

fear of becoming victimized at school (Snyder and Sickmund, 1999). Involvement in violent crime appears to be increasing among adolescents, across ages, genders, and racial groups (Tatem Kelley et al., 1997).

Students are not the only victims of school-based violence. Of all violent crime perpetrated by adolescents, the hour immediately after school is the most common time for these events to occur (Snyder, 1999). A significant portion of these crimes target nonstudents. Victims often include members of the community, family, acquaintances, or nonstudent members of the school community. For example, researchers estimate that about 11 percent of teachers experience victimization by students (Friday, 1996; Hranitz and Eddowes, 1990).

Dozens of reports by the CDC, Department of Education, and Department of Justice detail the amazing scope of the problem. Few dispute the severity of the problem and many agree on the need to treat this disease. To accomplish this, we must have a good understanding of the etiology of the disease.

RISK FACTORS FOR SCHOOL VIOLENCE

Hundreds of studies and reports have attempted to understand the risk factors for school violence. In a comprehensive review of 66 studies examining the predictors of youth violence, Hawkins et al. (2000) reported that adolescent violence was related to

- *individual factors* such as pregnancy and delivery complications, low resting heart rate, internalizing disorders, hyperactivity, concentration problems, restlessness, risk taking, aggressiveness, early involvement in violent behavior, involvement in other antisocial behavior, beliefs and attitudes favorable to deviant or antisocial behavior;
- *family factors* such as parental criminality, child maltreatment, poor family management practices, low parental involvement, poor family bonding, family conflict, parental attitudes favorable to substance abuse and violence, parent-child separation;
- *school factors* such as academic failure, low bonding to school, truancy, withdrawal from school, frequent school transitions;

- *peer-related factors* such as delinquent siblings or peers, gang membership; and
- *community and neighborhood factors* such as poverty, community disorganization, availability of drugs and/or firearms, neighborhood adults involved in crime, and exposure to violence and racial prejudice.

Perhaps more important, Hawkins et al. (2000) empirically examined the relative importance of all these factors, concluding that the most significant predictors of adolescent violence included a lack of social ties, connections with antisocial peers, school attitudes and performance, parent-child relationships, and being male. Although the report by Hawkins et al. (2000) did not identify race as a specific predictor of adolescent violence, other studies, such as the 1999 National Report on Juvenile Offenders and Victims (Snyder and Sickmund, 1999) report that Latino and non-Latino blacks are more likely to perpetrate school violence than whites.

As with most human behavior, violent behavior, whether in school or out of school, is determined multiply. Examining the long list of risk factors provided previously, such factors can generally be categorized into one of two groups—factors amenable to intervention, and factors not amenable to intervention. Race, gender, family and community environment, behavioral background, and neonatal history are generally immalleable. From a treatment-and-prevention point of view, factors that are amenable to intervention (either prevention or treatment) are of the most interest. As such, these factors will become the focus of this paper. Many of the factors identified by Hawkins et al. (2000) as the most important predictors of violent behavior (lack of social ties, connections with antisocial peers, school attitudes and performance, and parent-child relationships) are also likely candidates for intervention because they tend to be amenable to intervention.

This chapter focuses on what Hawkins et al. (2000) called "bonding to school." The concept of bonding to school, which has been dealt with in the education and psychological literature as *school engagement* and *identification with academics,* is a psychological factor that has the power to determine (and be determined by) important adolescent outcomes, including the participation in deviant and violent behaviors. It provides a clear path toward intervention in preventing unwanted outcomes, such as school violence and dropping out.

WHAT IS IDENTIFICATION WITH ACADEMICS?

Identification with academics refers to the extent to which an individual defines the self through his or her role and performance in the academic domain. It is a special case of domain identification, the extent to which an individual defines the self through a role or performance in a particular domain. If you were asked to list the five most important things you would want another person to know about you, what would they be? For many, aspects of the self, such as job/career, relationships (wife/husband, parent, friend), hobbies or passions (painter, musician, artist, chef, craftsperson, athlete), personality traits, and religiosity rise to the top. Not all domains are important to all people, however. The extent to which one identifies with a particular domain can vary. The aspects of the self that people identify as important, or central, to the self, are important in self-esteem theory. Thus, there is good reason to believe that identification with a domain can provide significant insight into performance in that domain.

Adolescents are forced to deal with a certain array of domains in one way or another—schooling, extracurricular activities, peer relationships, romantic relationships, family/parental relationships, appearance, social status, and religiosity, to name a few. However, not all adolescents view all aspects as equally important. For some, their looks and appearance are strongly tied up with how they feel about themselves, whereas others do not live or die on whether they perceive themselves as attractive or not. Some are strongly involved with the student role, doing well in academics, whereas others care very little about academic outcomes, not seeing the student role as important. Some put a lot of emphasis on athletics, music, or art, whereas others care little about these pursuits.

The concept of identification with a domain is rooted in the symbolic interactionist perspective on self-esteem (see Figure 2.1), although many self-esteem theories acknowledge the concept. Throughout the history of self theory, from William James ([1890] 1981), through Cooley (1902) and Mead (1934) to the present, the symbolic

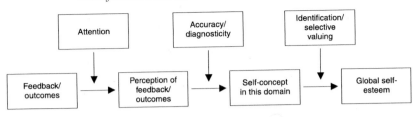

FIGURE 2.1. This diagram represents identification with academics.

interactionist view of the self posits that people base their self-esteem largely on feedback from their environment. This feedback, if attended to, is perceived and interpreted. If the feedback is deemed accurate or valid, it is incorporated into the self-concept. If that facet of the self-concept is viewed as central, or important (and thus, an individual is *identified* with that domain), then the changes in the self-concept will affect an individual's self-esteem (Marsh, 1993, 1995; Pelham, 1995a,b; Pelham and Swann, 1989).

According to this model, if an individual does not value a particular domain, does not view that domain as important to the self (and thus is considered not identified or *disidentified* with that domain), then feedback in that domain will ultimately have little effect on that individual's self-esteem. Note that although the focus is on the symbolic interactionist perspective to frame this discussion, this is not the only self-esteem theory that posits academics as a source of self-esteem (for a more thorough discussion of this point see Osborne, 1995), nor is this perspective the only perspective that includes the notion that different areas of life can have different levels of relevance to the self (Pelham and Swann, 1989; Rosenberg, 1979; Tesser, 1988).

An important point here is that although all individuals assign relative weights to different aspects of their lives, and thus are differentially identified with different domains, these weights are by no means static or permanent. Several decades worth of research have argued that the relative importance of a domain can fluctuate over time. Authors such as Rosenberg (1979) have argued that the various facets of the self are weighted, hierarchized, and combined according to individual needs and conditions. Tesser and Campbell (1983) and Tesser (1988) have explicitly posited the notion that individuals maintain their self-esteem by variously increasing and decreasing the importance of different domains of the self, depending on the quality of the outcomes in those domains. Tesser (1988) details several studies that show support for this hypothesis that relative importance of a domain can fluctuate in response to outcomes in a domain. Although Tesser (1988) outlines these processes primarily in older adolescents and adults, Harter (1986) detailed these same processes in children. Other authors have also reported on this phenomenon (Allport, 1943; Crocker and Major, 1989; Epstein, 1973; Greenwald, 1980; Major and Schmader, 1998; Taylor and Brown, 1988).

Much of the research and discussion in this area examines identification with a domain as a function of outcomes in that domain, yet it is possible to argue that domain identification, the relative importance of a domain to the self, can also influence performance in that domain (in fact, it is likely that both processes operate circularly and iteratively).

Taking a simple operant conditioning point of view, domain identification should be related to outcomes in a domain. Assuming that a positive self-view is important and rewarding to the self, and that a negative self-view is undesirable, aversive, or punishing to the self, an argument supported by many self theorists (Greenberg et al., 1999; Steele, 1988; Tesser, 1988), individuals should be motivated to behave in ways that maximize the probability of positive outcomes in domains that are considered important and identified with. For students who are identified with academics, good performance should be rewarding (higher self-esteem, leading to more positive emotions), whereas poor performance should be punishing (lower self-esteem, leading to negative emotions). In contrast, students who are not identified with academics should have little motivation to succeed because little contingency exists between academic outcomes and self-esteem—good performance is not intrinsically rewarding, and poor performance is not intrinsically punishing. Thus, in the case of domains that are important to the self, poor outcomes will harm self-esteem, a punishing event, whereas positive outcomes will boost self-esteem, a rewarding event. Conversely, students have little motivation to expend efforts in pursuit of positive outcomes in domains that they are not identified with, because poor outcomes in those domains do not harm the self, and positive outcomes do not boost the self.

Further, students who incorporate academic success into their self-concept are also likely to have possible/future selves that are fundamentally different than those students who are not identified. As Markus and Nurius (1987) point out, these possible selves and future goals can be powerful motivators, and can also impact behavior substantially (see also Miller et al., 1996). Goal theory tells us that students' goals can impact motivation significantly. Students who have stronger learning goals (e.g., increasing competency, understanding, and appreciation for the topic being studied) tend to engage in more self-regulated learning (Ames, 1992; Pintrich and De Groot, 1990) and tend to believe that effort is the key to academic success and failure (Pintrich and Schunk, 1996). Further, although researchers generally believed that students holding strong performance goals tended to be less motivated, research shows that students who have a competitive orientation (performance/approach goals [Elliot and Harackiewicz, 1996], which involves seeking success relative to peers, such as outperforming other students, or siblings) put considerable time and effort into their academic work. Both of these goals are completely consistent with a strong identification with academics, and research (Elliot and Harackiewicz, 1996) shows both increased motivation and better academic outcomes as a result of holding these goals.

Many other perspectives on achievement motivation are compatible with this argument. For example, psychologists have known for years that motivation to achieve in a domain or work toward a goal is a function of the value of the goal and the perceived likelihood of attaining the goal (Atkinson and Feather, 1966; Eccles, 1987). Although many individuals have the ability or potential to attain particular goals in particular domains, individuals cannot expend effort on achieving all possible goals. They work toward goals that are meaningful and valuable to them in the domains they are identified with.

In summary, clear theoretical rationale exists for expecting identification with a domain to lead to more positive outcomes, whereas a lack of identification with a domain should be related to a lack of positive outcomes or increased negative outcomes.

A COMPREHENSIVE MODEL

Given this basis, we can develop a more comprehensive model of identification with academics, the relationship of identification with academics to academic outcomes, and the relationship of identification with academics and various nonacademic outcomes, most particularly violent, aggressive, or deviant behavior in school. An outline of this model is presented in Figure 2.2. We will start with a discussion of identification with academics and academic outcomes. Academics is a large part of most adolescents' lives, for better or worse, and as such must be the starting point for later discussions of identification with academics and violence.

As with any other psychological variable, a variety of background or exogenous factors influence identification with academics, such as race or group membership (Osborne, 1995, 1997b; Steele, 1992), school climate (Finn, 1989), and family or community environment, e.g., the extent to which parents, peers, and the community value schooling and support excellence (Ogbu, 1992). Prior academic outcomes also are likely to play a role in the level of identification at any particular point in time (Tesser, 1988). Note that this is not meant to be an exhaustive list. These starting points will influence some initial level of identification with academics.

At this point, the student's motivation to achieve enters the equation. Students who are more strongly identified with academics should be more strongly motivated to succeed academically and persist longer in the face of frustration or failure than those who have

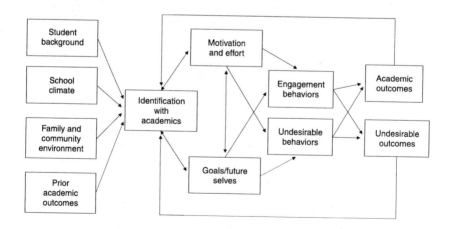

FIGURE 2.2. This diagram represents precursors and consequences of identification with academics.

disidentified because their self-esteem is more strongly influenced by academic performance. The level of motivation should then lead to behaviors that will increase the possibility of positive outcomes in the domain, such as attending class, doing homework, studying, coming to class prepared, monitoring and self-regulating learning, engaging in extracurricular activities, and so on. These behaviors arguably increase the probability of desirable academic outcomes, such as receiving good grades, receiving relatively high standardized test scores, remaining in school, graduating, attending college, etc. Further, this motivation to succeed should *decrease* other, undesirable behaviors, such as truancy, rebelliousness, or acting out in class, and perhaps even violent or aggressive behaviors, which then predispose students toward poor academic outcomes and other outcomes that are undesirable, such as suspension from school, withdrawal from school, and so on (this point is expanded upon later). Note that these relationships are not always unidirectional, as indicated in Figure 2.2. Also note that this model has been stripped to its essential elements for expediency. At every step in Figure 2.2, other potential variables mediate relationships or contribute to a particular outcome. Thus the gist of the model is presented in a relatively simple fashion while acknowledging the complexity of the issue at hand.

Given this argument, we begin to build an image of students as variously identified or disidentified with academics. Those who are disidentified are likely to be at much higher risk for adverse academic outcomes because of their lack of motivation in the academic realm. They will find school irrelevant to their needs, and will endure it while forced to, or while it does not interfere with their esteem-seeking efforts in other areas. As soon as they are not forced to endure schooling, however, or when schooling becomes a particular impediment to the activities necessary for self-esteem, school will be abandoned. Thus, a theoretical link exists between domain identification, motivation, behaviors, performance in academics, and other less desirable outcomes, such as violent or deviant behavior.

EVIDENCE FOR THE LINK BETWEEN IDENTIFICATION WITH ACADEMICS AND ACADEMIC OUTCOMES

Management research has long focused on workers' identification with work (valuing, defining the self through work, etc.), with the common conclusion that highly identified workers tend to perform better than less-identified workers (Kanungo, 1979; Rabinowitz and Hall, 1977). In the marriage-and-family literature (Pasley, Futris, and Skinner, 2002), a father's identification with the fathering role predicts behavior and outcomes related to fathering, such as involvement in child-related activities. Similarly, the few studies investigating the link between identification with academics and academic outcomes indicate that increasing identification with academics is likely to increase the probability of positive outcomes in that domain.

Osborne (1997a) reported that, among community college students, identification with academics prospectively predicted important academic outcomes over a two-year period. Those higher in identification with academics on their first day of classes after enrolling ended with significantly higher grade point averages. They were also more likely to receive academic honors (e.g., dean's list), and were significantly less likely to receive adverse academic outcomes (e.g., dismissed for academic cause, placed on academic probation).

Identification with academics has also been shown to be related to important academic outcomes in secondary students. Voelkl (1997) reported significant relationships between identification with academics and academic achievement and classroom participation. Osborne and Rausch (2001) followed a cohort of students from the time they enrolled in high school (the summer between eighth and ninth grade) through the end of tenth grade. Identification with academics was measured prior to their matriculation into ninth grade. As expected from the previous discussion, the results of this study showed that identification with academics was related to motivation to succeed, goals, and academic outcomes. Significant correlations existed between identification with academics and indicators of motivation or effort in the domain—the amount of deep ($r = .62, p < .001$) and shallow cognitive processing of course material ($r = .51, p < .001$), and self-regulation ($r = .63, p < .001$). Identification with academics was found to be related to goals as well, with significant correlations between identification with academics and learning goals ($r = .71, p < .001$), performance goals ($r = .36, p < .001$), and future goals ($r = .38, p < .001$). Identification with academics was also related to important academic outcomes, such as GPA ($r = .52, p < .001$), and important nonacademic outcomes, such as the number of behavioral referrals ($r = -.20, p < .05$) and absenteeism ($r = -.27, p < .02$) after two years.

Osborne (2002) examined these hypotheses in the National Education Longitudinal Survey of 1988 (NELS88), a nationally representative database of 24,599 secondary students gathered by the National Center for Educational Statistics. Similar to the results reported in Osborne and Rausch (2001), student identification with academics was related to motivation, engagement and undesirable behaviors, and academics outcomes. Specifically, the more highly identified students tended to spend significantly more time on homework outside of school, were more likely to come to class prepared for the lesson, were less likely to cut classes, had fewer absences, and were less likely to withdraw from school prior to graduation, relative to less strongly identified students.

Although no studies prior to Osborne (1997a) and Voelkl (1996) defined and operationalized identification with academics in this fashion, other researchers have reported relationships between academic outcomes and similar constructs. For example, Trusty and Dooley-Dickey (1993) reported a relationship between alienation from school and reading and mathematics achievement, and Goodenow and Grady (1993) reported relationships between feelings of belongingness in school and engagement, motivation, and persistence in academic tasks.

In summary, the available literature provides evidence supporting the basic model presented in Figure 2.2 linking identification with the domain of academics to outcomes in that domain. Given this starting point, it is relatively straightforward to posit relationships between identification with academics and deviant and violent behavior.

The First Path to School Violence: Disidentification with Academics

Many researchers report links between academic outcomes and school violence. It seems intuitive that the best-performing students are less likely to engage in violent or deviant behavior than the worse-performing students, but why? Given what we know of the self, and the arguments presented relating to identification with academics, one hypothesis as to why this relationship might exist is that identification with academics is a factor in both outcomes.

In this section two scenarios relating identification with academics to school violence will be developed. Both involve a student who is disidentified or who has a relatively low level of identification with academics.[1]

Scenario #1: Academic Disidentification and Identification with Peer Relationships

In self-esteem theory, it is explicitly assumed that people are identified with at least one, and usually several domains, although the specific domains and the number of domains might change. Although no theorists have put forth a compelling argument for whether there is a universal critical number,[2] what the range of identified domains might be, and so on, the expectation is that if an individual disidentifies from a domain (eliminates outcomes in that domain as a source of self-esteem) then that individual will generally find another domain to identify with, another set of outcomes on which to base self-esteem. Without this replacement strategy an individual might end up with no domains on which to base self-esteem, which does not make sense from most theoretical perspectives.

This tiny, commonsense assumption is the foundation of the first mechanisms for linking identification with academics with school violence. Should a student be doing poorly, or see no utility in pursuing academics, the logical step from a self point of view is to disidentify with academics. Many researchers have argued that individuals devalue or disidentify with domains in which they receive relatively poor outcomes (Crocker and Major, 1989; Major and Schmader, 1998; Steele, 1997; Tesser, 1988), and dozens have reported results supporting these hypotheses.

If a student has disidentified from academics, on what can that student base his or her self-esteem? Given the developmental stage of the students we are talking about, common domains might include peer or romantic relationships, appearance, or participation in extracurricular activities, such as sports, music, or the arts.

However, it is difficult to find evidence concerning this hypothesized transference of identification to other domains with more reward potential. Finn (1989) argued convincingly that it should occur, and that it explains why researchers have failed to find self-esteem differences between dropouts and nondropouts—namely that dropping out is a process during which students change the basis of their self-esteem from academics to another domain, probably completing this transference prior to or concomitantly with the dropping out.

Osborne (1997b, 2002) reported some evidence of this phenomenon, both in the context of analyses of the NELS88 data set. Osborne (1997b) tested Steele's (1992, 1997) hypothesis that African-American students would disidentify from academics in response to continued exposure to the negative stereotype of intellectual inferiority. Not only did this study show support for Steele's argument (particularly among African-American males), but also showed some evidence supporting Finn's (1989) argument about transference of identification. In this case, Osborne (1997b) showed evidence of increasing identification with peer relationships and athletics as identification with academics was decreasing.

Osborne (2002) examined identification with five areas in his first study: math and reading achievement, family, same-sex, and opposite-sex relationships among tenth-graders. The findings demonstrated that those withdrawing from school had lower identification with academics than those not withdrawing, across all race and gender groups. However, this study also showed that dropouts tended to identify with parent and same- or opposite-sex peer relationships at the same or higher level as nondropouts. This suggests that social relationships might be one area of focus for those disidentifying with academics.

This focus on relationships is certainly adaptive, and makes sense intuitively, as one of the tasks of adolescence is to practice creating and maintaining adult relationships (Erikson, 1968; Hill, 1987). However, depending on the peers or family, this increased emphasis on these relationships can have dramatically different effects. If the peers are strongly interested in socially desirable activities, such as sports, music, or art, for example, the student is more likely to be drawn into participating in socially desirable activities. However, if the peers are strongly interested in socially undesirable activities, this increased identification with peer relationships might draw the student into behaving in undesirable ways, particularly into violent or antisocial behavior, thus explicating one of the links between identification with academics and school violence. The mechanism should work similarly for family relationships. If the student is more identified with family relationships than academics, and family members (particularly siblings, but also parents and extended family or community members) encourage violent or antisocial behavior, those behaviors become more likely if the student is to maintain self-esteem.

To summarize, one hypothesized link between identification with academics and school violence is that, for students who have disidentified with academics, it is a strong possibility that social relationships take on heightened importance, and therefore behavior becomes increasingly motivated by maintaining the esteem of the social group that is most important to the student. To the extent that violent, disruptive, or antisocial behavior is necessary to maintain positive feedback from these relationships, adolescents will become increasingly likely to perform these behaviors.

This scenario depends on the following conditions: (1) as the student is reducing the levels of identification with academics, the student becomes more strongly identified with, or maintains a strong identification with, peer, opposite-sex, family, or community relationships; (2) the people in those relationships have positive attitudes toward violent, aggressive, and/or antisocial behavior; and (3) there is no other factor that would significantly affect the student's willingness to participate in these sorts of activities (i.e., there is no identification with another domain, such as religion or parent/family relationships that would counteract the effect of peer pressure).

Some evidence supports this hypothesis, as researchers have identified peer and family relationships as significant factors in adolescent violence. For example, Saner and Ellickson (1996) reported that students with strong peer support were *more likely* to exhibit deviant and rebellious behavior, and Hawkins et al. (2000) report that students with deviant peers (including but not limited to gang membership) or deviant siblings were more likely to engage in deviant behavior than those without these relationships.

Scenario #2: Academic Disidentification and Frustration at Being Forced to Remain in the School Setting

The frustration-aggression hypothesis (Miller, 1941) is a well-known psychological theory. Briefly, psychologists proposed that frustration (inability to attain a desired goal) resulted in aggressive behavior. Indeed, many aggressive acts are instrumental in achieving goals when frustrated, as they often remove the source of frustration. They thus represent a certain class of coping strategy, although a generally socially undesirable one. As later research has pointed out, not all aggression appears to stem from frustration, and not all frustration leads to aggression. Yet there are clear cases when frustration does lead to aggression, although in some cases the frustration can be displaced and targeted on an object that is not the source of the original frustration. With this point in mind, let us then assume that sometimes frustration will lead to aggression, hostility, or violence, although not always targeted at the source of the frustration. There are at least three cases in which identification with a domain can either diffuse the frustration and tendency toward aggression and violence, or exacerbate it. The first example of how identification and frustration intersect occurs when a student has disidentified with academics (for whatever reason), and yet is forced to keep attending school, leading to significant levels of frustration.

Schools tend to be fairly restrictive environments. Ironically, although school is where adolescents spend most of their waking hours, it is also (often) the most rigid environment where the students have little perceived or actual control over their lives. Laws and parents dictate that they must attend, counselors tell them what classes to take, bells and schedules indicate where they are to be at any particular time, teachers and other faculty tell them what to do at any particular time, and peers rigidly enforce codes of conduct and dress. There is little time or opportunity for students to feel free to choose any course of action for themselves. It is not surprising that students might come to feel like prisoners in a penal system. In many cases, they might have less actual freedom than inmates in penal institutions. All these factors might combine to precipitate significant feelings of frustration among some (or perhaps, a majority) of students.

Students who are strongly identified with academics are not as likely to perceive this situation as negatively as those who have disidentified. Although most students probably perceive the school environment as unnecessarily restrictive and desire more control, for those heavily identified with the process of schooling, and with achieving success in academics, it is probably little more than a source of aggravation or annoyance. However, it must be tremendously frustrating to a student who has mentally withdrawn from school but who is forced to be physically present and endure this restrictiveness and lack of control often present in the school environment. Thus, students who have disidentified might be at risk for significant levels of school-related frustration.

These high levels of frustration might predispose academically disidentified students to rebel against these conditions in aggressive or violent ways, leading to higher levels of aggression or violence independent of the influence of the peer group discussed in the first scenario. In this case it is not peer esteem that is driving behavior, but rather frustration at being forced to remain in school despite schooling not being desirable or important to the student. For these students, violence, aggression, antisocial, and destructive acts are instrumental, as their goal is to escape the situation, and these types of acts produce the highest probability of their escape, through suspensions, expulsions, transfers to other types of environments, and even arrests.

In both scenarios presented thus far, the process of disidentification precipitates situations in which violent or aggressive behavior is instrumental to achieving important goals. In the first scenario, the goal is the positive regard of select members of a social network, and when valued members of the social network value and reward violent, aggressive, or delinquent behaviors the student is going to be motivated to behave in this way. In the second scenario, the goal is escape from an aversive situation—an overly restrictive environment that has little to offer the self, and contains perhaps many negative outcomes for the self. Escape can be arranged through absenteeism, truancy, and skipping classes, but there may be external factors that limit the success of these strategies. Thus, aggressive, violent, or delinquent behavior can be instrumental in ensuring the student is removed from the aversive situation.

Evidence for These Hypotheses

Aside from the evidence that identification with peer relationships might become stronger as identification with academics weakens, Osborne (2002) found in his second study that a variety of undesirable behaviors were associated with disidentifying from academics.

As mentioned, those students reporting mildly undesirable behaviors (being unprepared for class, cutting classes, and having many absences) tended to be lower in identification with academics than those not exhibiting these behaviors.

However, more deviant and undesirable behaviors were also more common among those with lower identification with academics. Those who reported being in physical fights with other students more than two times during the previous semester had significantly lower identification with academics than those reporting never having been in a physical fight with another student. Furthermore, those students suspended (out of school) more than two times in the previous semester had significantly lower identification with academics than those never suspended. A similar pattern was observed for students transferred to different schools for disciplinary reasons, and those students reporting being arrested—in both cases, students with the less socially desirable outcomes had lower identification with academics.

Note that in both scenarios an important condition is met: academics is no longer an important part of the self. Students who are strongly identified with academics would not just have an absence of a significant incentive to engage in these behaviors, but rather might have a powerful disincentive. Social control theorists (Liska and Reed, 1985) have pointed to a lack of identification as a precursor to delinquent behavior, as students are less likely to commit acts of violence or aggression in a place where they have intimate ties and attachments. From a psychological view, this makes a great deal of sense for two reasons. First, to the extent that a domain, place, or activity is an important aspect of the self, aggressive or violent acts against that domain, place, or activity are difficult. From a psychological point of view, if the school is part of the self, then an act of violence against the school is an act of violence against the self, not generally an adaptive or desirable thing. Second, all students are aware that the consequences of violent, aggressive, or antisocial behavior might include separation from the school environment and other undesirable outcomes. For a student strongly identified with academics, this potential separation and other negative outcomes in that domain would be a strong disincentive. These two points flow directly from William James' ([1892] 1968) notion of an "empirical self" wherein individuals extend the self to incorporate external aspects of the environment, thus experiencing positive or negative outcomes as a result of the outcomes experienced by the external entities.

Although the first two scenarios represent a significant portion of school violence, there are two other scenarios in which identification with academics is related to school violence. These scenarios involve specific sources of frustration, and how strong identification with academics can either fuel or diffuse the impulse to use aggression and violent behavior as a coping strategy for dealing with the frustration.

The Second Path to School Violence: Frustration and Inappropriate Levels of Domain Identification

Scenario #3: Unattainable Goals and Inappropriately Strong Identification with Academics

Although strong identification with academics is, in general, an important ingredient in positive outcomes for students, one universal truth about psychology is that in psychology there are no universal truths. This scenario shows how certain students need to reduce their levels of identification with academics under certain conditions or be at risk for school violence.

Occasionally, students might have certain expectations for performance that they are consistently unable to meet. There are two possibilities as to why this occurs. It could be that the student is engaging in a self-handicapping strategy of setting unrealistically high performance goals in order to have an excuse for not achieving those goals (Covington, 2000). This particular case is not of concern in the context of this chapter.

The other possibility is that some entity holds and communicates unrealistically high performance goals (in this case, an unrealistic performance goal is a level of performance that is far beyond or outside past performance or is unreasonable given prior preparation). Furthermore, the student has received the message that these goals are reasonable and attainable. It could be that the student has internalized unrealistically high standards for the self, that the teachers or parents have standards that the student is consistently unable to meet, or it could be peer standards for academic performance that the student is unable to meet. There may be some external entity setting standards that the student is not able to meet, such as when a student has the goal of going to Harvard but cannot attain the GPA or SAT scores necessary to be competitive.

The evidence in the literature from decades of research suggests that humans are fairly sophisticated at managing various factors to protect a positive self-view. Researchers (discussed previously) have proposed that "healthy" individuals are able to strategically manage their self-concepts so that they devalue domains where they rarely receive positive outcomes and value domains where they commonly receive positive outcomes. Of course, this strategic management of domains is (from a self-perspective) a desirable and usual outcome. In the case where it is not possible to alter the unrealistically high expectations, devaluing and disidentification are alternative self-protective strategies.

It might not be possible to devalue or disidentify with a domain due to situational or environmental constraints. For example, in American society, physical attractiveness is a domain that is difficult to devalue, particularly for girls and women. Affluence and socioeconomic status is another. At particular developmental stages, such as adolescence, certain domains might become particularly important, and difficult to disidentify with, such as same- or opposite-sex relationships. Another reason might be more proximal—it is possible that a student's family or peer group does not allow the student to devalue a particular domain. Thus, some factor prevents devaluing or disidentification with a domain despite the presence of chronic, negative outcomes in that domain.

Although the "normal" or "adaptive" reaction to this situation from a self-perspective would be to disidentify with academics and identify with a different domain in which the self has better prospects for success, if a student cannot disidentify with academics, then that student is placed in an intractable situation. The student is required by whatever standards to perform at a particular level, yet the student is consistently unable to perform at that level. The result must be an increasingly severe level of frustration. In this case a strongly identified student will be strongly motivated to (1) seek assistance to meet the standards through remediation or other support from various sources, (2) use cheating or other antisocial methods to achieve the desired goal, or (3) exhibit increasingly aggressive, destructive, or violent behavior as the frustration from the elusive goal builds with no resolution in sight. Ironically, under this scenario, strongly identified individuals will be most at risk for violence, although it is only those who are maladaptively highly identified.

Scenario #4: Peer Derogation and Exclusion
and Inappropriately High Identification
with Peer Relationships

In a review and synthesis of a number of theories and studies of school crime Kulka, Klingel, and Mann (1980) argued that a significant lack of person-environment fit can contribute to school violence. Specifically, they argued that when students do not fit into the schooling environment (i.e., when there is a lack of person-environment fit for a variety of reasons, from academic to behavioral and social), that student will feel devalued, alienated, frustrated, and hostile.

In any social group or organization there appears to always be some emergent social hierarchy. No matter the nature of the social hierarchy, there is almost always some individual or group that is derogated, subject to abuse, harassment, and even attack. Socioeconomic status, race, physical attributes (such as obesity or physical disability or deformity), sexual orientation (actual or perceived), social aptitude, and other characteristics can mark individuals or groups as targets of prejudice, discrimination, and/or abuse. Unfortunately, teachers and faculty can pick up on the social hierarchies and may be influenced in the way they treat students, so that in some schools, students receive abuse and derogation from all corners.

In this scenario a student receives substantial amounts of negative outcomes and frustration from significant others in the social domain (same- or opposite-sex peers, parents, teachers, etc.). One adaptive and self-protective solution might be to change who the significant others are in the social milieu. Another would be disidentification with social outcomes and increasing identification with another domain (such as academics), although given the issues surrounding adolescence, devaluing the social domain is difficult.

Although there are many aspects of the academic domain that are perceived to be out of students' control, academic outcomes are perceived as more controllable than social outcomes. Members of derogated or excluded groups have virtually no power to change their lot in the social hierarchy, yet with effort most can achieve some significant measure of academic success, particularly where learning goals and mastery orientations prevail. Thus, the ability to devalue social outcomes and to identify with another domain, such as academics, might be a critical coping strategy for these individuals. Failure to do that will, as in the third scenario, result in an increasing spiral of negative outcomes and frustration, leading to aggression and hostility against the agents of social exclusion or derogation (Twenge et al., 2001), or perhaps aggression and hostility displaced to another target. In this case, then, developing or maintaining a strong identification with academics might be self-protective, diffusing the frustration and aggression by providing an alternate source of self-worth, and reducing the likelihood of violence.

Three of the four scenarios link decreased violence and delinquent behavior to a high level of identification with academics (the third scenario being a rather unique case). Given this, it is possible that these mechanisms help to explain the well-documented link between school violence and academic outcomes such as poor achievement and withdrawal from school.

TYPES OF VIOLENCE IN SCHOOL

We must be careful in discussing such a broad category of behaviors as "violence" or "antisocial behaviors." Given the scenarios and factors just discussed, it is possible to construct more specific hypotheses about the types of behaviors most and least likely to be exhibited in a given scenario. For the purposes of this chapter, school violence is being considered broadly as a group of undesirable behaviors that result in a significantly negative outcome for another student or entity (such as the school building itself). These behaviors can include

1. acts against objects, such as theft, vandalism, and arson;
2. acts against same-sex peers, such as intimidation, bullying, assault, battery, and homicide;
3. acts against opposite-sex peers, such as sexual harassment, sexual assault, intimidation, bullying, and rape;

4. acts against staff and faculty, such as intimidation, bullying, assault, battery, theft, sexual offenses of various types, and homicide; and

5. other deviant or undesirable behaviors that are "victimless," such as truancy, and skipping classes.

This is not meant to be an extensive or complete cataloguing of possibilities but merely a framework for thinking about different types of acts that tend to get lumped together as violence.

In light of this simple taxonomy of "violent behaviors" we can propose the following hypothesized links between identification with academics and specific types of school violence.

Scenario #1: Disidentification with Academics and Identification with Peer Relationships

The first paths to school violence previously presented posited the notion that if a student decreases the level of identification with academics (for any of a variety of reasons) then that student is likely to increase identification with another domain. Often, (for a variety of reasons) the esteem of a segment of the social network (peers, opposite-sex peers, family members, community members, etc.) is likely to become or remain one of the domains that comes to the fore when academics fades as an important source of self-esteem.

As discussed, many students who disidentify with academics and identify with social relationships will not exhibit violent, aggressive, or delinquent acts. It is the particular nature of that social network that will determine the nature of the behavior that the peers will motivate. The question here is what sort of behaviors would be seen as "cool" or desirable to a particular group? Let us assume that the most common situation is that the student is looking to the peer group for esteem and social rewards. There are several groups of behaviors that are likely in this case. First, because students gravitate toward those that they perceive as similar, these peers are likely to also be disidentified with academics and probably exhibiting delinquent behavior. Wanting to fit in, the student will want to behave in ways that telegraph and communicate similar values (especially academic disidentification). Behaviors that demonstrate this perceived unimportance are likely, such as truancy and skipping classes, vandalism of school facilities, and other acts of "coolness" (as discussed in Majors and Billson's [1992] notion of cool pose). Second, given that these students are semioutcasts in the schooling environment, it is likely that a class of behaviors that derogate and intimidate other students are likely, as these behaviors will provide favorable social comparison outcomes. This class of behaviors will include bullying and other aggressive acts against peers, and sexual harassment and assault against opposite-sex peers (if the students are male; this behavior appears less commonly in girls).

Extreme violence against students is not likely unless that is what is valued by the peers. Also, teachers and faculty are not likely to be common targets under this scenario, as they are not easy targets to the same extent that inanimate objects, lower-status peers, and girls often are. However, it is difficult to form generalizations here, unless one knows the particulars of the social networks, and what behaviors they will or will not reward. If they are particularly antiteacher, or have a particular vendetta against a member of the faculty, then violence against teachers becomes more likely.

Scenario #2: Academic Disidentification and Frustration at Being Forced to Remain in the School Setting

In this scenario, a student has disidentified with academics (for whatever reason) yet is forced to remain in the restrictive environment of the school, an aversive situation to be sure. In this case, the most likely behaviors are those that are instrumental in achieving escape from the aversive situation. Students in this situation are likely to participate in the nonviolent behaviors of absenteeism and truancy, skipping classes, and/or any behavior that would lead to being removed from the environment, such as vandalism of school property. Should these behaviors be sufficient to escape the situation, no further action on the part of the student will be necessary, as the goal has been achieved. However, if those behaviors fail to achieve the goal of not being forced to be in school, other more violent behaviors might manifest as a result of the increased frustration or in an attempt to find behaviors that will allow escape. In this case, it is likely that students will exhibit increasingly deviant behaviors until they find one that meets the goal. Furthermore, there is often no single agent of frustration, and therefore the escalating frustration could be displaced to peers, teachers, or administrators, or even the facilities. However, it is likely that few cases get to this point. Most students in this situation are likely to achieve their goal of being removed from the school situation through less violent means.

Scenario #3: Unattainable Goals and Inappropriately Strong Identification with Academics

In this scenario a student is caught in an intractable situation—a consistent failure to achieve desired levels of performance coupled with a strong identification with academics—a familiar recipe for frustration. As discussed, there are at least three possible outcomes from this situation, if the student is unable to alter the expectations or the identification with academics: (1) the student will seek assistance to improve performance to meet the standards through remediation or other support from various sources; (2) the student will artificially raise performance to meet the standards through cheating or other undesirable methods of achieving the desired goal; or (3) the student will exhibit increasingly aggressive, destructive, or violent behavior as the frustration from the elusive goal builds with no resolution in sight. In the last case, this student will be seeking a target on which to vent frustrations. If there is a specific teacher or administrator who is seen as causing the frustration (i.e., the student is failing math, but meeting expectations in other areas) then violence against that teacher or in the context of that class is increasingly likely. If there is more of a global failure to meet expectations, harassment, aggression, and violence against other peers (both same and opposite sex), including sexual violence, becomes more likely as well. This is probably not a situation where vandalism of school property, or other delinquent acts, such as truancy or skipping classes will be likely behaviors, as they have little instrumentality to relieve the frustration, and may actually work against the student achieving his or her goals of academic performance (especially behaviors that remove the student from the classroom, such as truancy or skipping class).

Scenario #4: Peer Derogation and Exclusion and Inappropriately High Identification with Peer Relationships

This final scenario is, unfortunately, a common one in the U.S. education system, and one that might be related to some of the most spectacular and disturbing displays of school violence, such as those of Columbine High School. Although derogation, "pecking orders," and social exclusion are common social processes, generally, in the "real world" people can escape these situations by modifying where they live, the types of jobs they seek, the people they socialize with, the churches they attend, and so on. The educational system does not allow for easy escape, however, as students are mandated to attend schools until a particular age, and it is not commonly easy to switch classes, schools, or social environments. Furthermore, the faculty members in the schools are often unwilling or helpless to intervene in this process. Nevertheless, many students in this situation cope through a variety of self-protective strategies, such as devaluing social outcomes, altering the individuals who represent significant others in this domain, and so on. Unable to cope through these avenues, the situation becomes bleak.

One coping strategy for this situation is to decrease exposure to this aversive situation by increasing absenteeism and skipping classes, making this class of behaviors a likely outcome under this scenario through simple instrumentality. Unfortunately for these students, external factors often limit their ability to escape these social situations. Parents, school officials, and law enforcement agencies can work to limit truancy. In these cases, a student or group of students receive significant levels of negative outcomes in a domain, an inability to devalue these outcomes, and an inability to escape these outcomes. The most likely reaction at this point is for students to strike back at the source of the frustration, their peers who are the agents of derogation or exclusion. As with the third scenario, it is possible that the aggression can be displaced onto another target, particularly if that target is seen as facilitating the situation (as teachers and administrators sometimes inadvertently reinforce or facilitate these social processes). In this case, other behaviors, such as vandalism against school facilities are only likely if there is instrumentality, such as when burning down the school will result in time off from school, and thus escape from the aversive situation.

PREVENTING SCHOOL VIOLENCE

Given this perspective, it is of paramount importance that we deal with the underlying causes of the undesired behavior rather than create punishments or deterrents. In the first two cases just presented, inappropriately low levels of identification with academics is hypothesized to contribute to inappropriate behavior. One obvious solution is to either prevent academic disidentification or to facilitate identification with academics. There are many ways to attempt this, but the successful strategy will depend on the particular details of the student's background, present situation, and the reasons for disidentification.

If the disidentification is due to significant levels of negative outcomes in the academic domain, increasing the levels of positive outcomes would be effective in assisting to increase identification with academics. This can be done through providing remediation, training, and practice in the use of metacognitive strategies, providing additional resources, helping the student to manage his or her idea of what success and failure is, and so forth. In addition, fostering a "change from baseline" approach to evaluation should help tremendously. Many students compare their performance to the top students, consistently falling short and thus receiving consistently negative outcomes. However, in many other areas of life people are encouraged to evaluate themselves based on their growth from a particular point in time. Thus, asking students to evaluate their progress or level of performance relative to their starting point makes it more likely that more students can perceive their performance positively. Mastery learning orientations and criterion-referenced assessments can facilitate that process, while competitive grading schemes (such as curving) and norm-referenced assessments tend to exacerbate this issue.

Another common cause of disidentification is the perception that academic success has little value for meeting the student's goals. There are many areas throughout the United States where getting a high school diploma or college degree does not significantly improve important outcomes, such as job attainment, income, or esteem in the community. If academics is not seen as a route through which one can achieve one's goals, there is little reason to identify with the domain. Thus, another way to attack this problem is to identify and highlight the ways in which strong academic performance can be instrumental in achieving student goals.

For students trapped in "lower" or "slower" or "remedial" academic tracks, disidentification is probably a significant problem. When curricula are slowed down, and then the difficulty level of work is reduced, students often find little to keep their interest. With no challenge, there is little reward of successfully completing a task or course, and thus little reason to remain identified. Although it is certainly true that not all students can work at the same level, it is true that all students can make progress from their baseline level of performance. All students should be challenged appropriately so that they have initial successes (to increase perceived efficacy in the area) and increasing gradually so that they do not always succeed at a task, but can succeed with a little assistance or practice. This strategy will both keep students identified with academics through consistent, real successes in the domain, but also assist students who have disidentified to reidentify.

In some cases, school systems need to rethink how they manage schooling, particularly at the secondary level. Not all students should be expected to want or need a college-preparatory track, but many schools have no real alternative for the students to value. The explicit message in many schools is that the college preparation track is the valued track, and the rest of the tracks are for students who cannot manage the work. Vocational education should be a viable alternative for these students, but too often vocational programs are dumping grounds for disenfranchised or hopeless students, rather than being challenging programs with real value. To the extent that schools can provide alternatives to the college preparation track that have real value, the students can continue to have academics as a valuable source of self-esteem and remain identified with academics.

For students who are at risk for violent or undesirable behavior because they are too highly identified with academics yet not receiving acceptable outcomes in the domain (Scenario #3), it is critical that the faculty and staff at the school assist the students to either improve performance to meet their goals, through increased access to resources, remediation, extra practice, and so on, or to assist the students in forming alternate expectations and goals that are realistic. Of course, simply dumbing down the goals without allowing the student to value and feel good about the new expectations and goals is unproductive.

Of course, not all students are disidentifying due to poor academic outcomes. Some discussion indicates that students who are African

American, Latino, or Native American are particularly prone to disidentification (Ogbu, 1992, 1997; Osborne, 1995, 1997b, 2001; Steele, 1992, 1997). In this case, the causes of the disidentification might be different from those previously discussed, as will the remedies. Osborne (2001) synthesizes several lines of research on this topic, providing some specific recommendations on how to reduce disidentification from this perspective.

In summary, there are many reasons why a student might reduce or eliminate academics as a source of self-esteem. Teachers and school faculty (school counselors can be particularly important here) must be vigilant for signs of this, and must take the effort to understand why a student might be going through this process if they are to take effective measures to prevent or thwart the process. No one remedy will always work for all students, but some of the remedies can go a long way toward preventing many students from disidentifying.

CONCLUSIONS, CAVEATS, AND FUTURE DIRECTIONS

The goal of this chapter was to present a psychological model that relates identification with academics (or, more accurately, academic disidentification) to undesirable outcomes, particularly (but not limited to) aggressive, violent, and deviant behavior in school. The model, presented in Figure 2.2, links identification with academics to both academic and nonacademic outcomes of this type. Some evidence exists for this model in the literature, especially concerning the link between identification with academics and academic outcomes, but also between disidentification and undesirable outcomes.

From this, two possible scenarios developed that specifically linked inappropriately low identification with academics to violent or aggressive behavior (broadly defined). In the first case, students who removed academics as a source of self-esteem are likely to replace academics with peer relationships, which might facilitate undesirable behavior. In the second case, students who were academically disidentified would experience significant levels of frustration at being forced to continue attending school, which might lead to violent behaviors.

Two other special cases were also discussed in which inappropriately high identification with a domain might produce undesirable behavior. In the third case, it is possible that students are laboring under performance expectations that are unattainable given their background, preparation, or aptitude, which might lead to frustration and violent behavior. Finally, in the fourth case, it is possible that students who are members of socially derogated or excluded groups might experience intense levels of frustration, leading to violent behaviors if there is an inappropriately high level of identification with peer relations and an inappropriately low level of identification with academics (or any other domain).

These hypotheses will not explain all deviant and violent behavior, but this model goes a long way toward understanding a significant portion of these behaviors. Furthermore, this model gives explicit courses of action for teachers and school faculty to take to prevent or reduce the levels of school violence.

The model presented in this chapter is not intended to be comprehensive and a finished product, but rather a starting point for researchers. Much work needs to be done in this area. First, many of the hypotheses discussed have limited empirical support within limited populations or samples. The next step is to get researchers studying these issues, talking with students, and testing the goodness of these ideas. Second, as this model is meant to be a starting point rather than a finished product, researchers should think critically about the model, and about the four scenarios presented. There are certainly going to be ways to add to, or otherwise improve these ideas, and researchers should be thinking critically about how to do so.

One future direction school violence researchers need to take seriously is the careful consideration of proposed remedies to the problem. People in power to effect change are not always well trained in dealing with these issues, and they need to be informed by experts on the ramifications of proposed remedies. For example, as many schools contemplate zero-tolerance rules, installation of metal detectors, erosion of student privacy through random locker searches, and the creation of a more restrictive (i.e., jaillike) environment, researchers and experts in the field need to provide thoughtful and informed commentary on the likely ramifications of implementing these rules. As Skiba and Noam (2001) point out, well-intentioned policies can have unintended (or even harmful) consequences.

Finally, there may be some fundamental flaws in our notion of universal schooling and mandated attendance. Perhaps it is not the notion itself, but the implementation. One flaw relates to the perception of an abundant resource—few people value an abundant resource, particularly one that is forced upon them. If you were forced to drink five gallons of water a day, access to and consumption of water might not be viewed as desirable. In fact, you might come to dread and shun water whenever possible. But if you were living in a desert climate and your well constantly dried up, water would become a valuable commodity. From this psychology of scarcity and forced consumption we have created a climate in which we force individuals to partake of what we as a culture consider to be essential and extremely valuable. Yet by forcing all to partake, we might be causing many to loathe this valuable commodity. It is unlikely that our society would take the step of removing this mandated attendance, and most would argue that it is not even a step worth considering, regardless of the consequences. Yet there might be some way to change the perception of the school system and how it is run to eliminate this effect. Doing so might eliminate some of the factors that contribute to violent behavior.

A second flaw in the educational system is the unwillingness of many parties to remove students from the educational setting, even when that student is exhibiting substantial levels of violence and aggression. Parents are unwilling to have their children suspended, administrators are unwilling to fight to have a student removed (or do not feel empowered to do so, or do not feel the support of superiors to do so), students often are unwilling to "rat" on fellow students, teachers are unwilling to get involved, and so on. In the "real world" outside of schools, there are often significant and serious consequences for offenders. Few businesses would tolerate an employee who is violent or aggressive, yet educational institutions are often loath to take action. Although action might not be a deterrent, removing a student who has demonstrated a tendency toward violent, aggressive, or disruptive behavior is the only reasonable course of action, both to prevent reoccurrence of the violent behavior, but also to maintain the integrity of the educational enterprise. Education and learning cannot happen effectively when students are fearful, when lessons are disrupted, and when students see no repercussions for deviant behavior.

NOTES

1. The term, *disidentification,* coined by Claude Steele (1992), refers to someone who has detached his or her self-esteem from academic outcomes. This notion, and the notion of selective valuing, discussed by Crocker and Major (1989) were the genesis of many of the ideas presented in this chapter.

2. It is likely that there is an absolute range and then a "healthy" range of the number of domains identified with. For example, it is probably not psychologically healthy for an individual to be identified with only one domain. Having only one domain as a source of self-worth might result in significant instability in level of self-esteem, extreme reactions to negative outcomes, and so on. Conversely, it is probably not desirable to be highly identified with dozens or hundreds of domains. This could conceivably lead to too much diffusion of efforts, a lack of significant motivation to excel in any particular domain, and perhaps other undesirable psychological outcomes. There is probably some range (e.g., five to ten) that is optimal for healthy functioning. I am not aware of any research on this topic, however.

REFERENCES

Allport, G. W. (1943). The ego in contemporary psychology. *Psychological Review, 50,* 451-478.

Ames, C. (1992). Classroom goals, structures, and student motivation. *Journal of Educational Psychology, 84,* 261-271.

Atkinson, J. W. and Feather, N. T. (1966). *A Theory of Achievement Motivation.* New York: Wiley.

Cooley, C. H. (1902). *Human Nature and the Social Order.* New York: Scribner's.

Covington, M. V. (2000). Goal theory, motivation, and school achievement: An integrative review. *Annual Review of Psychology, 51,* 171-200.

Crocker, J. and Major, B. (1989). Social stigma and self-esteem: The self-protective properties of stigma. *Psychological Review, 94*(4), 608-630.

Eccles, J. S. (1987). Gender roles and women's achievement-related decisions. *Psychology of Women Quarterly, 11,* 135-172.

Elliot, A. J. and Harackiewicz, J. M. (1996). Approach and avoidance achievement goals and intrinsic motivation: A mediational analysis. *Journal of Personality and Social Psychology, 70,* 968-980.

Epstein, S. (1973). The self-concept revisited: Or a theory of a theory. *American Psychologist, 28,* 404-416.

Erikson, E. H. (1968). *Identity, Youth, and Crisis.* New York: Norton.

Finn, J. D. (1989). Withdrawing from school. *Review of Educational Research, 59*(2), 117-142.

Friday, J. C. (1996). Weapon-carrying in school. In A. M. Hoffman (Ed.), *Schools, Violence, and Society* (pp. 21-31). Westport, CT: Praeger.

Goodenow, C. and Grady, K. E. (1993). The relationship of school belonging and friends' values to academic motivation among urban adolescent students. *Journal of Experimental Education, 62,* 60-71.

Greenberg, J., Solomon, S., Pyszczynski, T., Rosenblatt, A., Burling, J., Lyon, D., Simon, L., and Pinel, E. (1999). Why do people need self-esteem? Converging evidence that self-esteem serves an anxiety-buffering function. In R. F. Baumeister (Ed.), *The Self in Social Psychology* (pp. 105-118). Philadelphia, PA: Psychology Press.

Greenwald, A. G. (1980). The totalitarian ego: Fabrication and revision of personal history. *American Psychologist, 35,* 603-618.

Harter, S. (1986). Processes underlying the construction, maintenance, and enhancement of the self-concept in children. In J. Suls and A. W. Greenwald (Eds.), *Psychological Perspectives on the Self,* Volume 3 (pp. 136-182). Hillsdale, NJ: Lawrence Erlbaum.

Hawkins, J. D., Herrenkohl, T. I., Farrington, D. P., Brewer, D., Catalano, R. F., Harachi, T. W., and Cothern, L. (2000). *Predictors of Youth Violence.* Washington, DC: Office of Juvenile Justice and Delinquency Prevention.

Hill, J. P. (1987). Research on adolescents and their families: Past and prospect. *New Directions for Child Development, 37,*13-31.

Hranitz, J. R. and Eddowes, E. A. (1990). Violence: A crisis in homes and schools. *Childhood Education, 67,* 4-7.

James, W. ([1890] 1981). *The Principles of Psychology.* Cambridge, MA: Harvard University Press.

James, W. ([1892] 1968). The Self. In C. Gordon and K. J. Gergen (Eds.), *The Self in Social Interaction,* Volume 1 (pp. 41-49). New York: Wiley & Sons.

Kanungo, R. N. (1979). The concepts of alienation and involvement revisited. *Psychological Bulletin, 86*(1), 119-138.

Kulka, R. A., Klingel, D. M., and Mann, D. W. (1980). School crime and disruption as a function of student-school fit: An empirical assessment. *Journal of Youth and Adolescence, 9,* 353-370.

Liska, A. E. and Reed, M. D. (1985). Ties to conventional institutions and delinquency: Estimating reciprocal effects. *American Sociological Review, 50,* 547-560.

Major, B. and Schmader, T. (1998). Coping with stigma through psychological disengagement. In J. K. Swim and C. Stangor (Eds.), *Prejudice: The Target's Perspective* (pp. 219-241). New York: Academic Press.

Majors, R. and Billson, J. M. (1992). *Cool Pose: The Dilemmas of Black Manhood in America.* New York: Lexington Books.

Markus, H. and Nurius, P. (1987). Possible selves: The interface between motivation and the self-concept. In K. Yardley and T. Honess (Eds.), *Self and Identity: Psychosocial Perspectives* (pp. 157-172). New York: John Wiley & Sons Ltd.

Marsh, H. W. (1993). Relations between global and specific domains of the self: The importance of individual importance, certainty, and ideals. *Journal of Personality and Social Psychology, 65,* 975-992.

Marsh, H. W. (1995). A Jamesian model of self-investment and self-esteem: Comments on Pelham (1995). *Journal of Personality and Social Psychology, 69,* 1151-1160.

Mead, G. H. (1934). *Mind, Self, and Society.* Chicago: University of Chicago Press.

Miller, N. E. (1941). The frustration-aggression hypothesis. *Psychological Review, 48,* 337-342.

Miller, R. B., Greene, B. A., Montalvo, G. P., Ravindran, B., and Nichols, J. D. (1996). Engagement in academic work: The role of learning goals, future consequences, pleasing others, and perceived ability. *Contemporary Educational Psychology, 21,* 388-422.

Nolin, M. J., Davies, E., and Chandler, K. (1996). Student victimization at school. *Journal of School Health, 66,* 216-221.

Ogbu, J. U. (1992). Understanding cultural diversity and learning. *Educational Researcher, 21,* 5-14.

Ogbu, J. U. (1997). Understanding the school performance of urban African Americans: Some essential background knowledge. In H. Walberg, O. Reyes, and R. Weissberg (Eds.), *Children and Youth: Interdisciplinary Perspectives* (pp. 190-222). London: Sage Publications.

Osborne, J. W. (1995). Academics, self-esteem, and race: A look at the assumptions underlying the disidentification hypothesis. *Personality and Social Psychology Bulletin, 21*(5), 449-455.

Osborne, J. W. (1997a). Identification with academics and academic success among community college students. *Community College Review, 25*(1), 59-67.

Osborne, J. W. (1997b). Race and academic disidentification. *Journal of Educational Psychology, 89*(4), 728-735.

Osborne, J. W. (2001). Unraveling underachievement among African-American boys from an identification with academics perspective. *Journal of Negro Education, 68*(4), 555-565.

Osborne, J. W. (2002). Relationships between identification with academics and important academic outcomes in secondary school students. Unpublished manuscript, North Carolina State University.

Osborne, J. W. and Rausch, J. L. (2001). "Identification with academics and academic outcomes in secondary students." Paper presented at the American Education Research Association (April), Seattle, WA.

Pasley, K., Futris, T. G., and Skinner, M. L. (2002). Effects of commitment and psychological centrality on fathering. *Journal of Marriage and Family, 64,* 130-138.

Pelham, B. W. (1995a). Further evidence for a Jamesian model of self-worth: Reply to Marsh (1995). *Journal of Personality and Social Psychology, 69,* 1161-1165.

Pelham, B. W. (1995b). Self-investment and self-esteem: Evidence for a Jamesian model of self-worth. *Journal of Personality and Social Psychology, 69,* 1141-1150.

Pelham, B. W. and Swann, W. B. J. (1989). From self-conceptions to self-worth: On the sources and structure of global self-esteem. *Journal of Personality and Social Psychology, 57,* 672-680.

Pintrich, P. R. and De Groot, E. V. (1990). Motivational and self-regulated learning components of classroom academic performance. *Journal of Educational Psychology, 82,* 33-40.

Pintrich, P. R. and Schunk, D. H. (1996). *Motivation in Education: Theory, Research and Applications.* Englewood Cliffs, NJ: Prentice-Hall Merrill.

Rabinowitz, S. and Hall, D. T. (1977). Organizational research on job involvement. *Psychological Bulletin, 84,* 265-288.

Rosenberg, M. (1979). *Conceiving the Self.* New York: Basic Books.

Saner, H. and Ellickson, P. (1996). Concurrent risk factors for adolescent violence. *Journal of Adolescent Health, 19,* 94-103.

Skiba, R. J. and Noam, G. G. (2001). *Zero tolerance: Can Suspension and Expulsion Keep School Safe?* San Francisco: Jossey-Bass.

Snyder, H. N. and Sickmund, M. (1999). *Juvenile Offenders and Victims: 1999 National Report.* Washington, DC: Office of Juvenile Justice and Delinquency Prevention.

Steele, C. M. (1988). The psychology of self-affirmation: Sustaining the integrity of the self. In L. Berkowitz (Ed.), *Advances in Experimental Social Psychology,* Volume 21 (pp. 261-302). San Diego, CA: Academic Press.

Steele, C. M. (1992). Race and the schooling of black Americans. *The Atlantic Monthly* (April), 68-78.

Steele, C. M. (1997). A threat in the air: How stereotypes shape intellectual identity and performance. *American Psychologist, 52*(6), 613-629.

Tatem Kelley, B., Huizinga, D., Thornberry, T. P., and Loeber, R. (1997). *Epidemiology of Serious Violence.* Washington, DC: Office of Juvenile Justice and Delinquency Prevention.

Taylor, S. E. and Brown, J. D. (1988). Illusion and well-being: A social psychological perspective on mental health. *Psychological Bulletin, 103,* 193-210.

Tesser, A. (1988). Toward a self-evaluation maintenance model of social behavior. In L. L. Berkowitz (Ed.), *Advances in Experimental Social Psychology,* Volume 21 (pp. 181-228). San Diego, CA: Academic Press.

Tesser, A. and Campbell, J. (1983). Self-definition and self-evaluation maintenance. In J. Suls and A. G. Greenwald (Eds.), *Psychological Perspectives on the Self,* Volume 2 (pp. 1-31). Hillsdale, NJ: Lawrence Erlbaum.

Trusty, J. and Dooley- Dickey, K. (1993). Alienation from school: An exploratory analysis of elementary and middle school students' perceptions. *Journal of Research and Development in Education, 26,* 233-243.

Twenge, J. M., Baumeister, R. F., Tice, D. M., and Stucke, T. S. (2001). If you can't join them, beat them: Effects of social exclusion on aggressive behavior. *Journal of Personality and Social Psychology, 81,* 1058-1069.

Voelkl, K. E. (1996). Measuring students' identification with school. *Educational and Psychological Measurement, 56,* 760-770.

Voelkl, K. E. (1997). Identification with school. *American Journal of Education, 105,* 294-318.

PART II:
PREVENTION OF SCHOOL VIOLENCE

The Cornish Test of Insanity comprised a sink, a tap of running water, a bucket, and a ladle. The bucket was placed under the tap of running water, and the subject was asked to bail the water out of the bucket with the ladle. If the subject continued to bail without paying some attention to reducing or preventing the flow of water into the pail, he or she was judged to be mentally incompetent. (Morgan and Jackson, 1980, p. 99)

The flow of violent acts and abusive behaviors at schools across the world will not be reduced until teachers, school administrators, school counselors, and other education personnel work deliberately with law enforcement, mental health services, and other community agencies to develop prevention programs to head off violence. These prevention programs will necessarily involve the domains of human functioning that Lazarus (1981) identified with the acronym BASIC ID: behavior, affect, sensation, imagery, cognition, interpersonal relations, and diet and physical functioning.

The following is a cursory examination of how each domain helps in guiding the prevention of school violence.

Behavior

The prevention of violent and abusive behavior often begins in the classroom. Teaching is a challenging and difficult process. It is especially difficult when teachers experience problems with classroom management that spill over into problem behaviors outside the classroom. Students who are not managed well in the classroom often lose a sense of disciplined behavior that results in chaotic conditions beyond the classroom. School administrators working in collaboration with counselors, school psychologists, and other behavior specialists need to make group discussion and workshop opportunities available to teachers whereby they can explore various behavior management strategies to deal with the ever changing behavior challenges they face in the classroom. These group opportunities make teachers vigilant and help them support one another in behavior management. These groups allow teachers to focus on

1. new ways to reinforce appropriate classroom behaviors consistently with a variety of reinforcers,
2. appropriate ways to ignore and discount disruptive and abusive behavior in the classroom that often brings inordinate attention to troublemakers, and
3. ways to improve instructional activities that hold students' attention and interest.

Obviously, school administrators and law enforcement officials also need to find effective means beyond the classroom using the most sophisticated technology and threat assessment techniques to prevent egregious behaviors, including the bringing of weapons and other instruments of destruction into the school.

Affect

Prevention programs will also necessarily involve listening activities and other techniques that are designed to help children feel worthy as persons and as students, recognize their feelings about themselves and others, and feel comfortable about expressing these feelings openly and honestly. Teachers and support personnel in the schools who engage in deliberate listening activities with individuals and with groups of students have the opportunity to enhance students' sense of self-worth and in so doing help to eliminate one reason for violence at school.

Sensation and Imagery

In a world of unrelenting sensory stimulation and violent images, teachers and others need to help students discover the value of calm and peaceful reflection. The students we serve are often the products of troubled homes and violent communities where hope seems faint at best. Teachers who are strong in character themselves need to challenge students with times of quiet reflection. This challenge is especially important in an educational world that demands high test scores and other evidence of achievement with little regard for self-reflection. Teachers and counselors, for example, who allow students the opportunity to keep personal journals to record reactions to troubling circumstances help to free students' minds from the violent images that often lead to escape through alcohol and drugs or to unmanageable bursts of abusive and violent acts—many of which are never observed or documented but which add discontent to daily life at schools throughout the world. The new Internet program, Succeeding in School (Gerler, 2001), offers students the opportunity to reflect on and to record their reactions to what they experience at school.

Cognition

Students in today's schools face intellectual and moral dilemmas that cause unrelenting confusion and restlessness. Teachers and support personnel in the schools need to create opportunities for students to discuss the dilemmas they face. Teachers need to challenge students to confront these dilemmas with courage and with increasingly advanced thinking. Teachers also need to support and comfort students in the face of intellectual and moral challenges. These challenges encompass the very core of students' existence particularly during adolescence when students are confronted with loneliness and alienation for not following the will of the crowd in such matters as sexual activity and alcohol use.

Similarly, teachers need to help students explore reasoned and rational thinking that leads to productive emotional reactions and sensible behavior in the face of difficult circumstances. Helping students face these dilemmas will reduce the likelihood that students will react violently to the pressure created by intellectual and moral challenges.

Interpersonal Relations

In his classic book *Reason and Emotion in Psychotherapy,* Albert Ellis (1971) noted that one of the irrational ideas we confront from childhood on is that it is a "dire necessity . . . to be loved or approved by virtually every significant other person" (p. 61). He noted that this goal is unattainable, that this goal requires us to worry constantly about maintaining the approval of others. Students, particularly adolescents, who seek the approval of others constantly and who most often fail miserably in the search often become bullies and proceed to victimize weaker individuals among their peers. Schools need to provide educational opportunities (e.g., community volunteer experience) for students to extend love and care to others rather than to foster the demand for approval seeking. As Ellis (1971) stated so poignantly, "Loving, rather than being loved, is an absorbing, creative, self-expressing occupation. But loving tends to be inhibited rather than abetted by the dire need to be loved" (p. 62). Approval seeking leads to frustration and to a sense of failure that may in turn lead to abusive acts. Schools can create solid programs to prevent the cycle that leads to abusive behavior.

Diet and Physical Functioning

Substance abuse among students is one of the prime contributors to violence inside and outside of school. Educators need to offer substance abuse prevention programs that students take seriously and which offer students more than information about drugs. Substance abuse among adults is also a leading contributor to violence. Schools need to have programs available or make available community programs that address the needs of alcoholic parents, whose abusive and erratic behavior at home leads to confusion and resentment in children, likely precursors to school violence.

An Overview of Part II

Part II examines only a few means of preventing school violence but begins with a comprehensive meta-analysis of school violence prevention programs that were published during the last decade of the twentieth century. This meta-analysis was first published in the *Journal of School Violence* (Scheckner et al., 2002) and appeared in print and online at the journal's Internet site.

This meta-analysis in Chapter 3 is the foundation for the other chapters in Part II of the handbook. Dewey G. Cornell's chapter, "Student Threat Assessment," first reviews the Federal Bureau of Investigation and Secret Service/Department of Education reports that recommended threat assessment for schools and then describes how schools can set up threat assessment teams, based on a field-test project conducted in 35 schools by the Youth Violence Project at the University of Virginia. As Cornell points out, "threat assessment represents a promising new approach to school violence prevention."

Chapters 5 and 6 focus on peer mediation as a means of violence prevention in schools. Helen Lupton-Smith's chapter, "Peer Mediation," addresses the background for the development of peer mediation programs and the various logistics involved in program setup. Maura Dillon's chapter, "Lessons from the Field: Balancing Comprehensiveness and Feasibility in Peer Mediation Programs," presents a substantial review of the peer mediation literature as well as the result of a qualitative study on peer mediation which explores the practical perspectives of five middle school counselors involved in coordinating peer mediation programs. This chapter also includes many of the supporting research materials and documents needed to conduct a qualitative study.

The chapter by Laura Kallus, "Because No One Ever Asked: Understanding Youth Gangs As a Primary Step in Violence Prevention," emphasizes human compassion and understanding as a primary means of gang and youth violence prevention. The chapter combines the real voices of gang members from a Washington, DC, community with current research in the field of youth violence and delinquency. Gang members share the experiences in their families, schools, and communities that led from childhood to gang membership.

Part II of the handbook concludes with David C. May's chapter, "Weapons in Schools." This chapter reviews much of what we know about the incidence and prevalence of weapons in schools and examines how reducing weapons in schools will reduce the violence perpetrated with those weapons on school grounds.

As more books appear in this series on school violence published by The Haworth Press, scholars will address other means of preventing school violence. In addition, as the *Handbook of School Violence* Internet site evolves, practitioners, graduate students, and other scholars will be able to go online to critique and build on what is presented here on preventing school violence. Individuals may follow the evolution of the handbook's Internet site at the following address: <http:// genesislight.com/hsv%20files/>.

REFERENCES

Ellis, A. (1971). *Reason and emotion in psychotherapy.* New York: Lyle Stuart.

Gerler, E. R. (2001). Succeeding in School. Available online: <http://genesislight. com/web%20files/>.

Lazarus, A. A. (1981). *The practice of multimodal therapy.* New York: McGraw-Hill.

Morgan, C. and Jackson, W. (1980). Guidance as a curriculum. *Elementary School Guidance and Counseling, 15,* 99-103.

Scheckner, S., Rollin, S. A., Kaiser-Ulrey, C., and Wagner, R. (2002). School violence in children and adolescents: A meta-analysis of the effectiveness of current interventions. *Journal of School Violence, 1(2),* 5-33.

Chapter 3

School Violence
in Children and Adolescents:
A Meta-Analysis of the Effectiveness
of Current Interventions

Stacey Scheckner
Stephen A. Rollin
Cheryl Kaiser-Ulrey
Richard Wagner

INTRODUCTION

Certainly learning is a lifelong and challenging process. Learning in public schools can be an even greater trial due to underfunding, large classroom sizes, teacher shortages, and everyday problems inherent in being a growing child. But imagine how much of a struggle learning would be for a child in an environment that feels unsafe—where a child is uncertain as to whether he or she will witness or be involved in an act of violence at school. Violence has thus grown to become a major educational problem.

Particularly illustrative is the report in the National Center for Educational Statistics (NCES) of the annual survey of public school principals. According to principals, during the 1996-1997 school year, there were 210,160 reported violent crimes that occurred in their schools. These student-perpetrated crimes included rape, sexual battery, robbery, and physical attack/fights both with and without a weap-

This chapter originally appeared as an article of the same name in the *Journal of School Violence* 1(2) in 2000.

on. During that same year, 64 of every 1,000 12- to 14-year-old students and 35 of every 1,000 15- to 18-year-old students experienced a violent or seriously violent crime at or en route to school. Furthermore, 2 percent of elementary schools, 12 percent of middle schools, and 13 percent of high schools reported to the police at least one occurrence of fighting with a weapon in that same school year (NCES, 1999).

Not only are principals, teachers, parents, and the community fearful of the violence that occurs in schools but students also perceive threats to their safety (Cirillo et al., 1998). Between the years of 1989 and 1995, adolescent students' fear of being attacked at school rose by 33 percent (NCES, 1998). During that same time frame adolescent students' reports of avoiding one or more places in schools that were perceived as unsafe increased by 33 percent (NCES, 1998). The question remains: what are the most efficacious strategies that can be implemented in schools to reduce the rate of violence?

Many different school violence prevention programs have been researched in an effort to determine best practices. Parsing programs down and looking at the effectiveness of each component therein would allow for greater efficacy in the creation of a worthwhile and potentially successful violence prevention program. Cirillo et al. (1998) have identified that violence has significant effects on the psychological and physical abilities of children to thrive, and therefore, results in devastating effects to the school at large. Some researchers suggest that to thwart school violence, it is more effective to prevent school violence rather than to manage the problem via remediation (Krug et al., 1997).

Early intervention (elementary level) has been identified as key to breaking this potentially pernicious chain of events that lead to violence (Grossman et al., 1997; Krug et al., 1997; Coie, 1994; Greenwood, 1995; Kazdin, 1987; Patterson, Reid, and Dishion, 1992; Reid, 1993; Walker et al., 1998). According to Walker and colleagues (1998), the longer a child is exposed to such risks as violence, the more likely he or she will experience deleterious outcomes, such as avoidance, fear, retaliation, drug use, and the like (Krug et al., 1997; Lochman, 1992). Based upon this concept, Hawkins, Von Cleve, and Catalano (1991) stated that prevention programs which focus on reducing aggression during early grades hold the most promise for preventing delinquency in adolescence (Krug et al., 1997; Walker et al., 1998; Lochman, 1992).

Because school is one of the focal points for socialization of children and a venue where violence occurs, it seems logical that violence prevention programs take place in the school setting. Krajewski et al. (1996) go deeper to categorize school violence as a public health concern, which should thus be managed in the public sector. Hawkins et al. (1999) further state that school-based interventions can increase bonding to school and academic success. Walker et al. (1998) identified that violence interventions implemented in the school teach prosocial behavior patterns that support effective interactions between teachers, students, and peers. Adding parents as partners in this process further facilitates growth and success (Walker et al., 1998).

METHOD

Meta-Analysis

Due to strong interest in school violence prevention programs and lack of information regarding successful programs that have been implemented within the past ten years, a decision was made to conduct a meta-analysis of programs developed within the past ten years. The results of an earlier meta-analysis of violence prevention programs in schools (Howard, Flora, and Griffin, 1999) was qualitative in nature and thus, inconclusive as far as any truly statistical useful information. Therefore, a decision was made to conduct a statistically rigorous meta-analysis of all school-based violence prevention programs appearing in the literature between 1990 and 1999; weighted effect sizes and a taxonomy that classifies components of a successful program were studied as features of the meta-analysis. Studies included in this meta-analysis were school-based programs who used a control group and who implemented an experimental design.

Studies Reviewed

Criteria for Selection

Studies eligible for review consisted of reports of empirical studies appearing from 1990 through 1999 that examined the topic of school violence prevention programs. Samples were diverse in terms of selection and assignment criteria, size, and content, including gender, age of cohort explored, and other characteristics. Treatment inoculation varied as well, with programs lasting anywhere from a few weeks to a few years. Program leaders received training in most of the studies explored. Numerous outcome measures (e.g., Child Behavior Checklist, Social Skills Rating Scale, etc.) were used throughout each of the studies to assess a variety of specific program effects (e.g., violence, prosocial behaviors, etc.).

Search Procedures

Three procedures were used to search for studies. First, computer searches were conducted using the following databases: PsychInfo, Social Sciences, ERIC, First Search (e.g., Wilson Select), Socio-Abstracts, and MEDLINE. Key words, such as "violence," "prevention," "intervention," "schools," "children," and "adolescents" were used during each of these searches. Second, the contents of the current issues of the following 15 journals were manually examined for relevant studies:

> *Journal of Adolescent Health*
> *Psychology in the Schools*
> *Journal of Community Psychology*
> *American Journal of Preventative Medicine*
> *American Journal of Public Health*
> *Education and Urban Society*
> *Child Psychology and Human Development*
> *Journal of Applied Developmental Psychology*
> *Child Development*
> *Journal of Counseling and Clinical Psychology*
> *Journal of Family Violence*
> *Journal of Interpersonal Violence*
> *Adolescence*
> *Society for Adolescent Medicine*
> *Applied and Preventative Psychology*

Third, the reference lists from each initially included study were examined.

Search procedures identified approximately 80 articles evaluating school violence prevention programs. Twenty-seven articles were initially chosen and examined closely based on the following criteria: used an experimental or quasi-experimental methodology and implemented a school violence prevention program with at least one aspect located directly in a school. A few of the interventions took place both in the school and also in other settings. Of those 27, a final 16 articles, which met all criteria *as well as* reported postintervention data necessary to calculate effect sizes, were selected for use in the final analysis.

Description of Studies

Table 3.1 is an overview of the 16 articles reviewed in this study. Descriptors fell into six categories: intervention theory, intervention setting, intervention age group, leader training, intervention duration, and random assignment. Intervention theory fell into three subgroups: cognitive, behavioral, and cognitive-behavioral orientations. Cognitive theory was defined as using mainly instructional interventions with a minimum of behavioral practicing. Behavioral theory was described as interventions using a reinforcement schedule. Lastly, cognitive-behavioral theory was defined as interventions combining both cognitive and behavioral procedures previously delineated.

Most interventions took place solely in the school, while a few combined the school setting with parent and/or community settings (Table 3.2). Each intervention group was characterized as elementary (kindergarten through fifth grades), middle (sixth through eighth grades), and high (ninth through twelfth grades). More elementary interventions were evaluated than middle or high school. Leader training was denoted as simply yes or no, with most studies including leader training as part of their intervention. Intervention duration was depicted as short (less than a few weeks), moderate (less than a few months), and long (about a year). Each of these categories was equally represented by the studies examined. Random assignment was also simply denoted as yes (+) or no (−), with most studies using random assignment.

TABLE 3.1. School-Based Violence Prevention Interventions: Overview

Author (year)	Sample/School (Grade/Ethnicity)	Treatment/Control (R+/-)	Intervention Duration	Statistic Measures
Walker et al. (1998)	46 subjects/1 school, kindergarten/NR	T: 24 subjects C: 22 subjects/ +	12 weeks	Average Effect Size =.86 (range of .26 to 1.17)
Farrell and Meyer (1997)	978 subjects/6 schools, sixth grade/>90% AA	T: 348 subjects C: 350 subjects/–	45 minutes a session for 18 sessions for one semester health class for each group	ANOVA and ANCOVA
Grossman et al. (1997)	790 subjects/12 schools, second/third grades/427 m, 363 f, 626 W, 57 AA, 66 A, 30 H, 9 NA, 2 O	T: 346 subjects C: 303 subjects/+	35 minutes each lesson for 30 lessons for 16-20 weeks	Change in scores before and after intervention, Generalized Estimating Equation (GEE), and Regression Analysis
Krug et al. (1997)	6,292 subjects/9 schools, kindergarten-fifth grades/1,873 H, 1,438 W, 588 NA	T: 2,393 subjects C: 1,506 subjects/–	School year	Compared logs from year before to year after intervention, t-Test and ANCOVA
Shechtman (1999)	10 subjects/1 school, fourth grade/10 m /NR	T: 5 males C: 5 males/+	45 minute sessions for ten sessions	Compared pre- and post-measures of aggression and other constructive behaviors
Dolan et al. (1993)	864 subjects/19 schools, first grade/423 m, 441 f, 553 AA, 251 W, 60 O	T1: 182 subjects C: 107 subjects T2: 207 subjects C2: 156 subjects Ext. C: 212 subjects/+	T1: 3 times a week for ten minutes up to three hours and then varied T2: throughout reading program during the year	ANCOVA

86

Author (year)	Sample/School (Grade/Ethnicity)	Treatment/Control (R+/-)	Intervention Duration	Statistic Measures
Lochman (1992)	145 subjects/1 school, fourth-sixth grades/145 m NR	T1: 31subjects C: 52 subjects C: 62 subjects (12 subjects from T1 received booster interventions)/–	45-60 minute sessions for 12-18 sessions for 4-5 months (booster sessions were held the following year twice a week for 12 sessions lasting six weeks)	MANCOVA and ANCOVA
Krajewski et al. (1996)	239 subjects/2 schools, seventh grades/NR 189 W, 50 O	T1: ~ 120 subjects, T2: ~ 92 subjects (used as control group)/–	Ten consecutive health classes for two weeks	Mann-Whitney U Test
Bosworth, Espelage, and DuBay (1998)	81 subjects/1 school, seventh grade/ 45 f, 36 m, 72 W, 5 AA, 3 H, 1 O	(use own control)	Four-week pilot program, 40-minute class period	Chi-square Statistics and Paired t-Tests
Hilton et al. (1998)	350 subjects/4 schools, eleventh grade/60 m, 63 f/NR	T1: 123 subjects C: 227 subjects/–	One-hour long assembly and two one-hour workshops	Repeated measures and between group designs, compared pre- and posttests
Cirillo et al. (1998)	43 subjects/1 school, ninth-twelfth grades/ 22 m, 21 f, 19 W, 13 AA, 10 H, 1 O	T: 22 subjects C: 21 subjects/+	Ten, two-hour weekly sessions for ten weeks	Compare before and after (follow-up also); 2-Way ANOVA with Repeated Measures and t-Tests
Avery-Leaf et al. (1997)	193 subjects/1 school eleventh/twelfth grades/106 m, 87 f, 154 W, 21 H, 8 AA, 10 A	T: 102 subjects C: 91 subjects/+	Five consecutive health class sessions during fall semester of school year	Chi-Square Analyses, Pearson Product-Moment Correlations, MANOVA, t-Tests, and Box/Whiskers Method

TABLE 3.1 *(continued)*

Author (year)	Sample/School (Grade/Ethnicity)	Treatment/Control (R+/-)	Intervention Duration	Statistic Measures
DuRant et al. (1996)	225 subjects/2 schools, sixth-eighth grades/109 m, 116 f, 189 AA, 22 W, 2 N-A	T1: 151 subjects T2: 74 subjects/+	Ten, 50-minute sessions held twice a week over five weeks in classroom format in health classes	ANOVA, Kruskal-Wallis ANOVA, Chi-Square, and Repeated Measures ANOVA
Hawkins, Von Cleve, and Catalano (1991)	458 subjects/8 schools, first-second grades/ 218 m, 240 f, 20 NA, 76 A, 143 AA, 10 H, 209 W	T: 285 subjects C: 173 subjects/+	Parent training was offered on seven consecutive weekly sessions to parents of children in treatment group/at the beginning of each year (two-year program)	MANOVA and ANOVA
Shechtman and Nachshol (1996)	117 subjects/3 schools, sixth-eighth grades/NR	T: 18 subjects C: 38 subjects/+ (yr 1) T1: 42 subjects C: 19 subjects/+ (yr 2)	15 weekly one-hour sessions for two years during social class sessions	ANOVA and t-Tests
O'Donnell et al. (1993)	Numerous subjects 8-18 schools, first-sixth grade/NR	T: 75 subjects C:102 subjects T: 44 subjects C: 62 subjects/+	Children in the intervention group were given training in the first and sixth grades; parent training classes were offered during their child's first, second, third, fifth, and sixth grades	Independent group t-Tests and ANOVA

Note: m = male, f = female; NR = not reported or breakdown not given; W = White, AA = African American, H = Hispanic, A = Asian, NA = Native American, M = mix, O = other; +/− = random assignment to intervention.

TABLE 3.2. School-Based Violence Prevention Interventions: Meta-Analysis Summary Results

Author (Year)	Theory	Setting	Age Group	Leader Training	Duration	Random (+/-) Assignment	Strength	Effect Size
Walker et al. (1998)	Beh	S and P	Elementary	Yes	Med	+	*Str	.85
Farrell and Meyer (1997)	Cog	S	Middle	Yes	Med	–	Sm	.09
Grossman et al. (1997)	Cog	S	Elementary	Yes	Med	+	Sm	.03
Krug et al. (1997)	Cog-Beh	S and P	Elementary	NR	Long	–	*Str	1.49
Shechtman (1999)	Cog	S	Elementary	Yes	Short	+	*Str	.84
Dolan et al. (1993)	Cog-Beh	S	Elementary	Yes	Long	+	Sm	.16
Lochman (1992)	Cog	S	Middle	NR	Med	–	Mod	.53
Krajewski et al. (1996)	Cog	S	Middle	Yes	Short	–	Mod	.45
Bosworth, Espelage, and DuBay (1998)	Cog	S	Middle	NR	Short	NA (own control)	*Str	.96
Hilton et al. (1998)	Cog	S	High	Yes	Short	–	Sm	.24

TABLE 3.2 *(continued)*

Author (Year)	Theory	Setting	Age Group	Leader Training	Duration	Random (+/-) Assignment	Strength	Effect Size
Cirillo et al. (1998)	Cog	S and C	High	Yes	Med	+	Mod	.39
Avery-Leaf et al. (1997)	Cog	S	High	Yes	Long	+	Sm	.10
DuRant et al. (1996)	Cog	S	Middle	Yes	Short	+	Sm	.30
Hawkins, Von Cleve, and Catalano (1991)	Cog-Beh	S and P	Elementary	Yes	Long	+	Sm	.32
Shechtman and Nachshol (1996)	Cog	S	Middle	Yes	Long	+	Mod	.69
O'Donnell et al. (1995)	Cog-Beh	S	Elementary	Yes	Long	+	Sm	.28

Note: Setting: P = parent, S = school, C = community; age group: elementary = kindergarten-fifth grades, middle = sixth-eighth grades, high = ninth-twelfth grades; leader training: yes or not reported (NR); duration: short < a few weeks, med < a few months, long = a year or more; +/− = random assignment to intervention; composite effect sizes are reported above: Sm = Small ($\sim .20$), Mod = Moderate ($\sim .50$), *Str = Strong ($\sim >.80$) and calculated according to the following equation in order to compare each study with the others and to use in the meta-analysis regression procedure: ces = sum of each g^u from a study/square root of [the correlation among g^us times (the number of g^us) squared plus (one minus the correlation) times the number of g^us] (Cooper and Hedges, 1994).

Effect Sizes

The effect sizes for each study were computed using two different formulas. The main formula employed is called Hedges' g (Cooper and Hedges, 1994) and is defined in Table 3.3. The other formula, also indicated in Table 3.3, was used when the article did not provide the necessary information needed in order to calculate Hedges' g. These equations are considered interchangeable (Cooper and Hedges, 1994). Two studies (Hilton et al., 1998; Walker et al., 1998) reported effect sizes without references to the types of equations used. Therefore, the formula for Hedges' g is assumed due to its common use in social sciences (Cooper and Hedges, 1994).

Due to the variety of sample sizes used in each of the different studies, an unbiased effect size was calculated in order to adjust for small sample size (Cooper and Hedges, 1994). Biased effect sizes would be slightly larger than they should due to sample sizes less than 50 (Cooper and Hedges, 1994). The unbiased version of Hedges' g is defined in Table 3.3.

Effect sizes reflect the relative magnitude of the intervention effect in terms common across studies (Table 3.3). In other words, the effect size shows the degree of success of a treatment. Table 3.3 denotes the strength of each effect size as calculated.

Composite Effect Sizes

In order for appropriate comparatives to be achieved, it was necessary to calculate one composite effect size for each independent sample. Table 3.2 indicates the formula used to obtain the composite effect size for each study (Cooper and Hedges, 1994).

FINDINGS

Studies with Strong Effect Sizes

As demonstrated in Table 3.2, four studies were identified as having strong effect sizes. In Tucson, Arizona, a school-based violence prevention program called PeaceBuilders geared toward elementary students was implemented during the 1994-1995 school year (Krug

TABLE 3.3. School-Based Violence Prevention Interventions: Effect Sizes

Author (year)	Theory	Effect Sizes of Intervention vs. Control (Scales)	Strength	Formula Used
Walker et al. (1998)	Beh	.85 (antisocial behavior patterns)	*Str	Article reported
Farrell and Meyer (1997)	Cog	.04 (violent behavior scale)	Sm	Hedges' $g = \dfrac{X_T - X_C}{\text{Square root of: } \dfrac{(N_T - 1)S_T^2 + (N_C - 1)S_C^2}{(N_T + N_C - 2)}}$
		.04 (been in a fight in which someone was hit)	Sm	
		.13 (threatened or injured by someone with a weapon)	Sm	
		.09 (problem behavior scale)	Sm	
		.11 (drug use scale)	Sm	
Grossman et al. (1997)	Cog	.00 (interpersonal skills)	Sm	Hedges' g
		.00 (self-management skills)	Sm	
		.01 (hostile-irritable)	Sm	
		.05 (antisocial-aggressive)	Sm	
		.01 (demanding-disruptive)	Sm	
		.01 (aggressive behavior)	Sm	
		.04 (delinquent behavior)	Sm	
		.00 (acting out)	Sm	
		.00 (assertive social skills)	Sm	
		.06 (peer social skills)	Sm	
		.05 (aggressive behavior)	Sm	
		.08 (delinquent behavior)	Sm	

Author (year)	Theory	Effect Sizes of Intervention vs. Control (Scales)	Strength	Formula Used
Krug et al. (1997)	Cog-Beh	.49 (rates of visits to school nurses)	Mod	Hedges' g
		.89 (rates of injury-related visits to school nurses)	*Str	
		2.58 (rates of confirmed fighting-related injuries)	*Str	
Shechtman (1999)	Cog	.58 (self-report aggressive behaviors)	Mod	Hedges' g
		1.10 (teacher report aggressive behaviors)	*Str	
Dolan et al. (1993)	Cog-Beh	.03 (teacher-rated aggressive behavior)	Sm	Hedges' g
		.02 (teacher-rated shy behavior)	Sm	
		.14 (peer-rated aggressive behavior)	Sm	
		.08 (peer-rated shy behavior—too shy)	Sm	
		.15 (peer-rated shy behavior—play alone)	Sm	
		.21 (peer-rated shy behavior—few friends)	Sm	
		.19 (reading achievement)	Sm	
Lochman (1992)	Cog-Beh	.45 (substance use)	Mod	Hedges' g
		.17 (general behavior deviance)	Sm	
		.48 (self-esteem)	Mod	
		.38 (social problem solving)	Mod	
		.10 (off-task classroom behavior)	Sm	
Krajewski et al. (1996)	Cog	.41 (knowledge)	Mod	$^\wedge g = z$ times square root of: $\dfrac{N_T + N_C}{N_T \times N_C}$
		.36 (attitudes)	Mod	

TABLE 3.3 (continued)

Author (year)	Theory	Effect Sizes of Intervention vs. Control (Scales)	Strength	Formula Used
Bosworth, Espelage, and DuBay (1998)	Cog	.41 (self-knowledge)	Mod	$^\wedge g$ = t times square root of: $\dfrac{N_T + N_C}{N_T \times N_C}$
		.49 (prosocial behavior)	Mod	
		1.59 (intentions)	*Str	
		.02 (confidence)	Sm	
		.38 (trouble behavior)	Mod	
Hilton et al. (1998)	Cog	.43 (key points score for workshops attended)	Mod	Article reported
		.08 (target item score)	Sm	
		.03 (key points score for workshops not attended)	Sm	
Cirillo et al. (1998)	Cog	.48 (general students/violence avoidance beliefs)	Mod	$^\wedge g$ = square root of F times square root of: $\dfrac{N_T + N_C}{N_T \times N_C}$
		.33 (drugs/alcohol students/violence avoidance beliefs)	Sm	
		.32 (physically violent students/violence avoidance belief)	Sm	
		.33 (verbally threatened/violence avoidance beliefs)	Sm	
Avery-Leaf et al. (1997)	Cog	.10 (male-to-female aggression)	Sm	Hedges' g
		.01 (male-to-male aggression)	Sm	
		.02 (male aggression)	Sm	
		.01 (female aggression)	Sm	
		.26 (male jealousy)	Sm	
		.10 (female jealousy)	Sm	

Author (year)	Theory	Effect Sizes of Intervention vs. Control (Scales)	Strength	Formula Used
DuRant et al. (1996)	Cog	.45 (use of violence in hypothetical situation)	Mod	Hedges' g
		.14 (avoidance of violence)	Sm	
		.09 (frequency of use of violence scale)	Sm	
		.39 (frequency of fighting)	Mod	
		.11 (frequency of injury during a fight requiring medics)	Sm	^g listed above (for an F statistic)
Hawkins, Von Cleve, and Catalano (1991)	Cog-Beh	.18 (anxious)	Sm	
		.18 (social withdrawal)	Sm	
		.16 (unpopular)	Sm	
		.32 (self-destructive)	Sm	
		.14 (obsessive-compulsive)	Sm	
		.14 (inattentive)	Sm	
		.18 (nervous-overactive)	Sm	
		.24 (aggressive)	Sm	
		.21 (external/antisocial)	Sm	
		.20 (internal/antisocial)	Sm	
Shechtman and Nachshol (1996)	Cog	1991/1992	Mod/Mod	^g listed above (for an F statistic)
		.46 (attitudes for aggression)/.69 (attitudes for aggression)		
		.49 (aggressive behavior)/.77 (aggressive behavior)	Mod/*Str	
		.40 (acting out)/.05 (acting out)	Mod/Mod	
		.63 (withdrawal)/.55 (withdrawal)	Mod/Mod	

TABLE 3.3 (continued)

Author (year)	Theory	Effect Sizes of Intervention vs. Control (Scales)	Strength	Formula Used
		.19 (distractability)/.26 (distractability)	Sm/Sm	
		.43 (disturbed peer relations)/.53 (disturbed peer relations)	Mod/Mod	
O'Donnell et al. (1995)	Cog-Beh	.37 (immaturity)/.39 (immaturity)	Mod/Mod	Hedges' g
		.14 (social interaction)	Sm	
		.37 (prosocial skills)	Mod	
		.17 (bonding)	Sm	
		.04 (–opportunities)	Sm	
		.31 (drug use)	Mod	
		.25 (+opportunities)	Sm	
		.11 (+rewards)	Sm	
		.06 (antisocial behaviors)	Sm	
		.03 (–rewards)	Sm	
		.22 (delinquency)	Sm	

Note: ^ = equations are interchangeable (Cooper and Hedges, 1994), Sm = Small (~.20), Mod = Moderate (~.50), *Str = Strong (~=.80). Effect Sizes: N = sample size, X = mean, S = standard deviation. Unbiased Effect Sizes are reported above calculated according to the following equation to adjust for small sample sizes: $g^u = c(m)g$, where m = $N_T + N_C - 2$ and $c(m) = 1 - [3/4(m)-1]$ (Cooper and Hedges, 1994).

et al., 1997). PeaceBuilders is a program that teaches prosocial behaviors. Activities were designed to improve daily interactions among students, teachers, other school staff, and parents. Students were taught to praise people, avoid put-downs, seek wise role models, correct hurts, and right wrongs. Teachers and parents provided positive reinforcement via rewards and feedback for prosocial behaviors observed in the students. A randomly selected sample of 2,393 students in treatment schools and 1,506 students in control schools (mostly low socioeconomic status and minority students in both schools) were assessed for increases in visits to school nurses' offices via this qualitative analysis. These schools were chosen due to the high rate of crime in their demographic area and randomly matched as treatment and control in pairs of two (four matched pairs).

Outcome data were collected by examining the school nurses' logs and measuring the rate of student visits. Researchers postulated that if less fighting occurred, less injury-related fighting would also occur. In addition, they felt that some children often visited the school nurse to escape bullying and therefore to be in a safe environment. Treatment success was indicated by a drop in the number of injury-related visits secondary to fights. After one year, overall visits to the nurse decreased by about 13 percent in the intervention schools compared to an increase of about 3 percent in the control schools. Similar success was demonstrated for injury-related nurse visits. Rates of fighting-related injuries did not change significantly in the intervention schools, but increased 56 percent in the control schools. The researchers concluded that in the intervention schools, injuries and visits to the school nurse decreased over the two-year period in part due by PeaceBuilders. They also indicated that visits to the school nurse may be a useful tool to evaluate some types of elementary school-based violence prevention programs.

Bosworth, Espelage, and DuBay (1998) used a multimedia, computer-based school intervention program called SMART Talk: Students Managing Anger Resolution Together. This four-week pilot study implemented in Tucson, Arizona, consisted of 40-minute class periods in which students had access to the program through the use of an available computer in the classroom. A diverse socioeconomic sample of 119 seventh-grade students (mostly Caucasian) volunteered for participation in this pretest/posttest design. There was no traditional control group employed in this model, however the pretest condition was used as a comparison against the posttest condition. Participants were used as their own control. Students learned through games, simulations, cartoons, and other interactive methods about nonviolent strategies to resolve conflict, manage anger, identify violent intentions and behaviors, and learn prosocial skills.

After each use, students completed a short questionnaire that inquired about their satisfaction and any improvement suggestions. In addition, 98 seventh graders completed a pretest (Teen Conflict Survey), although only 81 participated in a posttest. The 65-item survey was used to collect data about a range of issues such as the following: knowledge and attitudes regarding nonviolent and violent strategies of conflict resolution, self-efficacy as it relates to conflict resolution and anger management, intentions to use nonviolent strategies in conflict situations, self-reported caring and noncaring behaviors, and self-esteem, impulsivity, nonviolent role models, and peer influence. Most items were taken from previously standardized tests, although some questions were added by the researchers from their own literature review. Results indicated that SMART Talk was popular among students of both genders and that its use produced the following significant effects: self-knowledge increased from 43 to 77 percent, pro-social behavior increased from 15 to 30 percent, intentions increased from 10 to 67 percent, and trouble behavior decreased from 6 to 54 percent. The researchers concluded that the program engaged the students as well as increased their declarative knowledge. Furthermore, they suggested that the computer-mediated program should be considered a viable tool in school violence prevention.

Shechtman (1999), in Haifa, Israel, conducted a school-based violence prevention program utilizing group bibliotherapy as the primary intervention with fourth-grade males. Bibliotherapy was proposed in order to mediate relevant literature between the reader/listener and his or her difficulties. The program consisted of the use of short stories, poems, films, and pictures associated with issues of aggression. The primary purpose of this program was to reduce aggressive behavior in maladjusted adolescents. The criterion-referenced sample for this pretest/posttest-designed study consisted of five treatment and five control group students (eight-year-old boys). Treatment inoculation consisted of ten 45-minute sessions. Two special education teachers who were trained in working with aggressive children implemented the intervention.

Outcomes measured included behavioral aggression as well as level of empathy, insight, self-disclosure, and responsiveness to the media presented and were measured via self-report and teacher report utilizing the Child Behavior Checklist (CBCL) and Teacher Report Form (TRF). Results indicated reduced aggression and increased constructive behaviors exhibited by the treatment students, as compared to no change in the control students. The author did not indicate the percentage increases or decreases in change. Researchers suggested that in the future, bibliotherapy should be further investigated in the prevention of aggression and school violence.

In Eugene, Oregon, Walker et al. (1998) implemented a program, First Step to Success, which intervened at the point of school entry (kindergarten) to prevent antisocial behavior patterns. First Step to Success was developed as a way of combating the risk factors and family conditions associated with antisocial behaviors. The program targeted children who started school with early signs of aggression due to identified risk factors. This program lasted twelve weeks and used school staff, as well as parents, in teaching alternatives to violence to this criterion-referenced sample of twenty-four identified at-risk, treatment group students. Twenty-two control students did not receive the intervention. The intervention was coordinated and delivered by a school professional whom served as a consultant to teachers and parents.

The outcome measures of this pretest/posttest-designed study demonstrated a decrease in antisocial behavior patterns as indicated through teacher rating measures, including the Child Behavior Checklist. Through the next year, 80 percent of the behavioral improvements continued to be maintained. This study was replicated (Golly, Stiller, and Walker, 1998) on a new sample of 20 at-risk kindergartners in an effort to assess social validity and study reproducibility. Results indicated a very high level of satisfaction and behavioral level changes that mirrored the original study. However, the authors did not report the percentage of behavioral change. The researchers suggested that intervening at the point of school entry is necessary in order to divert at-risk children from antisocial behavior patterns.

Studies with Moderate Effect Sizes

Four studies contained intervention outcomes that produced moderate effect sizes (Table 3.1). Shechtman and Nachshol (1996) implemented the same bibliotherapy prevention program in Shechtman (1999), but used a larger sample size consisting of 117, criterion-referenced, male middle school students enrolled in special education who were randomly assigned into treatment and control groups. Graduate students, special education teachers, and school counselors received training in order to conduct fifteen, one-hour weekly sessions for a period of two years during students' social studies classes. This program was designed to help children effectively deal with emotions associated with aggression and aggressive behavior through storytelling, poems, and films. The intervention was based on the belief that learning is not only a rational process but also incorporates strong, emotionally charged experiences.

Outcome characteristics reported by the Walker Problem Identification Checklist measured behavioral problems as evaluated by teachers. Other measures included a projective technique designed to report responses to frustration and the Peer Assessment Inventory in order to determine aggressive behavior. Results from this study were inconsistent; the program was implemented and evaluated twice. The second-year results were found to be significantly more effective than the first-year results in reducing aggression as well as other maladjusted social behavior. Specifically, withdrawal behavior was consistently affected. The control group showed increased endorsement of beliefs that support aggression and actual aggressive and acting-out behavior. In addition, the program also reduced attitudes that supported aggressive behavior in the intervention group.

Lochman (1992) conducted a longitudinal study using a cognitive-behavioral intervention specifically focusing on coping with anger in aggressive middle school boys. A criterion-referenced sample of 145 middle school boys was selected for participation in this pretest/posttest-designed study. Students were not randomly assigned to groups, although two control groups were used as a comparison in this study (aggressive and nonaggressive boys). Twelve to 18 intervention sessions lasting 45 to 60 minutes occurred during a four- to five-month period. The program consisted of taking aggressive boys who were referred by classroom teachers as highly disruptive and teaching them effective skills to cope with anger. This group was compared to the two control groups three years later to examine the long-term preventive effects of a school-based intervention.

Outcome data were collected through portions of the National Youth Survey questionnaire, the Coopersmith Self-Esteem Inventory, and the Behavior Observation Schedule for Pupils and Teachers. Results indicated that boys who received the anger-coping program reported lower rates of substance use and deviant behavior as well as higher levels of self-esteem and prosocial skills. Interestingly, these boys were not shown to be significantly different from the control group of nonaggressive boys in terms of rates of drug and alcohol involvement, self-esteem, and social problem-solving skills. Also, the overall intervention did not have any long-term effects on delinquency or future classroom behavior for most of the intervention subjects. However, some students who did receive booster sessions maintained behavioral improvements over time. The researcher concluded that there should be an intensification of cognitive-behavioral interventions in regard to reducing aggression in boys and long-lasting effects.

Two prevention programs that focused specifically on violence-free relationships were implemented and evaluated by Krajewski et al. (1996). These programs taught a sample of 239 seventh-grade, health education students about violence in relationships. The programs were administered in a predominately Caucasian, midsized, midwestern city in a middle school by the health education teacher along with the help of a counselor from a battered women's shelter. Skills for Violence-Free Relationships, the name of the program, lasted ten consecutive health classes for a period of two weeks.

Outcomes in this pretest/posttest-designed study were measured by an inventory specifically developed for this curriculum. An analysis revealed that one week after the interventions were implemented, significantly higher knowledge and positive attitude scores resulted. In addition, more changes in these variables occurred in female students. However, a five-week follow-up did not indicate any significant differences between treatment and control groups. No percentage changes in pre/posttesting were reported. The authors concluded that reinforcement or booster sessions are required to maintain change.

In College Station, Texas, a study was conducted to investigate the effects of a social-cognitive group intervention on violence avoidance beliefs among at-risk high school students (Cirillo et al., 1998). Forty-three diverse students were randomly assigned to a treatment or control group. The intervention group participated in small/large group discussions, role-playing, journaling, and group and individual feedback sessions. The intervention was conducted for ten, two-hour weekly sessions. These activities focused on decision-making abilities, prosocial behaviors, and empathy skills. A licensed counselor who developed the program along with ten adult leaders served as mentors for the children in the program. Results of this intervention were assessed utilizing a pretest/posttest methodology.

Questions from the Student Health Survey helped researchers examine the effects of their program. Findings showed that the intervention did not result in any significant differences between groups on violence avoidance beliefs. This may have been due to the small sample size. On the other hand, students who used drugs and alcohol, and fought, did have significantly lower scores than students who did not engage in those behaviors. It was hypothesized that these students believed in using violence as a coping technique more than students who were not involved in those negative activities.

Studies with Small Effect Sizes

Eight studies resulted with program outcomes that produced small effect sizes (Table 3.1). DuRant et al. (1996) compared the effectiveness of two previously developed violence prevention curricula for a sample of 225, criterion-referenced middle school adolescents (mostly African American): the Violence Prevention Curriculum for Adolescents, and Conflict Resolution: A Curriculum for Youth Providers. The first curriculum focused on teaching adolescents about the risk factors associated with violence, positive ways to express anger, and alternatives to fighting. The second curriculum focused on conflict resolution skills. Researchers hypothesized that the conflict resolution curriculum would be more effective in reducing occurrence of self-reported violence due to a focus on conflict-resolution skills. Both curricula lasted for ten, 50-minute sessions held twice a week over five weeks during students' health class. The same instructor taught all curricula. The instructor was trained in both curricula and was an experienced mental health counselor with a background in group instruction.

Outcomes for this study consisted of self-report questionnaires administered in a pretest/posttest study design format. Results from each program were compared, although no percentages were indicated. Both curricula demonstrated success in significantly reducing three indicators: use of violence in hypothetical conflict situations, frequency of use of violence in the past 30 days, and frequency of physical fights in the past 30 days. The conflict resolution curriculum was more successful than the violence prevention program in reducing the frequency of more severe fights. However, both interventions were shown to have significant positive outcomes upon completion of the program. They were also not shown to be significantly different from each other.

In Long Island, New York, Avery-Leaf et al. (1997) assessed a high school dating-violence prevention program and its impact on students' attitudes toward justified aggression. A sample of 193 criterion-referenced junior and senior students (predominantly Caucasian) were assigned to treatment or control groups by class. Health teachers who were trained by the researchers for eight hours one week prior to program implementation conducted five consecutive program sessions, held during the fall semester of 1994. The program focused on increasing student knowledge about and skill enhancement in the management of dating violence.

Postprogram assessment, using the modified Conflict Tactics scale, indicated that there were significant decreases in overall attitudes justifying the use of dating violence. Those who were not exposed to the program did not exhibit this attitudinal change. However, another scale that measured these types of attitudes did not result in similar findings. Other behavioral measures were not evaluated and change percentages between pretest and posttest were not given. Researchers concluded that the curriculum shows promise if future research is performed to determine whether the observed attitude change is also linked to reduction in aggressive behaviors.

In another intervention, two classroom-based prevention programs were evaluated for short-term impact on aggressive and shy behaviors and poor achievement in a criterion-referenced, randomly selected sample of 864 first-grade students separated into treatment and control groups. Dolan et al. (1993) trained eight teachers for forty hours to implement this program in two different ways, by using either the Good Behavior Game or Mastery Learning. The first game was meant to teach students nonaggressive or good and nonshy behaviors. The game lasted anywhere from ten minutes to three hours three times per week and then varied throughout the rest of the year. The second method also lasted throughout the year and consisted of teaching better reading skills.

Measures used for analysis included the Teacher Observation of Classroom Adaptation-Revised, the Peer Assessment Inventory, and the California Achievement Test-Reading. Both interventions were shown to have statistically significant effects on the outcomes measured in this study. A significant reduction (no percentages revealed) was found in aggressive behavior among the children who were involved in the Good Behavior Game. An increase in reading achievement was found for children who participated in the Mastery Learning program. Overall, the Good Behavior Game appeared to have a greater impact in reducing aggressive behavior among identified aggressive children. Female high achievers benefited more from the Mastery Learning program than female low achievers. On the other hand, male low achievers benefited more than male high achievers. The researchers concluded that future research should investigate whether decreasing aggressive or shy behavior improves achievement or if increasing achievement improves aggressive or shy behavior.

Farrell and Meyer (1997) evaluated the effect of a curriculum adapted from the Violence Prevention Curriculum for Adolescents. Again, this program was designed mainly to increase knowledge about the nature of violence. Four prevention specialists trained in conflict resolution implemented the program to a randomly selected sample of 978 sixth graders. The program lasted for 45 minutes a session for 18 sessions during one semester of health-education classes.

Outcome measures (behavioral frequency scales) assessed through self-report included changes in students' experience with violence, antisocial behaviors, and drug use. Overall, there were no significant differences between the intervention and control groups. Significant decreases in violent behaviors were found for boys, but not for girls. Researchers indicated that this may have been due to the program's use of male instructors. Researchers also concluded that the program may be generalized for prevention in school use for reducing violent tendencies among sixth-grade male students, although no percentage changes were noted.

O'Donnell et al. (1993) conducted an investigation about the long-term effects of a school-based prevention program on a criterion-referenced sample of 106 low socioeconomic status, urban youth. This program lasted a total of six years and entailed a modification of classroom teacher practices along with a provision of child social skills training and parent training. Teachers were trained in specific instructional methods and other school staff were trained to give corrective feedback. Children in the intervention group were given training in the first and sixth grades, while parents of those children who were in the intervention group were offered classes when their child was in every grade except fourth.

Outcomes in this pretest/posttest study were assessed via student self-report and the Teacher Report Form of the Child Behavior Checklist. Many variables were analyzed, such as prosocial and antisocial behaviors. Children in the treatment group showed significant enhanced school commitment and class participation secondary to their participation in the program. In addition, the program demonstrated gender differences. Treatment group girls demonstrated lower rates of substance use initiation. On the other hand, treatment group boys exhibited an increase in social skills and schoolwork completion.

A classroom-based intervention called Second Step: A Violence Prevention Curriculum was implemented by Grossman et al. (1997) in six matched pairs of elementary schools to a sample of 790 randomly selected second- and third-grade students, predominantly Caucasian. This program was used to teach students social skills (e.g., anger management, empathy, and impulse control), via discussion, role-playing, and other interactive activities. Trained teachers implemented the program's 35-minute lessons for 16 to 20 weeks. The goal of this program was to assess reduction of aggressive behaviors and increase prosocial behaviors secondary to participation in the program in this randomized controlled trial. Assessment results reported no change in parent/teacher observations of student behaviors between the control and intervention groups. However, other measures did indicate a moderate decrease in aggressive behavior and increase in prosocial behaviors. Both of these occurrences were stable for six months following the program. Researchers admitted that this study only supported moderate effects of this program.

Hawkins, Von Cleve, and Catalano (1991) evaluated a primary prevention program targeting early childhood aggression. This study investigated the effects of social skills training on 458 randomly selected, mostly Caucasian first-grade students randomly assigned into treatment and control groups. Teachers and parents worked in tandem to administer this program. Teachers were trained in proactive classroom management and effective use of social skills. Parent training was offered on seven consecutive weekly sessions to parents of children in the treatment group at the beginning of each year (two-year program). The program was designed to enhance prosocial development, reduce aggressive and antisocial behaviors across settings, and reduce risk of delinquency and drug abuse through social bonding.

The short-term effects on early antisocial behavior were measured in this posttest-only design utilizing the Teacher Report Form of the Child Behavior Checklist. Significantly lower rates of aggressiveness were found for Caucasian boys in treatment classrooms compared with controls. There were no other differences found in terms of race for any measured variables. No gender effects were detected. Parents of 43 percent of the children attended at least one parent-training session. A significant relationship was found between parents who attended training and lower scores for female children in terms of exhibiting aggressive behaviors. Researchers admit that results present limited support for the program, although they assert that their study is part of ongoing longitudinal empirical research.

Hilton et al. (1998) evaluated antiviolence education in high schools to assess the knowledge students actually gain and retain from such programs. Intervention education included information about sexual assault, coping with and controlling anger, verbal aggression, date rape, etc. The sample selected for this study included high school juniors from a mixed urban/rural region for this pretest/posttest-designed study. A total of 123 students actually participated in all three assessment sessions (pretest, posttest, and follow-up). A one-hour assembly session and two one-hour workshops were led by trained counselors, police officers, and other project staff.

Knowledge of information presented in the intervention, self-reported physical and sexual aggression involving peers, and date rape were measured through an inventory developed for this study and used as program outcomes. Students with the least knowledge at pretest were least likely to attend the program. Students identified as perpetrators were found to know less information about violence than victims. Exclusive victims were more likely to be female. In addition, females had more favorable scores at pretest than males. Significant effects were found in specific workshop areas that students attended. A six-week follow-up showed significant improvement in all knowledge areas for students.

DISCUSSION

Empirical Support

Many components determined to affect program outcomes are empirically supported by school violence intervention literature. Theoretical orientation, intervention settings, and age group are discussed specifically in the literature with respect to program outcomes. Cognitive-behavioral therapy (CBT) is supported in the end when directed at social-cognitive deficits and cognitive distortions in aggressive children (Lochman, 1992). Many controlled studies using cognitive-behavioral strategies have shown classroom behavioral improvements along with improvements in self-esteem and perceived social competence in aggressive children (Lochman and Curry, 1986; Lochman et al., 1989). Some controlled studies using cognitive-behavioral programs also found reductions in parents' ratings of aggression (Kazdin et al., 1989; Kazdin et al., 1987a,b; Lochman and Curry, 1986).

Due to the abundance of significant outcomes in decreasing child aggressive behavior resulting from cognitive-behavioral therapies, it was hypothesized that this analysis would mete out similar results. On the contrary, this analysis did not show that theoretical orientation contributed significantly to program effect size as only one of the four programs resulting with a strong effect size employed a cognitive-behavioral strategy (Krug et al., 1997). Two other programs (Bosworth, Espelage, and DuBay, et al., 1998; Shechtman, 1999) used strictly cognitive techniques while Walker et al. (1998) applied a behavioral approach. Although the results of this analysis did not co-incide with prior conclusions delineated in the literature, it does not negate the importance of those findings. This may have been due to the small sample size of studies used in this analysis that met the inclusion criteria or the compounded effect of other program components. In addition, the specific theoretical labels and definitions chosen for this study could also have affected results as another researcher might have used different labels and definitions.

Other empirical research lends support to the idea that interventions covering a variety of settings are the most effective in decreasing antisocial behaviors in children (Howard, Flora, and Griffin, 1999). This is because children at risk for violent behaviors usually experience multiple risk factors, such as in peer, family, school, and community settings (Friedman and Rosenbaum, 1988; Sampson and Lauritsen, 1994; Tolan and Guerra, 1994). Therefore, school violence intervention programs should be implemented across settings to address risk factors in a multisystemic fashion (Morrison, Robertson, and Harding, 1998). Two of the four programs resulting with strong effect sizes in this study (Walker et al., 1998; Krug et al., 1997) were implemented in multisettings.

Last, some school violence intervention research supports prevention at the point of school entry as opposed to secondary and tertiary intervention after the child is already in middle and high school (Walker et al., 1998). According to the literature, the longer a child is exposed to risk factors, the more likely the child will acquire aggressive behaviors (Patterson, Reid, and Dishion, 1992). A pattern of negative consequences may then result, such as school dropout, delinquency, and adult criminality. Thus, early intervention is strongly suggested in order to achieve more successful outcomes (Coie, 1994; Greenwood, 1995; Kazdin, 1987; Patterson, Reid, and Dishio, 1992). Three of the four studies resulting with strong effect sizes (Walker et al., 1998; Krug et al., 1997; Shechtman, 1999) were employed at the primary prevention level (elementary school). Bosworth, Espelage, and DuBay's (1998) program was conducted in a middle school.

Intuitive Support

Several components hypothesized to affect program outcomes in this study are not directly mentioned in school violence intervention literature. These components—random assignment, leader training, intervention duration—are supported intuitively by overall research methodology in most subject areas. However, due to threats to internal validity of the studies explored (e.g., nonequivalence of samples, nonrandom sampling and/or assignment, inappropriate or incorrect statistical analyses, history effects, etc.), it is inconclusive as to whether any particular intervention had a true effect. For instance, some of the evaluations were implemented in the mid-1990s at the peak of the school violence epidemic whereas some of the programs were put into practice during the later part of the 1990s when the country had a drop in youth violence. Without proper methods (such as randomly assigned groups and control schools), a historical drop in a particular school's violence rate may be erroneously attributed to the program.

A program might be more effective if the leaders of the program are adequately trained in the implementation and delivery of the specific intervention. Almost all of the studies reported some form of leader training. Although Bosworth, Espelage, and DuBay (1998) did not directly report leader training, due to the nature of the program (computer mediated), it is assumed that a qualified leader must have been employed. The other three studies resulting with a strong effect size (Walker et al., 1998; Krug et al., 1997; Shechtman, 1999) directly reported leader training.

One would think that the longer the program, the more significant the impact. The duration of treatment was evenly varied (long, medium, and short durations) among the programs reviewed in this study. In addition, Krug et al. (1997) was the only program that resulted with a strong effect size that conducted the treatment for a long duration. This may have been due to the small sample size of studies used in this analysis that met the inclusion criteria as well as the compounded effect of other program components.

Limitations to this analysis include inadequate sample size, which limited further statistical analysis (i.e., regression). In addition, as previously identified, inherent internal and external validity issues existing within each of the studies evaluated may have increased the possibility of Type 1 errors. This would help to explain why some of the programs were not shown to have a stronger effect. If the studies' results were biased themselves, it would be difficult to appropriately compare and evaluate them based on their effect size.

CONCLUSION

There is an abundance of empirical literature that supports the use of cognitive-behavioral therapies in school violence prevention programs (Lochman and Curry, 1986; Lochman et al., 1989). In addition, school violence literature lends support to the idea that interventions covering a variety of settings at the primary prevention level (elementary school) are the most efficacious in decreasing antisocial behaviors in children (Howard, Flora, and Griffin, 1999; Walker et al., 1998). It is also important to have adequately trained leaders implement and monitor the programs themselves as well as have reinforcement through longer program implementation. In addition to empirical findings, appropriate statistical procedures recommend that in order to see the true effect of a program, the researcher should start out with equal groups, random sampling and/or assignment, correct and appropriate statistical treatment, etc., and attend as much as possible to threats to internal validity in the methodology of the study.

As previously discussed, the small number of studies included in this study raises many important issues. First of all, after a decade of major investments in intervention projects, only a modest number of programs met minimal criteria of methodological rigor. Second, it appears as if only a few of these programs are employed in a significant number of schools. Given that there are millions of students in the United States alone, the percentage of students exposed to these types of structured interventions may well be below 1 percent. Therefore, future researchers should employ the appropriate statistical procedures as well as implement their treatment in multiple school settings to provide more reliable and valid information concerning their prevention program.

Additional suggestions for future researchers would include the utilization of a control group and proper quantitative methodology to correct for any biases. It is also important to note that most studies used ANOVA or MANOVA to conduct statistical analyses. Future researchers may want to use larger sample sizes in an effort to examine the multisystemic problem of school violence. For example, there are model national programs, such as the following: Big Brothers Big Sisters of America, Bullying Prevention Program, Functional Family Therapy, Life Skills Training, Midwestern Prevention Project, Multidimensional Treatment Foster Care, Multisystemic Therapy, PATHS

(Promoting Alternative THinking Strategies), Prenatal, and Infancy Home Visitation by Nurses, and Quantum Opportunity Program (Center for the Study and Prevention of Violence, 2001). The Center for the Study and Prevention of Violence at the University of Colorado indicates that these programs are "model" interventions due to the following criteria: used an experimental or quasiexperimental design, evidenced a statistically significant deterrent (or marginal deterrent) effect, replicated in at least one additional site with an experimental design and demonstrated effects, and evidenced that the deterrent effect was sustained for at least one year posttreatment. In such cases, structural equation modeling, logistical regression, hierarchical linear modeling, or growth curve analyses that allow for the exploration of direct and indirect effects could be employed (Tabachnick and Fidell, 1996).

REFERENCES

Avery-Leaf, M.A., Cascardi, M., O'Leary, K.D., and Cano, A. (1997). Efficacy of a dating violence prevention program on attitudes justifying aggression. *Journal of Adolescent Health, 21*(1), 11-17.*

Bosworth, K., Espelage, D., and DuBay, T. (1998). A computer-based violence prevention intervention for young adolescents: Pilot study. *Adolescence, 33*(132), 785-795.*

Center for the Study and Prevention of Violence (2001). *Examples of exemplary/promising programs.* University of Colorado, Boulder, CO: <http://www.colorado.edu/research/espv/blueprints>.

Cirillo, K.J., Pruitt, B.E., Colwell, B., Kingery, P.M., Hurley, R.S., and Ballard, D. (1998). School violence: Prevalence and intervention strategies for at-risk adolescents. *Adolescence, 33*(130), 319-330. *

Coie, J. (1994). *Antisocial behavior among children and youth.* Keynote address presented at the OSEP National Research Director's Conference. Washington, DC: U.S. Office of Special Education Programs.

Cooper, H. and Hedges, L.V. (1994). *Handbook of research synthesis.* New York: Russell Sage Foundation.

Dolan, L.J., Kellam, S.G., Brown, C.H., Werthamer-Larsson, L., Rebok, G.W., Mayer, L.S., Laudolff, J., and Turkan, J.S. (1993). The short-term impact of two classroom-based preventive interventions on aggressive and shy behaviors and poor achievement. *Journal of Applied Developmental Psychology, 14,* 317-345.*

DuRant, R.H., Treiber, F., Getts, A., McCloud, K., Linder, C.W., and Woods, E.R. (1996). Comparison of two violence prevention curricula for middle school adolescents. *Journal of Adolescent Health, 19,* 111-117.*

Note: References marked with an asterisk indicate studies included in the meta-analysis.

Farrell, A.D. and Meyer, A.L. (1997). The effectiveness of a school-based curriculum for reducing violence among urban sixth-grade students. *American Journal of Public Health, 87*(6), 979-984.*

Friedman, J. and Rosenbaum, D. (1988). Social control theory: The salience of settings by age, gender, and type of crime. *Journal of Quantitative Criminology, 4,* 363-382.

Golly, A., Stiller, B., and Walker, H.M. (1998). First step to success: Replication and social validation of an early intervention program. *Journal of Emotional and Behavioral Disorders, 6*(4), 243-250.

Greenwood, P.W. (1995). *The cost-effectiveness of early intervention as a strategy for reducing violent crime.* Paper prepared for the University of California Policy Seminar Crime Project. Santa Monica, CA: RAND.

Grossman, D.C., Necklerman, H.J., Keopsell, T.D., Liu, P., Asher, K.N., Beland, K., Frey, K., and Rivara, F.P. (1997). Effectiveness of a violence prevention curriculum among children in elementary school. *Violence Prevention Among Children, 20,* 1605-1611.*

Hawkins, J.D., Catalano, R.F., Kosterman, R., Abbott, R., and Hill, K.G. (1999). Preventing adolescent health-risk behaviors by strengthening protection during childhood. *Archive of Pediatric Adolescent Medicine, 153,* 226-234.*

Hawkins, J.D., Von Cleve, E., and Catalano, R.F. (1991). Reducing early childhood aggression: Results of a primary prevention program. *Journal of American Academy of Child Adolescent Psychiatry, 30*(2), 208-217.

Hilton, N.Z., Harris, G.T., Rice, M.E., Krans, T.S., and Lavigne, S.E. (1998). Antiviolence education in high schools: Implementation and evaluation. *Journal of Interpersonal Violence, 13*(6), 726-742.*

Howard, K.A., Flora, J., and Griffin, M. (1999). Violence-prevention programs in schools: State of the science and implications for future research. *Applied and Preventive Psychology, 8,* 197-215.

Kazdin, A. (1987). Treatment of antisocial behavior in children: Current status and future directions. *Psychological Bulletin, 102,* 187-203.

Kazdin, A.E., Bass, D., Siegel, T., and Thomas, C. (1989). Cognitive-behavioral therapy and relationship therapy in the treatment of children referred for antisocial behavior. *Journal of Consulting and Clinical Psychology, 57*(4), 522-535.

Kazdin, A.E., Esveldt-Dawson, K., French, N.H., and Unis, A.S. (1987a). Effects of parent management training and problem-solving skills training combined in the treatment of antisocial child behaviors. *Journal of American Academy of Child and Adolescent Psychiatry, 26*(3), 416-424.

Kazdin, A.E., Esveldt-Dawson, K., French, N.H., and Unis, A.S. (1987b). Problem-solving skills training and relationship therapy in the treatment of antisocial child behaviors. *Journal of Consulting and Clinical Psychology, 55*(1), 76-85.

Krajewski, S.S., Rybarik, M.F., Dosch, M.F., and Gilmore, G.D. (1996). Results of a curriculum intervention with seventh graders regarding violence in relationships. *Journal of Family Violence, 11*(2), 93-112.*

Krug, E.G., Brener, N.D., Dahlberg, L.L., Ryan, G.W., and Powell, K.E. (1997). The impact of an elementary school-based violence prevention program on visits to the school nurse. *American Journal of Preventive Medicine, 13*(6), 459-463.*

Lochman, J.E. (1992). Cognitive-behavioral intervention with aggressive boys: Three-year follow-up and preventive effects. *Journal of Consulting and Clinical Psychology, 60*(3), 426-432.

Lochman, J.E. and Curry, J.F. (1986). Effects of social problem-solving training and self-instructional training with aggressive boys. *Journal of Clinical Child Psychology, 5*(2), 159-164.*

Lochman, J.E., Lampron, L.B., Genner, T.C., Harris, S.R., and Wicker, A.W. (1989). Teacher consultation and cognitive-behavioral interventions with aggressive boys. *Psychology in the Schools, 26*(2), 179-188.

Morrison, G.W., Robertson, L., and Harding, M. (1998). Resilience factors that support the classroom functioning of acting out and aggressive students. *Psychology in the Schools, 35*(3), 217-227.

National Center for Educational Statistics (1998). Violence and discipline problems in the U.S. public schools: 1996-1997. Available online: <www.nces.ed.gov>.

National Center for Educational Statistics (1999). Indicators of school crime and safety. Available online: <www.nces.ed.gov>.

O'Donnell, J., Hawkins, D., Catalano, R.F., Abbott, R.D., and Day, E. (1995). Preventing school failure, drug use, and delinquency among low-income children: Long-term intervention in elementary schools. *American Journal of Orthropsychiatry, 65,* 87-100.*

Patterson, G.R., Reid, J.B., and Dishion, T.J. (1992). *Antisocial boys.* Eugene, OR: Castalia Press.

Reid, J. (1993). Prevention of conduct disorder before and after school entry: Relating interventions to developmental findings. *Development and Psychopathology, 5*(1/2), 243-262.

Sampson, R.J. and Lauritsen, J.L. (1994). Violent victimization and offending: Individual-, situational-, and community-level risk factors. In A.J. Reiss and J.A. Roth (Eds.), *Understanding and preventing violence: Social influences,* Volume 3 (pp. 1-114). Washington, DC: National Academy Press.

Shechtman, Z. (1999). Bibliotherapy: An indirect approach to treatment of childhood aggression. *Child Psychiatry and Human Development, 30*(1), 39-53.*

Shechtman, Z. and Nachshol, S. (1996). A school-based intervention to reduce aggressive behavior in maladjusted adolescents. *Journal of Applied Developmental Psychology, 17,* 535-552.*

Tabachnick, B.G. and Fidell, L.S. (1996). *Using multivariate statistics.* New York: HarperCollins College Publishers.

Tolan, P. and Guerra, N. (1994). *What works in reducing adolescent violence: An empirical review of the field (f-888).* Boulder, CO: University of Colorado, Boulder.

Walker, H.M., Severson, H.H., Feil, E.G., Stiller, B., and Golly, A. (1998). First step to success: Intervening at the point of school entry to prevent antisocial behavior patterns. *Psychology in the Schools, 35*(3), 259-269.*

Chapter 4

Student Threat Assessment

Dewey G. Cornell

How should schools respond to a student who threatens to commit an act of violence? Imagine the case example of a seventh-grade student named Bill who told a classmate that he is going to kill an eighth-grade student who rides the same school bus. The classmate heard about several highly publicized school shootings, so he told his teacher what Bill said. The teacher informed the principal, who had to decide how to proceed. Consider the hypothetical responses of three middle schools, A, B, and C.

In School A, the principal confronted Bill with the alleged threat, and he admitted making the statement. The principal then responded according to the school board's zero-tolerance policy. According to this policy, a student who threatens to kill someone must be suspended from school for the remainder of the school year. The principal called Bill's parents and asked them to come to the school immediately to pick up their son.

In School B, the principal also confronted Bill with the alleged threat, and again he admitted making the statement. The principal consulted an official list of warning signs used to identify violent students. The warning signs included items such as, "low school interest and poor academic performance," "social withdrawal," "excessive

This work was supported with a grant from the Jessie Ball duPont Fund. I appreciate the cooperation of the Albermarle County and Charlottesville City Public Schools, especially Frank Morgan and Ron Hutchinson, who made it possible to field test the guidelines for responding to student threats of violence. I also thank my colleague Peter Sheras and our graduate students, Andrea Levy, Sebastin Kaplan, David McDonville, Lela McKnight, and Julea Posey of the Virginia Youth Violence Project.

feelings of isolation and being alone," "excessive feelings of rejection," "feelings of being picked on and persecuted," and "uncontrolled anger" (Dwyer, Osher, and Warger, 1998). After consulting with Bill's teacher, the principal concluded that Bill fit the profile of a dangerous student. Bill was suspended from school and referred for placement in an alternative school.

In School C, the principal and other school staff had participated in threat assessment training. The principal interviewed Bill about the alleged threat, and when Bill admitted making the threat, the principal asked a series of questions about Bill's intent, including how and why he would carry out the threat. The school psychologist conducted a clinical interview with Bill and met with his mother. Other members of the threat assessment team interviewed the classmate who reported the threat, other students who rode the bus, and the intended victim of the threat. Based on all of this information, the principal concluded that Bill made the threatening statement in anger and frustration because he was being bullied at the school bus stop, but that he did not have a plan or serious intent to carry out the threat. Bill was apologetic and remorseful, and now recognized that there was a more appropriate way to cope with bullying. Bill was suspended temporarily from school until the threat assessment team met with Bill's parents and agreed on a plan for his safe return.

In this hypothetical situation, threat assessment offers a more comprehensive and discerning response to Bill's threat, and results in a course of action that is less punitive and disruptive to Bill's education than either zero tolerance or profiling approaches. Because threat assessment emphasizes investigation of the origin and context of the threat, it was possible for the school to identify and address a broader problem with bullying. Had Bill actually been planning to carry out his threat, the threat assessment investigation would have made it more likely that the serious nature of the threat would be recognized and curtailed. Threat assessment is a flexible approach that guides the school to respond based on the seriousness of the threat. In contrast, a zero tolerance policy involves little or no flexibility, and imposes severe consequences on a student even if the risk of violence is low. In high-risk cases, severe consequences such as long-term suspension or expulsion do not ensure safety since the conflict or grievance that underlies the threat is not addressed. The purpose of this chapter is to present an overview of threat assessment as a response to student threats of violence.

WHAT IS THREAT ASSESSMENT?

Threat assessment is an approach to violence prevention originally developed by the U.S. Secret Service based on studies of persons who attacked or threatened to attack public officials (Fein, Vossekuil, and Holden, 1995; Fein and Vossekuil, 1999). Threat assessment was soon recognized as a way to analyze potentially violent situations that had general law enforcement applications (Fein and Vossekuil, 1998). In response to the series of high-profile school shootings that occurred in the 1990s, Reddy and colleagues (Reddy et al., 2001) advocated the application of threat assessment to schools. In 2002, a joint report of the U.S. Secret Service and Department of Education recommended that schools train threat assessment teams to respond to student threats of violence (Fein et al., 2002).

A threat assessment is conducted when a person (or persons) threatens to commit a violent act, or engages in behavior that appears to threaten an act of violence. This kind of threatened violence is termed targeted violence. Threat assessment is a process of evaluating the threat, and the circumstances surrounding the threat, in order to uncover any facts or evidence that indicate the threat is likely to be carried out. What has made threat assessment more than a generic term for investigation of a potentially dangerous situation is the development of foundational principles and key questions that guide the threat assessment. Threat assessment in schools is predicated on six principles (Fein et al., 2002) which will be summarized as follows.

First, targeted violence is not a spontaneous, unpredictable event, but is the result of a deliberate and detectable process. Students who commit serious acts of violence do not suddenly "snap" and begin shooting at random; their behavior is preceded by days or weeks of thought and planning, and in many cases they shared their ideas and intentions with others (Vossekuil et al., 2002). This means that targeted school violence can be prevented if enough is known about the student's preparatory behavior.

Second, threat assessment must consider not only the student who makes the threat, but the situation, the setting, and the target as well. Students who commit serious acts of violence may have experienced significant situational stress, such as family problems, separations, or personal losses. Factors in their setting may encourage violence or discourage more appropriate ways of resolving problems or seeking help. For example, several of the school shooters were encouraged by antisocial peers to carry out their attacks. Characteristics or behaviors of the target may be perceived as provocative, abusive, or deserving of attack by the student who makes the threat. The threat assessment team attempts to construct a complete picture of the threat in context.

Third, school authorities investigating a threat must adopt a critical and skeptical mind-set that strives to accumulate reliable evidence and verify all claimed facts about the situation. Their approach must be fair and they must be willing to accept or reject hypotheses based on a careful analysis of all available information. This principle guards against the potential for school authorities to jump to conclusions that a student is dangerous based on rumors or unverified allegations.

The fourth principle is that conclusions must be based on objective facts and behaviors, rather than inferred traits or characteristics of the student making the threat. This principle explicitly contradicts the effort to make judgments based on a hypothetical profile of the violent student. There is no set of psychological characteristics that unequivocally indicate future violence in the absence of specific observations that the student is planning or threatening to commit an act of violence.

The fifth principle is that information should be gathered from multiple sources within and outside the school system. An integrated systems approach to investigation seeks cooperation with law enforcement, social service agencies, mental health providers, religious organizations, and other groups or organizations that comprise the community. This principle requires schools to look beyond their own boundaries and to make good use of all available resources rather than function as a closed and isolated system.

The final principle is that threat assessment is ultimately concerned with whether the student *poses* a threat, not whether the student has *made* a threat. Any student can make a threat, but relatively few will engage in behavior that indicates planning and preparation necessary to carry out the threat. Threat assessment attempts to identify those students who pose a threat, which is to say that they have an intent and means to carry out the threat. Threat assessment does not conclude when a student is found to have made a threat; rather, threat assessment aims to determine how serious the threat is and then what should be done about it.

HOW DOES THREAT ASSESSMENT DIFFER FROM PROFILING?

The FBI's National Center for the Analysis of Violent Crime conducted a study of schools where lethal shootings took place or plans for shootings were foiled by law enforcement intervention, in order to determine factors that might be useful in preventing similar acts in the future (O'Toole, 2000). Although the FBI's Behavioral Sciences Unit is renowned for its use of criminal profiling techniques, the FBI's profiling experts concluded that profiling was not appropriate for the prediction of school shootings. As the FBI report concluded:

> One response to the pressure for action may be an effort to identify the next shooter by developing a "profile" of the typical school shooter. This may sound like a reasonable preventive measure, but in practice, trying to draw up a catalogue or "checklist" of warning signs to detect a potential shooter can be shortsighted, even dangerous. Such lists, publicized by the media, can end up unfairly labeling many nonviolent students as potentially dangerous or even lethal. In fact, a great many adolescents who will never commit violent acts will show some of the behaviors or personality traits included on the list. (O'Toole, 2000, pp. 2-3)

Checklists and warning signs that have been used to construct a profile of the homicidally violent student contain many general risk factors common to large numbers of youths. For example, the warning signs used by the hypothetical principal of school B are taken from the list in the federal government's guide, *Early Warning, Timely Re-*

sponse: A Guide to Safe Schools (Dwyer, Osher, and Warger, 1998). Even though the guide cautions against improper use of the warning signs, there is no clear way to avoid misuse when a school official is confronted with a potentially dangerous student and examines such a list of student characteristics.

Other warning signs and checklists lend themselves to speculative profiling. The American Psychological Association's "warning signs" pamphlet sounds an ominous note with the statement, "If you see these immediate warning signs, violence is a serious possibility." The list of "immediate warning signs" includes "increase in risk-taking behavior," "increase in use of drugs or alcohol," and "significant vandalism or property damage," and "loss of temper on a daily basis." Most school authorities could identify students in their schools who appear to meet these signs. Similarly, the National School Safety Center (1998) promulgated a 20-item "checklist of characteristics of youth who have caused school-associated violent deaths." This checklist includes some very general items, such as, "has been previously truant, suspended, or expelled from school," "has little or no supervision from parents or a caring adult," and "tends to blame others for difficulties she or he causes." The items on these checklists may well describe the small group of youths who committed school shootings, but this does not make them useful, specific indicators of violence. Because the base rate for severe violence is low, checklists of student characteristics will invariably lead to the false-positive identification of a very large number of students who are not violent (Sewell and Mendelsohn, 2000). In contrast, threat assessment emphasizes the examination of specific behaviors directly linked to committing a violent act. Has the student made a statement of intent to harm someone? Has the student made specific plans to carry out the act? Has the student attempted to recruit accomplices or invited an audience to observe the violence? More general student characteristics that are described in typical profile checklists play a secondary or tertiary role in evaluating the potential for violence.

In the case of highly infrequent events such as school shootings, profiles are likely to generate huge rates of false-positive identifications. Since more than 99.9 percent of schools will not experience a school homicide, it seems highly unlikely that any profile or prediction formula will be accurate enough to be of practical value. For this reason, school authorities should be skeptical of any profile or check-list approach that claims to be able to identify homicidal students.

Retrospective profiling should be distinguished from prospective profiling. Retrospective profiling is a deductive approach to identifying the perpetrator of a crime that starts with investigation of the crime scene. Suspects can be investigated and ruled in or ruled out based on facts such as where they were at the time of the crime. In contrast, prospective profiling is an inductive attempt to identify someone who will commit a crime in the future. There are no facts or evidence concerning the crime because no crime has occurred. There is no way to rule out a suspect who appears to fit the profile. As a result, prospective profiling is much more speculative and more inclusive of suspects, and therefore more prone to error.

Perhaps the major weakness of student profiling is that it assumes that there is a single type of violent student and that these violent youths share a common set of characteristics or traits. Yet studies of violent individuals find a remarkable diversity that defies characterization by a single profile (U.S. Surgeon General, 2001). Research on juvenile homicide has consistently identified multiple patterns or groupings of offenders, including a large proportion of youths who are antisocial, some who act out of intense conflict, and a few who are severely mentally ill (Cornell, 1999).

HOW DOES THREAT ASSESSMENT DIFFER FROM ZERO TOLERANCE?

The highly publicized school shootings in the 1990s generated tremendous fear and concern in school officials. Educator anxiety was further inflamed by waves of false bomb threats and hit lists that troubled many schools. School authorities became so highly sensitive to any seemingly dangerous student behavior that many turned to radical measures. "Zero tolerance" became a widespread practice in which students are automatically expelled for violations of school safety rules. Skiba and Peterson (1999) traced the emergence of zero-tolerance policies to personnel drug abatement efforts of the U.S. Navy and U.S. Customs Service. The notion of absolute sanctions against drug use in the military became a model for schools that was applied to violence as well as drug use.

In 1994, the Gun-Free Schools Act required that schools expel for one calendar year any student found to be in possession of a firearm at school. Although the law permitted local school districts to modify the expulsion on a case-by-case basis, this provision was frequently overlooked in favor of less flexible policies that mandated automatic expulsion for all infractions. In addition, many schools expanded zero tolerance well beyond the arena of firearms or even lethal weapons. For example, the prohibition of weapons in many school divisions often included toy weapons and objects that appeared to be weapons. In one case, a ten-year-old boy was expelled from elementary school because he brought to school a one-inch plastic toy pistol that was an accessory to his G.I. Joe action figure. The boy discovered he had the tiny toy in his pocket when he checked to see if he had his lunch money. Skiba and Peterson (1999) documented numerous cases of excessive punishment, which they referred to as "the dark side of zero tolerance." Among the examples they cited:

- A five-year-old in California was expelled after he found a razor blade at his bus stop and carried it to school and gave it to his teacher.
- A nine-year-old in Ohio was suspended for having a one-inch knife in a manicure kit.
- A twelve-year-old in Rhode Island was suspended for bringing a toy gun to school.
- A seventeen-year-old in Chicago was arrested and subsequently expelled for shooting a paper clip with a rubber band.

From a threat assessment perspective, none of these cases would merit serious concern unless the student actually posed a serious danger to others. Threat assessment distinguishes a toy gun from a real gun, and distinguishes finding a razor blade from planning to use a razor blade to injure someone. The students in these cases apparently were punished severely for breaking a rule, but not because their behavior threatened to harm others.

An article in the *American Bar Association Journal* (Tebo, 2000) sharply criticized zero-tolerance policies as making "zero sense." Tebo contended that the central problem with zero-tolerance policies is that all threats of violence are treated as equally dangerous and deserving of the same consequences. For example, Ohio state law requires every school district to have a zero-tolerance policy that makes no exceptions (Tebo, 2000). These kinds of policies provide no latitude for school authorities to consider the seriousness of the threat or degree of risk posed by the student's behavior. Tebo (2000) described cases in which Ohio schools imposed severe consequences on students whom they recognized did not pose a danger to others, such as a student suspended for displaying a school election poster that contained humorous threatening language in parody of a popular movie. A Pennsylvania court overturned one school's expulsion of a seventh-grade student who inadvertently brought his Swiss Army knife to school, but in almost all cases the courts have been unwilling to interfere with zero-tolerance practices in schools (Tebo, 2000).

A 2000 report by the Advancement Project and The Civil Rights Project of Harvard University pointed out that zero-tolerance policies were originally intended to apply only to serious criminal behavior involving firearms or illegal drugs, but have been extended to cover many more types of behavior and circumstances. "Zero Tolerance has become a philosophy that has permeated our schools; it employs a brutally strict disciplinary model that embraces harsh punishment over education" (p. 3). The report raised concern that zero-tolerance policies were resulting in high levels of suspension and expulsion of minority students. In 1998, more than 3.1 million students were suspended from school; although African-American children represent 17 percent of the public school enrollment, they constituted 32 percent of the out-of-school suspensions.

The basic dilemmas school officials face is that they are very concerned about the potential for violence and must have some means of taking protective, preventive action, but many policies and practices fail to give them the means for making practical distinctions and informed judgments concerning the level of risk posed by different student behaviors. Threat assessment meets this need.

HOW CAN THREAT ASSESSMENT WORK IN SCHOOLS?

The FBI's report on school shootings (O'Toole, 2000) outlined a general framework for school-based threat assessment. Schools were advised to designate a threat assessment coordinator who would lead the school's response to student threats of violence. The threat assessment coordinator would chair a multidisciplinary team that included law enforcement and mental health professionals. When a threat came to the attention of school authorities, the team would conduct a four-pronged assessment to determine the seriousness of the threat and identify an appropriate course of action. The four prongs or assessment domains were: (1) personality traits and behavior; (2) family dynamics; (3) school dynamics; and (4) social dynamics. In each domain the team would attempt to identify characteristics that might increase the level of violence risk, such as a turbulent parent-child relationship or a peer group that encourages violent behavior. The team would also attempt to identify strengths or protective factors that could decrease the risk of violence. In more serious cases, the team would integrate all available information to plan an appropriate intervention to reduce the risk of violence.

The FBI report (O'Toole, 2000), as well as the Secret Service and Department of Education joint report (Fein et al., 2002), provided a compelling argument for schools to adopt a threat assessment model. Nevertheless, there remains a substantial gap between the conceptual framework for threat assessment and school-based practice. The available literature on threat assessment generally advises schools on what principles to follow, but not how to put them into practice. To bridge the gap between principle and practice, the Virginia Youth Violence Project of the University of Virginia's Curry School of Education, undertook a project to develop and field test practical guidelines for schools to follow in responding to student threats of violence (Cornell, 2001; Cornell et al., in press). The guidelines contained a decision tree for the team to follow in responding to different kinds of threats. Thirty-five schools participated in a yearlong field test of the guidelines and provided data on 188 student threats of violence that came to the attention of school authorities. The results of this field testing provide evidence for the viability of student threat assessment and guidance for other schools wishing to adopt this approach.

Guidelines were developed for threat assessment in collaboration with a work group representing two school divisions. The two school divisions encompassed a socioeconomically and ethnically diverse population of 16,400 students enrolled in four high schools, six middle schools, 22 elementary schools, and three alternative schools. The work group consisted of an assistant superintendent, principal, school psychologist, and school resource officer supervisor from each school division. An external advisory board consisting of state and national experts in school safety, law enforcement, and risk assessment served as consultants for the project. The shared objective was to develop guidelines that would respond effectively to the risk of violence posed by student threats, yet meet the day-to-day needs of educators to work in a practical and efficient manner.

The process of developing guidelines began by conducting telephone interviews with all of the school principals and psychologists in the two divisions. They were asked about the kinds of student threats that came to their attention in the past year, and about the process they used to respond to student threats and what kinds of guidelines or policies would help them respond most effectively. The principals reported that student threats to hurt someone were a relatively common event, although few threats were regarded as very serious. The most significant concerns were how to identify truly serious threats and how to respond to them. Principals from elementary, middle, and high schools all expressed concern that there were no standards or rules to rely upon in making decisions about student threats, and that they were forced to rely on their own intuition in making decisions about the seriousness of a student's risk for violence. The school psychologists expressed concern that they had no training in how to conduct psychological evaluations of students who made threats of violence. Furthermore, they noted an absence of school division policy or professional standards on the scope and purpose of such evaluations.

The concerns of principals and psychologists made it clear that threat assessment required a set of written guidelines to assist staff in making triage determinations of the seriousness of a threat and to specify how to undertake the more extensive evaluation of the most serious cases. It was recognized that an elaborate process of threat assessment would be burdensome to school authorities and that it would be necessary to design an efficient process that would quickly distinguish the commonplace threats that could be quickly and easily resolved from more serious threats that might require a more labor-intensive response. It was decided that the school principals would conduct the initial evaluation of a threat and make a triage decision, either resolving the threat immediately because it was not serious or initiating a more comprehensive team assessment if the threat was serious.

What constitutes a threat? In this study a threat was defined as any expression of intent to harm someone. Consistent with the FBI report (O'Toole, 2002) it was recognized that threats could be spoken, written, e-mailed, or expressed in some other way, such as through gestures. Threats could be made directly to the intended victim, communicated to third parties, or expressed in private writings. Possession of a weapon such as a firearm or knife on school grounds would be presumed to indicate a threat, unless subsequent investigation found otherwise. Unlike many zero-tolerance policies, toy guns were not treated the same as real guns, nor were common objects such as a nail file. Any potential weapon was judged based on the threat of injury it posed to others. How the student used the weapon or threatened to use it was most important.

When in doubt as to whether a student's actions constituted a threat, our guidelines called for the team to investigate the behavior as a threat. However, it was made clear that all forms of aggressive behavior would not necessarily indicate a threat of future violence. For example, if two students insulted each other or got into a shoving match or fight, their behavior would not be investigated as a threat unless one of them expressed intent to harm the other in the future. It was expected that schools would follow their regular discipline practices for disruptive behavior or fighting, and that threat assessment would function as an additional component of the school's response. Threat assessment is not an approach to student discipline, but a means of preventing future acts of violence.

To capture the fundamental difference between threats that are readily resolved and threats that constitute a continuing danger to others, a distinction was made between *transient* and *substantive* threats. Transient threats were defined as statements that do not express a lasting intent to harm someone and can be readily resolved. These were the threats that principals said that they encountered frequently and were able to address as a routine disciplinary matter. Transient threats reflect feelings that dissipate in a short period of time when the student thinks reflectively about the meaning of what he or she has said. Transient statements might be made in a moment of anger, but are retracted when the student calms down. Transient threats might be made as a tactic in an argument or during an exchange of insults, or they might be intended as jokes or figures of speech. The most important feature of a transient threat is that the student does not have a sustained intention to harm someone. Transient threats might merit a disciplinary response, but there is no need to take protective action to prevent a future act of violence because the threat is short-lived.

Substantive threats are serious in the sense that they represent a sustained intent to harm someone beyond the immediate incident or argument where the threat was made. If there is doubt whether a threat is transient or substantive, the team treats it as a substantive threat. Substantive threats may be identified by several features that are regarded as *presumptive* indicators. The presumptive indicators, derived from the FBI report (O'Toole, 2000), include:

- The threat has specific plausible details, such as a specific victim, time, place, and method of assault.
- The threat has been repeated over time or related to multiple persons.
- The threat is reported as a plan, or planning has taken place.
- The student has accomplices, or has attempted to recruit accomplices.
- There is physical evidence of intent to carry out the threat, such as a weapon, bomb materials, a map or written plan, or a list of intended victims.

Although the presence of any one of these features may lead the school official to presume the threat is substantive, none are absolute indicators and it is possible that with additional investigation other facts could indicate that the threat is transient. For example, a student who seeks an accomplice to help in carrying out a threat might be presumed to have a serious intent to harm someone. However, several cases were observed in which an angry student enlisted a classmate to help send a threatening letter to another student as an act of revenge or intimidation, but without intent to carry out the threat. Such an incident would be handled as a serious disciplinary matter, but not as a serious threat. In essence, threat assessment teams must always take into account the context of the threat and make reasoned judgments based on all the available information. The guidelines assist the team in its investigation, but do not provide a prescription or formula.

The distinction between transient and substantive threats captured an important difference in how schools can respond to student threats at the lower end of the risk continuum, but how should schools differentiate among threats at the higher end? A serious threat to shoot someone clearly warrants a more extensive response than a threat to hit someone. Therefore, a further distinction was needed within the category of substantive threats.

In this study, the legal distinction between simple assault and aggravated or felonious assault was used as a guide, and also the law in Virginia requiring school officials to report felonious assaults to law enforcement. Therefore, substantive threats to assault someone were designated as *serious* substantive threats, and substantive threats to commit an aggravated or felonious assault were classified as *very serious* substantive threats. Very serious threats would include all substantive threats to kill, sexually assault, or inflict very serious injury on someone. Threats to injure someone with a weapon also would be regarded as very serious, because of the potential to inflict severe injury.

The school principal was designated as the leader of the threat assessment team, since the principal has overall authority for school discipline matters as well as responsibility for school safety. In schools where the assistant principal had chief responsibility for disciplinary matters, the assistant principal similarly assumed leadership of the threat assessment team. The team leader is the person who receives the initial threat report and conducts the triage assessment to determine if the threat is transient or substantive. If the case is substantive, other team members become involved.

The school resource officer (SRO) is an essential team member (Fein et al., 2002; O'Toole, 2000). The SRO is a consultant on law enforcement and security matters, and responds to emergencies or crisis situations in which there is an imminent risk of violence. If a school does not have an SRO, then the school division should make arrangements for a liaison from the local police department.

In very serious cases, the SRO has legal duties and responsibilities as a law enforcement officer just as he or she would have if the threat situation took place outside of school. For example, an officer might investigate a suspected bomb plot by obtaining a search warrant for a student's home. In less serious cases, SROs might counsel students about the potential consequences of their actions. More generally, schools are encouraged to make use of their school resource officers for prevention purposes, consistent with the philosophy of community-oriented policing that seems so well-suited to school-based law enforcement (Atkinson, 1997). School resource officers can have a positive impact on the school climate by establishing high visibility in the school, maintaining positive relations with students, and taking an interest in school activities and events as another member of the school staff. They can adopt a problem-solving approach to crime prevention, identifying potentially volatile situations or brewing conflicts between students or groups of students before violent actions take place.

The school psychologist is the team member called upon to conduct a mental health assessment of students who make very serious substantive threats. However, this mental health assessment is not intended to render a prediction as to whether the student will or will not commit a violent act. The prediction of violence is a complex and highly uncertain task, and communications about violence risk are easily misstated or misinterpreted (Borum, 1996). Although evidence shows that clinicians can make reasonably accurate short-term predictions of violence in some situations (Borum, 1996), little is known about the prediction of student violence, particularly in the context of active school intervention aimed at preventing violence. The assessment we recommend is concerned first with identifying the student's mental health status and second, with elucidating the student's motivation in making the threat.

Ideally, the school psychologist will begin a mental health evaluation on the day the threat is made, to determine whether the student should be hospitalized or has other pressing mental health needs. In a small proportion of cases, the student may exhibit psychotic symptoms such as paranoid delusions or auditory hallucinations that concern the intended victim. More commonly, the student may be depressed and the threat represents an act of desperation. The level of depression bears careful assessment. In most of the high profile school shootings, the student was suicidal prior to the attack (Vossekuil et al., 2002). Some of these students either planned to shoot themselves or expected to be shot and killed by the police. The psychologist should screen all cases for suicidal as well as homicidal intent and make appropriate follow-up recommendations.

In addition to screening the student for mental health treatment, the school psychologist should investigate the student's feelings and attitudes toward the intended victim, and explore the grievances presumably underlying the threat. Guidelines include an interview protocol with key topics and questions to cover in a threat assessment. Particular attention is paid to the student's history of violence and access to weapons, and to identifying immediate situational factors, such as bullying and peer conflict, that increase the risk of violence. Although a clinician might not be able to delineate the precise risk of violence, he or she should be able to make recommendations aimed to reduce risk. For example, if a student threatened classmates who teased him, the school psychologist could recommend efforts to mediate or resolve the conflict. In the hypothetical case example, the school psychologist also might recommend that Bill no longer ride the school bus. All allegations of bullying deserve serious investigation, since students often perceive school authorities as overlooking this problem and this perception may contribute to a school culture that supports bullying (Unnever and Cornell, in press).

The school counselor has a leadership role in planning, coordinating, or implementing interventions for students who made threats. In relatively simple cases of transient threats, the counselor might educate students about appropriate language or help resolve a peer conflict. In more serious cases, the counselor might assist the family in seeking community-based treatment or establish an ongoing counseling relationship with the student.

Data were collected on 188 student threats from 35 schools in two school divisions that field tested these guidelines. Threats reported from a growing number of schools in Virginia and other states who have adopted these guidelines continue to be studied. As anticipated, the overwhelming majority of threats in the field-test sample were transient cases, about 70 percent of the total. Of the remaining 30 percent that constituted substantive cases, 21 percent were classified as serious and 9 percent very serious. However, these statistics concern threats reported to school authorities; undoubtedly there are many student threats that go unreported.

Just 16 students in 35 schools were identified as making very serious threats of violence, a rate of less than one case per thousand students. (Under careful review of the guidelines, three of these cases technically would not be considered very serious substantive threats, but the school authorities chose to respond to them in this way, largely because the student's behavior was so disruptive and disturbing to others.) The identification of these 16 students is noteworthy for two reasons. First, it is clear that schools were not inclined to overreact to student threats and identify a large number of students as highly dangerous. Many students who made references to shooting, killing, or seriously harming someone were classified as making transient threats, and the cases were resolved without the threatened outcome taking place.

Second, those students who made very serious threats received consequences that varied according to the nature and circumstances of their threat, as well as the student's age and discipline history. If the school had employed a zero-tolerance policy, these factors would not have mattered and all of the students would have been expelled. Instead, 11 of these 16 students were suspended from school, and only two were expelled. Five were placed in an alternative school setting. The cases receiving the most severe consequences had aggravating circumstances, such as brandishing a knife or assaulting the victim.

DIRECTIONS FOR FUTURE RESEARCH

Student threat assessment is a new and largely unstudied approach to violence prevention in schools, and so there are many research questions that merit careful investigation. The differentiation between transient and substantive threats is intended to capture an important practical distinction made routinely by school authorities, but the validity of these constructs is not yet established. What are the criteria that reliably distinguish transient and substantive threats, and are substantive threats more likely to result in a violent outcome? Of course, it will be difficult to show a differential outcome from substantive threats since schools will understandably make a concerted effort to prevent a violent outcome.

A related area for research is the effectiveness of various risk reduction or violence prevention strategies. To what extent does counseling a student or attempting to resolve a peer conflict prevent a threat from being carried out? Although evidence supports certain general forms of youth violence prevention (U.S. Surgeon General, 2001), such as conflict mediation and schoolwide bullying prevention programs, no studies have examined the impact of such strategies on student threats or student conflicts that have risen to the level of an articulated threat of violence.

More generally, little is known about the characteristics of students who make threats of violence or their victims. We do not know how threat making relates to other forms of aggressive behavior, and whether threatening others is associated with increased aggression or represents, perhaps in some students, an alternative to physical aggression. In some situations threats may represent an act of frustration by a student who lacks other means of dealing with a conflictual situation, but undoubtedly there are bullies who are skillful in using threats to their own advantage.

Finally, threat assessment is contingent upon threat reporting. We do not know how many threats go unreported or what distinguishes threats that go unreported from those that come to the attention of school authorities. How do students decide whether to report a threat? Is the nature of the threat most important, and if so, how do students evaluate threats by their peers? Or can schools identify characteristics of the school climate and their relationships with their students that influence whether students are comfortable coming forward to seek help? A recent study comparing bully victims who did or did not report being bullied (Unnever and Cornell, 2002) suggests that multiple factors could be involved. Among middle school students, more severe bullying was associated with higher victim reporting, but gender and age mattered, with female victims and younger victims more likely to seek help for bullying. However, students of both genders who perceived the school climate to be tolerant of bullying were less likely to report being bullied, suggesting that school policies and staff response to bullying were important. There was also evidence of family influences; high parental marital discord and use of coercive discipline were associated with lower reporting of bully victimization experiences. These findings bear investigation in students who are threatened with violence in bullying relationships and in other interpersonal contexts.

RECOMMENDATIONS FOR STUDENT THREAT ASSESSMENT

Although its methods and principles are practiced to some degree in many schools, threat assessment represents a promising new approach to school violence prevention. Threat assessment is not a substitute for other violence prevention efforts, but a means of investigation that leads directly to targeted interventions and attempts to deal with specific conflicts before they result in violence. Threat assessment presents a clear alternative to widespread practices such as zero tolerance and student profiling. Based on experience, training, and consulting with student threat assessment teams, the following are recommendations for establishing threat assessment teams:

1. Each school should form its own threat assessment team rather than rely on a single team to assess threats for an entire school division or group of schools. Teams based in the school are able to respond immediately to student threats and team members have a knowledge of the school and their students that is essential to making good decisions and developing risk reduction plans which are compatible with school functioning. Outside consultants can assist the team in special situations involving very serious substantive threats.

2. The threat assessment team should be led by the school principal or assistant principal. Principals have authority over student discipline and quite understandably would desire involvement in any serious threat of violence. It would be problematic for someone other than a principal to be in a position of authority in making decisions about a student who had made a serious threat of violence.

3. The threat assessment team should include the school resource officer (SRO) or some other law enforcement representative. If the school does not employ an SRO, the school should identify a liaison officer from the local police department.

4. The school psychologist or another school-based mental health professional should be available to conduct mental health evaluations of students who make very serious threats. Routine mental health eval-

uations for all students who make threats is not recommended. The purpose of these evaluations is to make mental health and risk reduction recommendations rather than absolute predictions of violence.

5. The first step in student threat assessment is to distinguish transient threats that can be readily resolved from more serious, substantive threats. Although there may be disciplinary consequences for making a transient threat, only substantive threats require protective action to prevent a violent act.

6. Very serious substantive threats merit a comprehensive evaluation addressing the areas covered in the FBI report (O'Toole, 2000) and following the principles recommended by the Secret Service and U.S. Department of Education (Fein et al., 2002). Both reports are available on the Internet (<www.fbi.gov> and <www.secretservice. gov>) and provide a wealth of useful information.

7. Threat assessment should extend beyond evaluation of the threat to development of a threat response. Threat management involves the implementation of strategies or interventions aimed at reducing the risk of violence. The school counselor and other members of the threat assessment team should make risk reduction their ultimate goal.

REFERENCES

Advancement Project and The Civil Rights Project (2000). *Opportunities suspended: The devastating consequences of zero tolerance and school discipline policies.* Boston, MA: Harvard Civil Rights Project. Available online: <http://www.law.harvard.edu/civilrights/conferences/zero/zt_report2.htm>.

American Psychological Association (1996). *Potential Warning Signs for Violence in Children.* Available online: <http://helping.apa.org/family/warning.html>.

Atkinson, A. (1997). *Virginia school resource officer handbook.* Richmond, VA: Virginia Department of Criminal Justice Services.

Borum, R. (1996). Improving the clinical practice of violence risk assessment: Technologies, guidelines and training. *American Psychologist, 51,* 945-956.

Cornell, D.G. (1999). Child and adolescent homicide. In Vincent B. Van Hasselt and Michel Hersen (Eds.), *Handbook of psychological approaches with violent criminal offenders: Contemporary strategies and issues* (pp. 131-152). New York: Kluwer Academic.

Cornell, D.G. (2001). *Guidelines for responding to student threats of violence.* Charlottesville, VA: University of Virginia.

Cornell, D.G., Sheras, P.L., Kaplan, S., Levy, A., McConville, D., McKnight, L., and Posey, J. (in press). Guidelines for responding to student threats of violence: Field test of a threat assessment approach. In M.J. Furlong, P.M. Kingery, and

M.P. Bates (Eds.), *Appraisal and prediction of school violence: Context, issues, and methods.* New York: Wiley.

Dwyer, K., Osher, D., and Warger, C. (1998). *Early warning, timely response: A guide to safe schools.* Washington, DC: U.S. Department of Education.

Fein, R.A. and Vossekuil, F. (1998). *Protective intelligence and threat assessment investigations: A guide for state and local law enforcement officials.* Washington, DC: U.S. Secret Service.

Fein, R.A., and Vossekuil, F. (1999). Assassination in the United States: An operational study of recent assassins, attackers, and near-lethal approachers. *Journal of Forensic Sciences, 44,* 321-333.

Fein, R.A., Vossekuil, F., and Holden, G.A. (1995). Threat assessment: An approach to prevent targeted violence. *National Institute of Justice: Research in Action,* 1-7 (NCJ 155000), Available online: <http://www.secretservice.gov/ntac.htm>.

Fein, R.A., Vossekuil, F., Pollack, W.S., Borum, R., Modzeleski, W., and Reddy, M. (2002). *Threat assessment in schools: A guide to managing threatening situations and to creating safe school climates.* Washington, DC: U.S. Secret Service and U.S. Department of Education.

O'Toole, M.E. (2000). *The school shooter: A threat assessment perspective.* Quantico, VA: National Center for the Analysis of Violent Crime, Federal Bureau of Investigation.

Reddy, M., Borum, R., Berglund, J., Vossekuil, B., Fein, R.A., and Modzeleski, W. (2001). Evaluating risk for targeted violence in schools: Comparing risk assessment, threat assessment, and other approaches. *Psychology in the Schools, 38,* 157-172.

Sewell, K.W. and Mendelsohn, M. (2000). Profiling potentially violent youth: Statistical and conceptual problems. *Children's Services: Social Policy, Research, and Practice, 3,* 147-169.

Skiba, R. and Peterson, R. (1999). The dark side of zero tolerance: Can punishment lead to safe schools? *Phi Delta Kappa.* Available online: <http://www/pdkintl.org/ kappan/kski9901.htm>.

Tebo, M.G. (2000, April). Zero tolerance, zero sense. *American Bar Association Journal.* Available online: <www.abanet.org/journal/apr00/04FZERO.html>.

Unnever J. and Cornell, D.G. (in press). The culture of bullying. *Journal of School Violence.*

Unnever, J. and Cornell, D. (2002). Middle school victims of bullying: Who reports being bullied? Unpublished manuscript, Radford University, Radford, Virginia.

U.S. Surgeon General (2001). *Youth violence: A report of the surgeon general.* Rockville, MD: U.S. Department of Health and Human Services.

Vossekuil, B., Fein, R.A., Reddy, M., Borum, R., and Modzeleski, W. (2002). The final report and findings of the *Safe School Initiative:* Implications for the prevention of school attacks in the United States. Washington, DC: U.S. Secret Service and U.S. Department of Education.

Chapter 5

Peer Mediation

Helen Lupton-Smith

Teaching all students how to negotiate and mediate will ensure that future generations are prepared to manage conflicts constructively in career, family, community, national, and international settings. There is no reason, however, to expect that this process will be easy or quick. It took over 30 years to reduce the rate of smoking in the United States. It took over 20 years to reduce drunk driving. It may take even longer to ensure that children and adolescents can manage conflicts constructively. Yet, the more years students spend learning and practicing negotiation and mediation procedures the more likely they will be to actually use those procedures skillfully both in the classroom and beyond the schoolhouse door. (Johnson and Johnson, 1996b, p. 334)

INTRODUCTION

This chapter will address the background behind the development of peer mediation programs, the process, and the various logistics involved in program setup. Differences involved in elementary, middle, and high school programs will be discussed as well as some examples of successful programs. The total school model and cadre model of peer mediation will be covered. Finally, a summary of research efforts delineating the specifics needed to create effective programs and also examining the benefits for students, staff, and families will be included.

HISTORY

Conflicts among students in the United States schools result in destructive outcomes with disturbing frequency. In many schools, outbreaks of violent behavior and the presence of weapons are very common with estimates indicating over 25,000 handguns enter schools daily (Stop the Violence, 1994). As the frequency and severity of conflicts in schools appears to be rising (Elam, Rose, and Gallup, 1994), children are frequently engaging in ineffective or destructive resolution strategies (Johnson, Johnson, Dudley, and Magnuson, 1995). Fighting, violence, and gangs are listed among the biggest problems facing public schools today (Rose and Gallup, 1999). Students who do not resort to violence report using maladaptive resolution strategies such as threats and withdrawal (Johnson, Johnson, Dudley, and Magnuson, 1995). The adolescent homicide rate has more than doubled in the past several years, and youth violence is currently the leading preventable cause of death for adolescents (Elliot, 1994). In response to the current epidemic of juvenile violence in our society, schools are instituting prevention efforts such as conflict resolution curriculum and peer mediation programs. This chapter will include an in-depth look at peer mediation programs.

Peer mediation began in the 1960s with the Teaching Students to Be Peacemakers Program (Johnson, 1970, 1991). The concept of peer mediation was derived from social interdependence theory (Deutsch, 1949; Johnson and Johnson, 1989) and focused on teaching all students in a school the nature of conflict, how to use an integrative negotiation procedure (win-win/mutual gains), and how to mediate peer conflicts. Peer mediation continued to evolve out of programs such as the Community Board Program (1987) in San Francisco and Resolving Conflict Creatively in the New York City public schools, which were developed by attorneys and child advocates in the mid-1970s (Lantieri and Patti, 1996). Peer mediation continues to receive much attention as an intervention to address conflict in the schools (Carruthers et al., 1996). The National Association for Mediation in Education estimated that in 1994 there were between 5,000 and 8,000 conflict resolution programs in the United States. As Johnson and Johnson (1996a) stated recently there is hardly a school that does not have a mediation program or is not anticipating the development of one. Peer mediation has a wealth of support from teachers, students, administrators, researchers, and politicians (Bey, 1996). Although some researchers and school staff are skeptical of its long-term benefits, faith in peer mediation programs is at an all time high. The programs are deemed capable of not only decreasing incidents of violence in schools and communities but of raising academic achievement and increasing test scores (Johnson and Johnson, 1996b). Research is needed to determine whether peer mediation results in effective outcomes and what processes influence the outcomes. Later in this chapter current research on peer mediation programs and results will be discussed.

PROGRAMS

What Is Peer Mediation?

Peer mediation, a method of conflict resolution, is the utilization of a third-person mediator to help settle a dispute (Johnson et al., 1992). The mediator acts as a neutral and impartial third party who helps facilitate a process wherein two or more people can negotiate an integrative (mutual gains/win-win) resolution to their conflict (Johnson and Johnson, 1991). In school peer mediation programs, student mediators serve to facilitate this step-by-step process of communication and problem solving that leads to the resolution between two parties in conflict (Schrumpf, Crawford, and Usadel, 1991). Student mediators often work in pairs serving as comediators (Araki, 1990). Peer mediators facilitate conflict resolution processes between peers who are close in grade level to the mediators. Usually, the mediator is the same age or older than the disputants involved.

Traditional interventions teach students that adult authority figures are needed to resolve conflicts. Casella (2000) declares that this approach does not empower students. Although adults may become more skillful in controlling students, students do not learn the procedures, skills, and attitudes required to constructively resolve conflict. With peer mediation they do.

Types of Peer Mediation Programs

Peer mediation programs are generally of two types: (1) the cadre approach, in which a small number of students are trained to serve as peer mediators for the whole school, and (2) the total school approach, in which all students in the school or class are taught how to manage conflicts constructively and have an opportunity to be a mediator.

The Cadre Approach

The cadre approach to peer mediation programs, which can be adopted relatively easily and inexpensively, is based on the assumption that a few specifically trained students can defuse and constructively resolve interpersonal conflicts among students (Johnson, Johnson, Dudley, and Magnuson, 1995). This model might include using mediators in a course such as an elective course (i.e., Peer Discovery) where peer mediation procedures and practices are taught as part of the class. This format provides a ready forum to conduct mediations, debrief, and receive ongoing support. The teacher of the course serves as the peer mediation coordinator. This structure could work well in a high school or magnet school that offers many electives. The advantages with this type of cadre approach are depth of training, ease of scheduling, and access to mediators. The weakness here is that only mediators are used who are enrolled in the course which may limit the number of students who will mediate as well as the diversity of mediators; and restrict the range of mediation times (Lupton-Smith et al., 1996).

Another cadre approach is the student club model that involves selecting students from the entire student body and bringing them together at a time and place outside their regular school curriculum. Training may be conducted after school or on weekends. Also, training can be done during lunchtime or homeroom time or be condensed into a one- or two-day period. Mediations are scheduled before school, during lunch, or after school when mediators and disputants have time free from class. This will minimize out-of-class time. This model permits more students to become involved with the possibility of recruiting a more diverse range of mediators. Some disadvantages here might be that the depth of training and frequency of support for mediators may not be as great as with the elective course model and coordinators may be confronted with space and scheduling issues (Lupton-Smith et al., 1996).

The Total School Approach

Johnson and Johnson (1994) advocate for the total school model in which all students are taught the principles and practices of conflict resolution and all have the opportunity to serve as mediators. The strength in this approach is that every student learns how to manage conflicts constructively and the experience of being a mediator reinforces and strengthens conflict management skills. However, there is also an increased chance that the severity and frequency of conflicts in school might decrease if everyone is trained (Lupton-Smith et al., 1996). The approach is based on the assumption that students are empowered to regulate their own behavior and resolve interpersonal conflicts when all the students in the school know how to negotiate integrative (mutual gains/win-win) agreements and to mediate conflicts. The school culture must support and promote this process of conflict management, which is evident in the fact that everyone is receiving training. As all students are rotated as mediators, everyone is responsible. Because training the whole student body in negotiation and mediation requires a fair amount of time and commitment from faculty and administration, it is relatively expensive (Johnson, Johnson, Dudley, Ward, et al., 1995).

Johnson and Johnson's (1996a) Teaching Students to be Peacemakers Program is an example of the total school approach. This program is a curriculum for grades 1 through 12 that presents the negotiation and mediation procedures in increasingly more sophisticated ways as the students grow and mature. Johnson and Johnson (1996b) state that a few hours of instruction is insufficient to train students to be at a high level of competence in managing their conflicts constructively. It takes years and years to acquire such competence but by implementing an incremental, schoolwide peer-mediation program students are increasingly empowered not only to solve their own problems but regulate their own and classmates' behavior. The Teaching Students to be Peacemakers Program maintains that schools need to be conflict positive where conflicts are encouraged and managed constructively. Conflict is inevitable and can be productive. If people express their feelings and needs in a positive and constructive way, it reduces anxiety and prevents the escalation of conflict. In conflict situations both parties can win. In this program, after all students are trained, teachers will select two class members on a daily basis to serve as mediators. The mediators are then rotated so that all students in the class or school serve as mediators an equal amount of time. The mediators work in pairs, wear official T-shirts, and are available to mediate any conflicts that occur in the classroom or school (Johnson and Johnson, 1996b).

The Peacemaker Program also stresses the importance of

1. giving each disputant adequate time to cool off before mediating;
2. convincing them to commit to the process (the mediator must introduce himself or herself, explain the process, and lay out the ground rules of conflict resolution);
3. helping the disputants negotiate through the problem-solving sequence; and
4. recording the negotiated agreement and routinely checking the status of the relationship.

If peer mediation fails, the teacher joins to serve as a mediator and if this fails the teacher must arbitrate the dispute. If the teacher arbitration fails then the principal is called on to serve as mediator and if this does not work the principal arbitrates the decision. Another part of this model is to integrate conflict resolution skills into academic lessons to continue building on students' skills (Johnson and Johnson, 1996b).

PROGRAM SETUP AND OPERATION

For the purposes of this chapter the process of developing and operating a school peer mediation program will be divided into the following stage sequence:

1. Orientation
2. Preparation
3. Operation
4. Follow-up and evaluation

Orientation

This stage involves obtaining support from the school administration, staff, students, parents, and community for starting a peer mediation program. Some schools create an advisory committee with individuals from these groups who can help make decisions related to introducing the material, training, and operation of the program. Staff and the general student population have to be oriented to peer mediation. With the staff this may be done through in-service or staff development training (a 10- to 20-hour program). With students this orientation might be accomplished through videotapes, assemblies, and the curricula (Lupton-Smith et al., 1996). Many schools hold assemblies by grade level educating the student body on the program using a video of a successful peer mediation (Thompson, 1996). When using curricula to help introduce conflict resolution and peer mediation, teachers can select the primary lessons and decide if they want to teach them independently or integrate the new concepts into the core curriculum. Parents might be informed through newsletters, assemblies, or by sitting on committees. The community may be educated about peer mediation through the media and presentations at organizations, etc. (Lupton-Smith et al., 1996).

Staff

Staff and administrative support for the program is crucial. Research by Bell et al. (2000) declared that securing the support of administrators and key people who are invested in peer mediation seems to be a vital factor for the longevity of the program. Carruthers et al. (1996) surveyed 40 schools operating peer mediation programs and found that program coordinators most frequently attributed the success or lack of success of their program to the involvement of their school administration.

Different ways exist to staff a mediation program and examples of the ways some schools have achieved this will be discussed later in this chapter. The responsibilities of peer mediation coordinators generally include pairing mediators, scheduling peer mediation sessions, locating the peer mediators for mediations, and staying in close proximity to the peer mediation area in case an adult is needed. Staff are expected to come in during a mediation only if called on for assistance by the participants. Staff may also be involved in the training, selecting, and ongoing training and supporting of peer mediators. Once the mediators are trained, the counselor or advisor schedules meetings with peer mediators to provide more training, debrief, and address concerns and success stories (Thompson, 1996). Other staff responsibilities include keeping records of mediation outcomes and conducting follow-ups with disputants to ensure that agreements worked out in mediation are valid and being honored. Public relations must be done with the administration and the community surrounding the program. The role of the coordinator may take 20 to 50 percent of an individual's time depending on factors such as size of the school, the model, and how long the program has been in operation (Lupton-Smith et al., 1996).

Preparation

Recruitment

Selecting mediators is a crucial step of the preparation stage if a cadre approach is to be used. Some researchers suggest that third and fourth graders can be trained as mediators and others have suggested that students as young as kindergarten could at least be taught how to take their conflicts to a mediator (Johnson et al., 1996). Lane and McWhirter (1992) described three means of identifying candidates for peer mediation: self nomination, peer nomination, and teacher nomination. Other authors such as Araki (1990) identified attributes of an effective mediator as an individual that is confident, directive, caring, and a good listener. Eisler, Lane, and Mei (1995) reported that sensitivity, maturity, self-confidence, trustworthiness, and the respect of other students are the personal attributes looked for in a mediator. The selection process with this cadre model of mediation varies by school—some schools use a screening or interviewing process, others select based on a first-come-first-serve application basis, etc.

To get a broad range of mediators, schools look for at-risk students as well as role models to serve as mediators. Schools should get a cross section of the school's population in terms of sex, race, ethnicity, culture, and neighborhood (Thompson, 1996). DeJong (1994) also indicated that mediators should be selected to represent a cross section of the student body as defined by gender, race, class, achievement level, and placement. Day-Vines et al. (1996) also supported the diversity program objective. Students need to see themselves reflected in the mediators. Students should have respect for their peers and speak the language of their peers.

Training

For training student mediators and staff, program coordinators may use community or school resources. Dispute resolution centers who work with court systems often assist schools with training and program implementation. School staff, a counselor, and a few teachers can work with a consultant of this sort and do training of staff and students. Using the cadre model, many schools start out with about 15 to 30 mediators. The time for training may vary between 10 and 20 hours. Most trainings are usually around 12 hours. How this training time is broken up depends on the school structure and if staff and/or students are being trained. Developmental elements must be considered when making decisions regarding training, i.e., elementary students will need shorter time periods with more concrete information (Lupton-Smith et al., 1996).

Training goals and curricula are generally consistent across grade levels including the teaching of basic conflict resolution principles, a description of negotiation and mediation, communication skills, and role-playing the different stages of mediation. Then a discussion will occur of how the program will run in the mediators' school (Lupton-Smith et al., 1996). Thompson (1996) adds that important peer mediation training areas include:

1. the role and qualities of the peer mediators,
2. understanding conflicts, sources, and styles,
3. communication skills such as active listening, and
4. the steps in peer mediation.

Thompson (1996) reports that ongoing advanced training needs to be scheduled to include caucusing, respecting differences, dealing with anger, and working with reflecting feelings. See Box 5.1 for a list of the stages of mediation; also, in the references, those marked with an asterisk are considered popular commercial peer mediation curricula (Lupton-Smith et al., 1996).

BOX 5.1. Stages of Peer Mediation

1. Open the session
   - Introductions.
   - State the ground rules.
   - Get a commitment to follow the ground rules: "Do you agree to follow the ground rules?"

2. Gather information
   - Ask each disputant for his or her side of the story and how he or she felt: "Please tell what happened."
   - Listen, summarize, clarify.
   - Ask if either wants to add anything, and listen, summarize, clarify.

3. Focus on common interests
   - Determine the interests by asking what each disputant wants and bring together by saying, "Both of you seem to agree or seem to want . . ."

4. Create options
   - State rules for brainstorming: Say any ideas that come to mind and don't judge.
   - Help with questions if needed.
   - Write ideas down on a brainstorming sheet.

5. Evaluate options and choose a solution
   - Ask which ideas seem to work best and circle on brainstorming sheet.
   - Evaluate the ideas: "What will happen if you do this?"

6. Write the agreement and close
   - Write down the agreement.
   - Ask each to sign, then mediator signs.
   - Shake hands and congratulate and ask disputants to shake hands.
   - Thank participants.

Source: Schrumpf, Crawford, and Usadel (1991).

Note: These stages and suggestions for each stage can be adapted to fit the age group using the model.

Operation

Scheduling

Which issues will be mediated? When will mediation sessions be held? How will the confidentiality of mediation be preserved? Who can refer someone to mediation and how does that referral process take place? These are all questions that will arise and need to be answered at this point (Lupton-Smith et al., 1996). Scheduling is an important but sensitive issue. Generally, mediations are scheduled during advisement time, lunch, elective courses, etc. Frequently, a high number of referrals and mediations may need to occur during class. With Thompson's (1996) program all mediators had to circulate a release form to all their teachers to obtain permission to be excused from class. As stated previously, peer mediators facilitate conflict resolution processes between peers who are close in grade level to the mediators. Elementary school students mediate with elementary students, middle school with middle school students, and high school students with high school students (Lupton-Smith et al., 1996). According to Thompson (1996) in her study of a mediation program, to ensure neutrality mediators were scheduled to mediate students one grade level below their own grade.

Generally, mediations can be self-referred, teacher, student, administration, and possibly parent referred. Usually a referral slip can be filled out and placed in a box in a classroom or outside the program coordinator's office—wherever it can be frequently checked by the coordinator.

Follow-Up and Evaluation

Concerns include promotion and maintenance of the peer mediation program, ongoing support and training for school staff, students, and mediators, and an evaluation of the program's effectiveness. Further training with student mediators includes ongoing support and skill building (Lupton-Smith et al., 1996). Data need to be collected and an evaluation of different aspects of the program needs to be conducted (i.e., number of mediations, number of successful resolutions, effect on school climate, effect on academic performance of mediators, and overall, etc.). In addition, the coordinator who is equipped with some data to support the efficacy of his or her program is in a much better position to convince those that are skeptical of the program's effectiveness and importance. Carruthers et al. (1996) have described a practical approach to program evaluation.

DEVELOPMENTAL PROGRAM CONSIDERATIONS

Preschool

Peer mediation programs are generally implemented at the elementary school level and higher. The closest program in the literature to peer mediation for preschool students is a program called Fussbusters. Fussbusters is a program that started in a Head Start preschool classroom. Here, negotiations take place at a Peace Table that has three chairs. If a conflict occurs the children go immediately to the Peace Table accompanied by a Fussbuster. The Fussbuster, a friend chosen by both participants, helps mediate the discussion at the Peace Table. The rules at the Peace Table include: no hitting; talk things over; one person talks at a time; take a helper; stay until the problem is solved; shake hands at the end; and get your spot back where you were playing. Students are told if they have a conflict that does not involve health or safety issues that they should talk it over first at the Peace Table. Because peer mediation has been limited at the preschool level, this program was offered as a related alternative. The results have been very positive, posing a helpful immediate solution for reducing classroom bullying (Wilson-Gillespie and Chick, 2001).

Elementary School

Coordinators of peer mediation programs should recognize that elementary grade mediators and disputants cannot handle as complicated a mediation process as can high school students. Children at the elementary level in grades three through five are advised to use a four-stage model. Coordinators should consider the following four stages:

1. Introduction and ground rules
2. Determining facts and feelings
3. Identifying possible solutions
4. Making an agreement (Lupton-Smith et al., 1996)

The training at the elementary level needs to match the development of the mediators. For example, Stichter (1986) suggests using simple words and concrete methods to convey the principles and practices of mediation. For training purposes it is also important to be aware of what kinds of conflicts an elementary student mediator will contend with. Araki (1990) found the highest occurrence of conflicts in elementary school concerned harassment in the form of verbal threats, bullying, and name-calling. Others included teasing, playground disagreements, access or possession conflicts, jealousy, and invasion of privacy (Araki, 1990; Burrell and Vogl, 1990). Johnson, Johnson, and Dudley (1992) found that the most frequent conflicts in elementary school involved put-downs and teasing, followed by playground conflicts and access or possession conflicts. In a study of third-through sixth-grade students in an elementary school, Johnson et al. (1994) found that before peer mediation training the most frequently used strategies for dealing with conflict were telling the teacher and withdrawal.

An example of a fairly typical elementary school mediation program that was highlighted in Lupton-Smith et al. (1996) included students from fourth and fifth grades who served as mediators for grades three through five at a magnet school with about 450 students. The school's guidance counselor was the program's coordinator. The school received a grant for the funding and then created an advisory council consisting of teachers, parents, the principal, and, of course, the counselor as coordinator. At the beginning of the fall semester all staff members and students were trained in conflict resolution principles and practices. Consultants with the court system were brought in to conduct a 12-hour training with school staff. Then each staff member taught lessons in conflict resolution to all classes over a two-month period. The lessons were separate from the core curriculum. Mediators here were selected from the fourth and fifth grades and were recommended by teachers. They were selected to represent a racially and ethnically diverse group. The counselor performed the training of mediators with a consultant from the court-based mediation program. The training was done through an elective course that met once a week for ten weeks. When training was complete an assembly was held for grades three through five to introduce mediation to the students who would be using it and mediation was also introduced to parents at a PTA meeting. The counselor met with the mediators' parents to describe the program to them. Mediators were usually paired by grade and again mediated conflicts for grades three through five. Mediations were conducted at lunchtime or before school. Two mediators were assigned for one week, then another two for the second week, and so on. Referral slips were kept in the homerooms with referrals to mediation usually being made by teachers, students, and occasionally parents. The coordinator sent out follow-up forms to the disputants to make sure the conflicts stayed resolved. Follow-up interviews with the disputants in the first year of operation indicated 62 out of 65 disputants expressed satisfaction with their mediation sessions and that their agreement had been honored by the other party in the conflict. In the second year of operation the time required to manage the program by the counselor was much less than in the first year (Lupton-Smith et al., 1996).

Middle School

For middle school students grades six through eight, some recommend that a five-stage model be used. For these students, a stage should be added for mediators—"Clarify interests and common grounds"—and placed after the "Determining the facts and feelings" stage (Lupton-Smith et al., 1996). Jones and Carlin (1994) stated that the majority of conflicts for middle school students involved verbal disagreements, physical fighting, and rumors. The duration of the conflicts ranged from very short to longer than one month. In Ohio schools the most frequently reported conflicts at this level involved friends, name-calling, dating rumors, and disrespect (Ohio Commission on Dispute Resolution and Conflict Management, 1993). Stern and Van Slyck (1986) found frequently occurring conflicts in middle school to be gossip and rumors, dating/friendship relationship issues, and harassment. Schrumpf, Crawford, and Usadel (1991) reported that out of 245 conflicts referred to peer mediators in a midwestern middle school of approximately 1,000 students, 26 percent involved name-calling, 23 percent involved rumors, 16 percent involved hitting and fighting, and the other 35 percent involved a wide variety of issues.

One noteworthy middle school program discussed in the literature had the in-school suspension coordinator serving as the peer mediation coordinator. In this case, the school's DARE (Drug and Alcohol Resistance Education) coordinator identified the need for the program and started an advisory council. The school staff was given 15 hours of training in conflict resolution and peer mediation. All sixth-grade students received ten days of instruction on conflict resolution during health class. The coordinator conducted mini-assemblies with all classes to inform them on peer mediation and parents were informed at an open house. The peer mediators were selected by a group of staff and all were diverse by race and gender but all had good listening skills and a concern for others. Mediators had 20 hours of training including attending an all-day workshop before the semester began and then met after school once per week during the semester. Role-playing was a major part of training. Experienced mediators helped train new students. Mediations occurred during the second half of fourth-, fifth-, and sixth-period lunches. There was a designated mediation room with the coordinator's office adjacent to the room and the door was left open between the two rooms and the coordinator was available in case adult supervision was needed. Two mediators conducted the mediations, taking turns working through the stages and they were always in the same or higher grade than the disputant. Mediators were instructed to read the bulletin board in the cafeteria every day to learn of their schedule for the day. In the first year of operation, 87 mediations were conducted and 84 resulted in an agreement (Lupton-Smith et al., 1996).

A special component of this program is how much time the coordinator spent with debriefing and practicing advanced skills with the mediators. The coordinator worked with mediators on how to build rapport or work with angry or resistant disputants. Also, if one person was really angry, the coordinator, as in-school suspension coordinator, was able to "hold" one of the disputants until he or she calmed down (Lupton-Smith et al., 1996).

High School

For high school students, a six-stage model has been suggested. For these students a stage called "Reflections" could be added at the end of the process which allows the mediators to probe deeper into the disputants' attitudes and beliefs about the conflict (Lupton-Smith et al., 1996). When training older students, Benson and Benson (1993) describe more advanced issues for continuing training including prejudice reduction, caucusing, uncovering hidden interests, and advanced role-playing. High school mediations generally take longer than elementary or middle school mediations. With high school students there are usually more hidden agendas and the students seem to need more time to articulate the nature of their problems (Lupton-Smith et al., 1996).

One high school program discussed in the literature had a social studies teacher serving as coordinator of the peer mediation program. She was trained as a court mediator. In the first year, 20 teachers and 20 students were trained by a community agency. Those trained prepared a video to train the rest of the staff and students. Mediators participated in a class format that met once a day before lunch and was led by the coordinator. Here the mediators could meet ongoing, debrief with the coordinator, and practice skills. Scheduled mediations lasted anywhere from 30 minutes to an hour. In the first year of operation the mediators conducted 80 disputes and 75 resulted in agreement (Lupton-Smith et al., 1996).

These school peer mediation program examples represent the cadre models. Many schools start with an elective class or student club model with the possibility of transitioning into a total school model in which everyone can function as mediators. The total school model is the more developed and comprehensive of the two models (Lupton-Smith et al., 1996).

RESEARCH

Much of the literature on peer mediation has been based on researcher judgment and opinion (Benson and Benson, 1993). More recently, investigators have moved toward outcome evaluations of peer mediation. Johnson and Johnson (1996b) noted that peer mediation studies, although lacking in methodological rigor, have consistently reported positive outcomes for individual mediations. Based on anecdotal data, many hundreds of schools have reported that student mediators help solve large numbers of disputes and the mediation agreements remain intact in the vast majority of cases (Roderick, 1988). Most studies in the literature report at least an 85 percent success rate—with the average being in the 90 percent range (Araki, 1990; Burrell and Vogl, 1990; Crary, 1992; McCormick, 1988). Most school peer mediation programs report that the overriding majority of mediations are successfully resolved.

Johnson and Johnson (1996a) in a major review of peer mediation programs state that several studies show that conflict resolution and peer mediation programs do have an impact on decreasing discipline problems, violence, referrals, detentions, and suspensions. Results from peer mediation schools consistently report reductions in principal referrals; reduction of physical violence in the classroom; decline in assaults; a decrease in the amount of misconduct slips; and a decrease in school suspensions (Johnson et al., 1992; Meek, 1992; Roderick, 1988; Roush and Hall, 1993; Sherrod, 1995; Singer, 1991). Advocates for peer mediation programs state that in addition to reducing suspensions and detentions, referrals to the principal, and absenteeism, these programs also increase students' self-confidence, academic time on task, and academic achievement (Araki, 1990; Davis, 1986; Marshall, 1987). Benson and Benson (1993) reported research by the National Association for Mediation in Education (NAME) which showed that peer mediation programs reduce administrators' and teachers' time in working with conflicts; reduce the level of violence and crime in the school; and enhance the self-esteem, grades, and attendance of the students trained as mediators. Several studies have shown that conflict resolution and peer mediation training result in increased self-esteem (Gentry and Benenson, 1993; Greenawald and Johnson, 1987; Metis Associates, 1990). With peer mediation, students learn the skills of problem solving through communication and critical thinking (Benson and Benson, 1993). In addition, Lane and McWhirter (1992) declare that parents and students in peer mediation schools report that conflict in the home is resolved in new and more productive ways.

Several recent quality research studies provide some information on what is and is not working with peer mediation programs.

Peer Mediation Programs Using the Cadre Approach

One study by Bell et al. (2000) investigated a peer mediation program in a rural school grades one through eight attended predominately by children from a low socioeconomic status. The program followed a cadre approach. The researchers investigated whether students selected as mediators realize more benefits than do other students in the school. Mediators were compared to a control group who did not receive peer mediation training. Pre-, post-, and follow-up testing showed that students achieved and maintained improvements in written responses to questions tapping their knowledge of conflict resolution and mediation skills after training. Results suggest that peer mediation training was successfully delivered and received. The students in this school performed 32 out of 34 successful mediations at the six-week follow-up which was 94 percent successful, similar to studies in urban and suburban settings (Johnson and Johnson, 1996b). Additional results show that the mediators may have realized behavioral improvements during the study. The peer mediators received significantly fewer office referrals during the intervention year compared to a group of matched controls. Peer mediators showed a decrease in their own office referrals from the previous year. This finding makes a beginning case for further investigation comparing the cadre and schoolwide approaches directly to sort out whether those who receive training receive additional benefits over those who merely attend mediations (Bell et al., 2000).

Another study by Johnson et al. (1996) examined the effectiveness of an inner-city peer mediation program at an elementary school. The researchers found that although conflicts were widespread through the student body, about 1.2 percent of the students accounted for 30 percent of the mediation conflicts. Using this research information to target these students for special training to learn how to manage their conflicts was an important element in significantly reducing discipline problems of the school. This study is unique because it involved kindergarten through fourth-grade students whereas other studies focused on grades four, five, and six. The study found that peer mediators successfully mediated conflicts 98 percent of the time. However, the majority of the solutions were agreements to avoid each other: "Stay away from each other"; "Don't sit by each other." These children did not resolve the issues through problem solving to achieve mutual gains. Instead, they decided to avoid each other in the future. A major implication of this study is that schools may wish to implement a conflict resolution program in which students are trained in a range of possible strategies for managing conflicts and agreements. In addition, Johnson et al. (1996) discovered that kindergarten children can learn to take their conflicts to a mediator so peer mediation programs can be brought to service that level.

Johnson, Johnson, Dudley, Ward, and Magnuson (1995) examined a peer mediation program in a midwestern, suburban elementary school. They found that there were significant differences between the strategies used before and after training in negotiation and mediation procedures. Before training the children used compromising, forcing, and withdrawal—strategies focused on one's goals while ignoring the relationship with the other person. After training, the children primarily used the integrative negotiation procedure—a strategy focused on achieving one's goals while maintaining a quality relationship with the other person. They also found that the negotiation and mediation procedures that students were taught did transfer to the home.

Another study by Humphries (1999) used playground observations and student interviews to examine the perceptions and experiences of a group of elementary student mediators. The interviews were conducted at the end of the school year after the participants had been peer mediators for around three months. Sixty-four percent of the mediators remembered the steps involved in the mediation process. The step most often missed was asking the disputant how he or she felt and why, and restating the problem. Children interviewed suggested that some of the training should occur on the playground so that the mediators could get a more realistic feel for the procedure and practice more realistic disputes.

Humphries (1999) reported that the greatest problems faced by being a mediator were: missing recess while on duty, not being able to help every situation, and having too many fights arise. In this study, most all of the children stated that they encountered some interpersonal problems with nonmediators while being a mediator, e.g., loss of friendship especially when they were mediating a problem involving a friend. This potential conflict of interest needs to be closely monitored by the coordinator when selecting who will mediate a particular conflict. Some were teased for being a mediator. Some children stated that if the mediator was not well liked then some disputants were unwilling to let the mediator help them resolve problems.

As a result of this study, Humphries suggested the following: ongoing practice sessions and carrying an outline of the process when on duty which may help with some of the mediation steps students said they forgot. Consistent findings have shown that mediators find it difficult to master skills involving the expressions of feelings at the elementary level so targeted additional training may help with this. More realistic scenarios need to be used during training. There is a need to educate the student body to a greater extent on mediation and let more children rotate through the year as mediators. Finally, providing rewards and recognition of mediators may be a way to increase student respect for mediation and the mediators (Humphries, 1999).

Johnson et al. (1994) studied a peer mediation training program that was conducted in four classrooms in a suburban middle-class elementary school and reported that from retention tests it was evident that students did learn the process of mediation. Training, therefore, was successful. They also investigated whether students could transfer their knowledge and skills to real-life conflicts. Simulated conflict scenarios were videotaped and showed that students knew the sequence of mediation and could use it in real conflicts over a period of four months. Also, observers were used to document how students managed conflicts in different settings to see if knowledge was transferred. Observations showed that the students were able to use the skills and regulate their behavior voluntarily and spontaneously. Self-regulation is an important aspect of cognitive and social development as well as socialization. Research also showed that after the training, teachers reported that conflicts were managed by the students with little adult involvement. The frequency of student conflicts that teachers managed dropped 80 percent and referrals to the principal were down to zero. Parents whose children were not part of the project requested that their children receive the training the following year and many parents wanted to receive the training so they could use the methods at home (Johnson et al., 1994).

These studies examining various peer mediation programs using the cadre model provide some profound implications:

1. Peer mediation training does work as is evidenced by students cognitively remembering the content as well as being able to demonstrate the skills up to four months after training in spontaneous situations.
2. Evidence suggests that these skills are transferred to the home as well as various settings at school.
3. When training elementary students, one needs to give concrete options for mediations and train using very real role-plays in real settings. Also, elementary students need to work on the expression of feelings aspect of mediation.
4. Students use different skills for handling conflict after training than were used before training.
5. Evidence shows that mediators may benefit more than those who do not receive the training (i.e., the disputants).

Peer Mediation Programs Using the Total School Approach

Findings from reports from student mediators and disputants suggest that while some students from the general school population may benefit from mediation, the students who gain the most from the programs are the peer mediators themselves (Van Slyck and Stern, 1991). McCormick (1988) stated that at-risk students who directly participated in a mediation program serving as peer mediators developed more prosocial attitudes toward conflict but those with only indirect exposure to the collaborative process (disputants) maintained the antisocial attitudes toward conflict. Peer mediators from across different mediation programs develop an improved ability to express problems, positive problem-solving skills, better communication patterns, and improved self-image (Lane and McWhirter, 1992; Roush and Hall, 1993; Stomfay-Stitz, 1994). Findings such as these and those that follow lend increasing support to the total school model as the optimal approach with maximum benefits for all students.

Johnson, Johnson, Dudley, and Magnuson (1995) tested the effectiveness of the total student body approach using the Teaching Students to be Peacemakers program of peer mediation with several different grade levels and classes. They wanted to determine if students conceptually learned the steps involved in mediation and reaching integrative agreements; were they able to describe how they would use mediation in actual conflict situations; and were they able to maintain this knowledge over time. Two hundred twenty-seven students participated in the study. A pretest and posttest design was used in which the experimental group was tested at three points—pretraining, posttraining, and at the end of the school year and the control groups were given the postmeasures immediately after training had ended. The peer mediation program was implemented once the training was done and each day the teacher chose two student mediators who wore special T-shirts and patrolled the playground and lunchroom. The students in the control group did not receive any peer mediation training and were administered only the postmeasure. The training included the teaching and practicing of the procedures for negotiation and mediation with the students.

Johnson, Johnson, Dudley, and Magnuson (1995) discovered that 94 percent of the students ranging from second to fifth grade in the experimental group recalled 100 percent of the steps of peer mediation after training had ended. This shows that students as young as second graders can learn these steps. Students were tested again at the end of the year to see if they had retained what they had learned about negotiation and mediation. Ninety-two percent of those who had been trained remembered all the steps of negotiation and mediation. Results of written and interview conflict scenario measures indicated that training had a significant positive effect on students' potential ability to use negotiation and mediation procedures in specific conflicts. The teachers and the principal believed the program reduced the incidence of destructively managed conflicts. Overall, the study confirms anecdotal evidence about the effectiveness of peer mediation in schools and validates the assumptions underlying the total student body approach to peer mediation (Johnson, Johnson, Dudley, and Magnuson, 1995).

Students appear to be able to learn the steps of peer mediation as well as to use and retain them over a period of months. The use of peer mediation can substantially change how students approach and settle conflicts (Peterson and Skiba, 2001). In one middle school, 83 percent of students trained in peer mediation reported win-win settlements whereas 86 percent of untrained controls reported that conflicts resulted in a win-lose outcome (Johnson and Johnson, 1996a). For the mediators themselves, learning the mediation process has been shown to increase self-esteem and even to improve academic achievement (Peterson and Skiba, 2001). As there are limited studies researching the total school approach to peer mediation, Johnson, Johnson, Dudley, and Magnuson (1995) recommend future research comparing the effectiveness of the two approaches to peer mediation, cadre and total student body, to delineate (1) their comparative strengths and weaknesses, and (2) the conditions under which each will have greatest effectiveness. Increasing evidence shows that the direct exposure of participating in mediation training and practice coupled with the responsibility and skills involved in being a mediator provide the peer mediator with distinct opportunities for growth and development as compared to those who indirectly participate in the program.

CONCLUSION

This chapter has provided an overview on where peer mediation began, what it is, and the basics of how a school can set up a program. Subtle differences do exist throughout program development for elementary, middle, and high schools and real examples were presented of programs across the grades to provide a sense of what works at different levels. An updated review of the research on peer mediation was provided with discussion of some specific implications as well as the need to look at both the cadre and total school models and what is more beneficial. Further work needs to be conducted on how to implement the total school model with the greatest efficiency and the least expense. Johnson et al. (1995) state that few schools have made the commitment to teach all students the procedures they need to constructively manage conflicts, and without direct training many students may never learn to do so. As managing conflicts is integrally related to one's quality of interpersonal relationships, social, cognitive, and moral development (Piaget, [1923] 1950; Berndt, 1984; Doise, 1985; Johnson and Johnson, 1992; Selman and Schultz, 1990; Smollar-Volpe and Youniss, 1982) the importance of these efforts cannot be stressed enough. The benefits of peer mediation programs for the individual, the mediator, school climate, and school staff have been addressed in this chapter. All these in turn benefit the community making peer mediation a program worth developing and nurturing throughout our schools.

REFERENCES

Araki, C.T. (1990). Dispute management in the schools. *Mediation Quarterly, 8*(1), 51-62.

Bell, S., Coleman, J., Anderson, A., Whelan, J., and Wilder, C. (2000). The effectiveness of peer mediation in a low SES rural elementary school. *Psychology in the Schools, 37*(6), 505-514.

Benson, A.J. and Benson, J.M. (1993). Peer mediation: Conflict resolution in schools. *Journal of School Psychology, 31,* 427-430.

Bey, T.M. (1996). *Making school a place of peace.* Thousand Oaks, CA: Corwin Press.

Berndt, T. (1984). The influence of group discussions on children's moral decisions. In J. Masters and K. Yarkin-Leven (Eds.), *Boundary areas in social and developmental psychology* (pp. 195-219). New York: Academic.

Burrell, N. and Vogl, S. (1990). Turf-side conflict mediation for students. *Mediation Quarterly, 7,* 237-250.

Carruthers, W., Sweeney, B., Kmitta, D., and Harris, G. (1996). Conflict resolution: An examination of the research literature and a model for program evaluation. *The School Counselor, 44,* 5-18.

Casella, R. (2000). The benefits of peer mediation in the context of urban conflict and program status. *Urban Education, 35*(3), 324-255.

The Committee for Children (1990). *Second Step—A violence prevention curriculum: Grades 6-8.* Seattle, WA: Author.

Community Board (1986). *Training middle school conflict managers.* San Francisco: Author.

Community Board Program, Inc. (1987). *Classroom conflict resolution training for elementary schools.* San Francisco: Community Board Program.

Crary, D. (1992). Community benefits from mediation: A test of the peace virus hypothesis. *Mediation Quarterly, 9,* 241-252.

Davis, A. (1986). Dispute resolution at an early age. *Negotiation Journal, 2,* 287-298.

Day-Vines, N.L., Day-Hairston, B., Carruthers, W., Wall, J., and Lupton-Smith, H. (1996). Conflict resolution: The value of diversity in the recruitment, selection, and training of peer mediators. *The School Counselor, 43,* 392-410.

DeJong, W. (1994). *Building the peace: The resolving conflict creatively program.* Washington, DC: U.S. Department of Justice, National Institute of Justice.

Deutsch, M. (1949). A theory of cooperation and competition. *Human Relations, 2,* 129-152.

Doise, W. (1985). Social regulations in cognitive development. In R. Hinde, A. Perret-Clermont, and J. Sevenson-Hinde (Eds.), *Social relationships and cognitive development* (pp. 238-262). Oxford: Clarendon.

Eisler, J., Lane, P., and Mei, L. (1995). A comprehensive conflict resolution training program. *ERS Spectrum: Journal of School Research and Information, 13*(1), 25-33.

Elam, S., Rose, L., and Gallup, A. (1994). The 26th annual Gallup poll of the public's attitudes toward the public schools. *Phi Delta Kappan, 76,* 41-56.

Elliot, D. (1994). *Youth violence: An overview.* Boulder: University of Colorado Center for the Study and Prevention of Violence.

Gentry, B. and Benenson, W. (1993). School to home transfer of conflict management skills among school age children. *Families in Society, 74,* 67-73.

Greenawald, D. and Johnson, G. (1987). Conflict resolution in the schools: Final evaluation report. Unpublished manuscript, Social Science Education Consortium, Boulder, CO.

Humphries, T. (1999). Improving peer mediation programs: Student experiences and suggestions. *Professional School Counseling, 3*(1), 13-19.

Johnson, D., Johnson, D., Mitchell, J., Cotton, B., Harris, D., and Louison, S. (1996). Effectiveness of conflict managers in an inner-city elementary school. *The Journal of Educational Research, 89*(5), 280-285.

Johnson, D. and Johnson, R. (1989). *Cooperation and competition: Theory and research.* Edina, MN: Interaction Book.

Johnson, D. and Johnson, R. (1991). *Teaching students to be peacemakers.* Edina, MN: Interaction Book.

Johnson, D. and Johnson, R. (1992). *Creative conflict: Intellectual challenge in the classroom.* Edina, MN: Interaction Book.

Johnson, D. and Johnson, R. (1994). Constructive conflict in the schools. *Journal of Social Issues, 50*(1), 117-137.

Johnson, D. and Johnson, R. (1996a). Conflict resolution and peer mediation programs in elementary and secondary schools: A review of the research. *Review of Educational Research, 66*(4), 459-506.

Johnson, D. and Johnson, R. (1996b). Teaching all students how to manage conflicts constructively: The peacemakers program. *Journal of Negro Education, 65*(3), 322-335.

Johnson, D., Johnson, R., and Dudley, B. (1992). Effects of peer mediation training on elementary school students. *Mediation Quarterly, 10,* 89-99.

Johnson, D., Johnson, R., Dudley, B., and Acikgoz, K. (1994). Effects of conflict resolution training on elementary school students. *Journal of Social Psychology, 134,* 803-817.

Johnson, D. W. (1970). *Social psychology of education.* Edina, MN: Interaction Book.

Johnson, D.W. (1991). *Human relations and your career* (Third edition). Engle-wood Cliffs, NJ: Prentice-Hall.

Johnson, D.W., Johnson, R.T., Dudley, B., and Burnett, R. (1992). Teaching students to be peer mediators. *Educational Leadership, 50,* 10-13.

Johnson, D., Johnson, R., Dudley, B., and Magnuson, D. (1995). Training elementary school students to manage conflict. *The Journal of Social Psychology, 135*(6), 673-686.

Johnson, D., Johnson, R., Dudley, B., Ward, M., and Magnuson, D. (1995). The impact of peer mediation training on the management of school and home conflicts. *American Educational Research Journal, 32*(4), 829-844.

Jones, T. and Carlin, D. (1994). *Philadelphia peer mediation program: Report for 1992-1994 period.* Philadelphia: Good Shepherd Neighborhood House and the Office of Desegregation of the Philadelphia Public School District.

Lane, P.S. and McWhirter, J.J. (1992). Peer mediation with middle school children. *Elementary School Guidance and Counseling, 27,* 15-23.

Lantieri, L. and Patti, J. (1996). *Waging peace in our schools.* Boston: Beacon Press.

Lupton-Smith, H.S., Carruthers, W.L., Flythe, R., Goettee, E., and Modest, K.H. (1996). Conflict resolution as peer mediation: Programs for elementary, middle, and high school students. *The School Counselor, 43,* 374-391.

Marshall, J. (1987). Mediation: A new mode of establishing order in schools. *Howard Journal, 26,* 33-46.

McCormick, M. (1988). Mediation in the schools: An evaluation of the Wakefield pilot peer mediation program in Tucson, AZ. Unpublished manuscript, University of Arizona, Bureau of Applied Research in Anthropology, Tucson.

Meek, M. (1992). The peacekeepers. *Teaching Tolerance* (Fall), 46-52.

Metis Associates (1990). *The Resolving Conflict Creatively Program: 1988-1989 summary of significant findings.* New York: Author.

Ohio Commission on Dispute Resolution and Conflict Management (1993). *Dealing with conflict in Ohio's schools.* Columbus, OH: Author.

Peterson, R. and Skiba, R. (2001). Creating school climates that prevent school violence. *The Clearing House, 74*(3), 155-163.

Piaget, J. (1950). *The psychology of intelligence.* New York: Harcourt, Brace, Jovanovich. (Original work published 1923).

Roderick, T. (1988). Johnny can learn to negotiate. *Educational Leadership, 45*(4), 86-94.

Rose, L. and Gallup, A. (1999). The 31st annual Phi Delta Kappa/Gallup poll of the public's attitudes toward public schools. *Phi Delta Kappan, 81,* 41-56.

Roush, G. and Hall, E. (1993). Teaching peaceful conflict resolution: *Mediation Quarterly, 11*(2), 185-191.

Sadalla, G., Holmbeg, M., and Halligan, J. (1990). *Conflict resolution: An elementary school curriculum.* San Francisco, CA: The Community Board Program.

Schmidt, F. and Friedman, A. (1991). *Creative conflict solving for kids.* Miami, FL: Grace Contrino Abrams Peace Education Foundation.

Schmidt, F. and Friedman, A. (1993). *Peacemaking skills for little kids.* Miami, FL: Grace Contrino Abrams Peace Education Foundation.

Schrumpf, F., Crawford, D., and Usadel, H.C. (1991). *Peer mediation: Conflict resolution in schools program guide.* Champaign, IL: Research Press.

Selman, R. and Schultz, L. (1990). *Making a friend in youth: Developmental theory and pair therapy.* Chicago: University of Chicago Press.

Sherrod, M. (1995). Student peer conflict management in California High Schools: A survey of programs and their efficacy as perceived by disciplinarians. *The Peer Facilitator Quarterly, 12*(4), 12-14.

Singer, D. (1991). Teaching alternative dispute resolution to America's children. *Arbitration Journal, 72*(December), 33-37.

Smollar-Volpe, J. and Youniss, J. (1982). Social development through friendship. In K. Rubin and H. Ross (Eds.), *Peer relationships and social skills in childhood* (pp. 279-298). New York: Springer.

Stern, M. and Van Slyck, M. (1986). Enhancing adolescents' self image: Implementation of a peer mediation program. Paper presented at the meeting of the American Psychological Association, Washington, DC, August.

Stichter, C. (1986). When tempers flare, let trained student mediators put out the flames. *The American School Board Journal, 173*(4), 41-42.

Stomfay-Stitz, A. (1994). Conflict resolution and peer mediation: Pathways to safer schools. *Childhood Education, 70,* 279-282.

Stop the Violence (1994). *Scholastic Update,* January, pp. 2-6.

Thompson, S. (1996). Peer mediation: A peaceful solution. *The School Counselor, 44,* 151-154.

Van Slyck, M. and Stern, M. (1991). Conflict resolution in educational settings: Assessing the impact of peer mediation programs. In K. Duffy, J. Grosch, and P. Olczak (Eds.), *Community mediations: A handbook for practitioners and researchers* (pp. 257-274). New York: Guilford Press.

Wilson-Gillespie, C. and Chick, A. (2001). Fussbusters: Using peers to mediate conflict resolution in a Head Start classroom. *Childhood Education,* summer, 192-195.

Chapter 6

Lessons from the Field: Balancing Comprehensiveness and Feasibility in Peer Mediation Programs

Maura Dillon

INTRODUCTION

Over the past ten years leaders in conflict resolution education have published extensively in response to a call for empirical proof of program effectiveness. They have made concerted efforts to establish best practices and ground these with sound research and evaluation. Although there is not unanimous agreement on all core elements of successful programs, most tend to agree that comprehensive programs are more effective for achieving long lasting, schoolwide objectives.

Despite the fact that comprehensive programs are the best researched and have the most far-reaching success, small cadre peer mediation programs tend to be the most frequent type of program implemented. These programs are appealing because they involve students in actively improving school environments, but also because they are cheaper and easier to implement.

Small peer mediation programs are beneficial to some extent, but the professional literature suggests that when they are implemented on a small scale, their benefits shrink as well. This leaves educators who value conflict resolution education in a quandary. On the one hand, no matter how successful comprehensive programs are proven to be they are of little use to schools if they are not feasible. On the other hand, conducting any program at all takes time and effort, and implementing an unsuccessful program can cause burnout, resentment, and mistrust.

This study focuses on practitioner assessment of some of the common research findings about what makes peer mediation programs successful. It investigates how five coordinators of middle school peer mediation programs estimate the importance of the recommendations made in the literature based on their experience. Looking at what they find important and effective about their programs and what they find important to the success of programs generally can offer preliminary ideas about how to create programs that are both realistic and capable of bringing the greatest benefits to schools.

LITERATURE REVIEW

Conflict resolution in schools is not a recent idea, but it was only in the past decade that it began to receive the serious attention of federal agencies such as the Department of Justice and the Department of Education (Bodine and Crawford, 1998). In the late 1960s and throughout the 1970s educators concerned with social justice began applying principles of cooperative conflict resolution in the classroom (Pilchard, 2000). Pioneer programs in the field, such as Children's Creative Response to Conflict (CCRC) and Teaching Students to Be Peacemakers Program (TSP), brought ideas of nonviolence and mutual understanding to public schools in the early 1970s (Johnson and Johnson, 1996). In the early 1980s, other pioneering organizations such as Educators for Social Responsibility (ESR) and the Peace Education Foundation (PEF) introduced broader curricula for training students and teachers to approach personal as well as community conflicts with constructive, nonviolent strategies (Bodine and Crawford, 1998). The New Mexico Center for Dispute Resolution (NMCDR) and the Community Board Program (CBP) were both founded in the mid-1980s and did a great deal to advance the development of peer mediation programs in schools (Bodine and Crawford, 1998).

In the early 1990s, new studies on school and youth violence revealed startling statistics. The National League of Cities reported that between 1990 and 1994, 33 percent of member cities had a significant increase in school violence (a student killed or seriously injured), and in 1993-1994, school violence increased 55 percent in large cities and 41 percent in cities of 100,000 or more (Stop the Violence, 1994). From 1984 to 1994, the homicide rate for adolescents doubled (Elliot, Hamburg, and Williams, 1998) and in 1992 homicide was identified as the third leading cause of death for children 10 to 14 years old (Fingerhut, 1992). Violence prevention suddenly became a national priority in education (Bodine and Crawford, 1998). At the same time that some schools hired security guards, installed metal detectors, and began to implement stricter disciplinary practices, others turned to conflict resolution education as a primary prevention strategy. When federal funds were made available to initiate more conflict resolution training for educators, the field was in a position to blossom, and, indeed, it has. The National Association for Mediation in Education (NAME)[1] estimated that there were approximately 50 school-based conflict resolution programs in 1984, the year of the organization's inception (Girard, 1995). By 1992 there were approximately 2,000 programs in U.S. public schools, and by 1994 somewhere between 5,000 and 8,000 (Johnson and Johnson, 1996). In 1998, the National Institute for Dispute Resolution (NIDR) estimated that there were 8,500 programs in schools, which would be approximately 10 percent of public schools in the United States (Bodine and Crawford, 1998). In 2000, the Conflict Resolution Education Network (CREnet) estimated that number at 10 to 15 percent (Pilchard, 2000).

Among conflict resolution programs peer mediation is the most popular (Baker et al., 2000; Cohen, 2001; Coleman and Deutsch, 2000; Pilchard, 2000). Peer mediation programs train the whole student body or a select group of students in mediation, a structured problem-solving process that aids disputants in working toward a mutually satisfactory agreement to a conflict. Trained students then mediate for their peers as conflicts arise in the classroom, playground, or overall school environment. Research on the benefits that have been associated with peer mediation programs tends to focus first, on the positive effects programs have on student mediators and second, on schoolwide benefits.

According to Schrumpf, Crawford, and Bodine (1997) the experience of being a mediator fosters student self-esteem, self-discipline, and leadership ability. The experience of being a mediator has also been correlated with increases in peer status, responsible behavior, academic improvement, and better resolution of problems at school and at home (Gentry and Benenson, 1993; Lane and McWhirter, 1992; Singh, 1995; Thompson, 1996). Peer mediators are thought to develop positive problem-solving and communication skills as well as the ability to transfer the use of these skills to their relationships at home and in the community (Gentry and Benenson, 1993; Johnson et al., 1995; Lane and McWhirter, 1992; Singh, 1995). In their 1996 review of the research, Johnson and Johnson conclude from many different studies on the subject that "the ability to resolve conflicts constructively tends to increase psychological health, self-esteem, self-regulation, and resilience" (p. 490).

At the schoolwide level there is evidence that mediation programs can reduce disciplinary referrals, detentions, and suspensions (Coleman and Deutsch, 2000; Daunic et al., 2000; T. S. Jones, 1998; Schrumpf, Crawford, and Bodine, 1997) and improve student and teacher perceptions of the school climate (Crary, 1992; T. S. Jones, 1998; Singh, 1995). Although school climate is a construct that has tended to be inconsistently defined and measured in the literature (Jones, Johnson, and Lieber, 2000), many researchers have asserted that providing students with a framework and a venue for solving conflicts at school can make classrooms more productive and peaceful (Benson and Benson, 1993; Deutsch, 1994).

Most of the schoolwide benefits associated with peer mediation are also associated with conflict resolution education in general (Johnson and Johnson, 1996). Peer mediation's dramatic popularity, however, is probably associated with a few of its more unique qualities. First, and arguably most significant, peer mediation creates a context in which students can practice and appreciate their new skills while improving school atmosphere. As Cohen (2001) states, "peer mediation encourages students to apply conflict resolution skills when it matters most—when they are in conflict." If students do not have the opportunity to practice the skills they are learning, they are far less likely to be able to use them in the heat of the moment (Cohen, 2001; Johnson and Johnson, 1996; Singh, 1995). Peer mediation programs are also popular because, depending on how they are structured, they can be the easiest and least expensive programs to implement (Coleman and Deutsch, 2000).

There are different ways of structuring peer mediation programs. While some programs are offered to students on a schoolwide basis—all students learn and practice conflict resolution and serve the school as mediators—other programs train only 20 to 30 students to mediate for the school. Johnson and Johnson (1995) distinguished between the former, "schoolwide," and the latter, "cadre programs." Some cadre programs are accompanied by schoolwide curricula that teach principles and skills of conflict resolution at each grade level, but many exist as the only form of conflict resolution education in the school. Thus, there are significant differences in the degree of comprehensiveness among peer mediation programs (Johnson and Johnson, 1996; Schrumpf, Crawford, and Bodine, 1997). Schoolwide conflict resolution curricula accompanied by schoolwide peer mediation programs would be the most comprehensive. Schoolwide conflict resolution curricula accompanied by a cadre peer mediation program would be somewhat less comprehensive, and cadre programs that exist without other forms of conflict resolution education would not be comprehensive at all. Even within these categories differences in comprehensiveness are associated with such things as staff training, time devoted to curricula, community involvement, and the extent to which conflict resolution principles guide the general operation of the school.

The effectiveness of various kinds of conflict resolution programs, especially peer mediation, was questioned soon after such programs became popular. Webster (1993) has been cited widely for questioning the broad implementation of programs that had yet to be evaluated (Johnson and Johnson, 1996; Sandy, Bailey, and Sloane-Akwana, 2000). Johnson and Johnson (1996) agreed that the anecdotal claims of conflict resolution and peer mediation's effectiveness had to be grounded with empirical and methodologically sound research to ensure their long-term viability. Trends come and go in education. Unless new programs can demonstrate dramatic benefits to schools and particularly an increase in student achievement, they tend to fall by the wayside (Gerber, 1999; Johnson and Johnson, 1996, 2001). Although it is notoriously difficult to conduct highly controlled research in school settings, many in the field have noted that evaluation studies are crucial to the development and maintenance of effective programs (Carruthers, Sweeney, et al., 1996; Johnson and Johnson, 1996; Kmitta, 2000). Over the past decade, scholars and educators have contributed to a growing body of research primarily documenting effectiveness of programs, overall benefits of programs, as well as best practices and elements of successful programs. Although the literature is far from comprehensive and exhibits a broad range of thoroughness and quality, there is also widespread agreement on certain topics.

The most vocal professionals in the field have consistently equated best practices with those that are most comprehensive. Johnson and Johnson's Teaching Students to Be Peacemakers Program (TSP), Bodine and Crawford's "peaceable schools," and Morton Deutsch's "systems approach" all recommend making conflict resolution principles and practices integral to classroom interactions and school culture in general. Many arguments for comprehensive programs are well documented in the research conducted over the past ten years.

First of all, many researchers have agreed that to be most effective peer mediation programs need to be accompanied by a substantial and developmentally appropriate conflict resolution curriculum (Crawford and Bodine, 2001; Coleman and Deutsch, 2000; Fitzell, 1997; Johnson and Johnson, 1995; P. Jones, 1998; Schrumpf, Crawford, and Bodine, 1997; Singh 1995). Carruthers, Carruthers, et al. (1996) asserted that while peer mediation programs have attracted nationwide attention, conflict resolution curricula "have the greater potential to effect lasting change in students' and staff members' knowledge, attitudes and behaviors" (p. 368). Johnson and Johnson (1995) contrast conflict resolution projects with violence prevention projects. If a program targets certain behaviors without providing a cooperative context and an understanding and appreciation for conflict in all students and staff members, it sets itself up for failure.

Second, there is widespread agreement that it is important for all students to have an opportunity to act as mediators. Even when cadre peer mediation programs exist alongside schoolwide conflict resolution training, many students miss the important practice and service opportunities that push their internalization and appreciation of mediation skills to another level. When all students are given the training and opportunity to apply their skills at school, chances are much higher that they will be able to use them in other life contexts. Singh (1995) and Johnson and Johnson (1996) have emphasized the extent to which students need to overlearn skills to be able to use them in the heat of the moment. This can be most easily achieved through a formal practice of mediation, in which students are using their skills to help others in real-life situations. Johnson and Johnson (1995) have argued that a few peer mediators with limited training are not likely to decrease the severity and frequency of conflicts in a school. They have strongly encouraged schools to allow all students to be trained in mediation and to apply their skills as school mediators. Casella (2000) has argued that if it is the mediation training and not having a conflict mediated that leads to decreased incidences of violence, the most effective strategy for violence prevention would be to train all students.

In contrast, the justification for cadre-type programs is that both the experience of being a mediator as well as the experience of going through mediation have positive and lasting effects that can spread throughout the school and community (Crary, 1992). Although they agreed with Johnson and Johnson (1996) that an ideal program would involve all students acting as mediators, Lupton-Smith et al. (1996) recognized the contributions that smaller programs make and asserted that involving all students would only be possible in a "very mature program." The Comprehensive Peer Mediation Evaluation Project (CPMEP) investigated the different effects of cadre and whole-school programs on students (T. Jones, 1998). Although the study confirmed other research indicating that schoolwide programs are more effective for achieving maximum benefits to the school, it also showed that cadre programs can result in better outcomes for individuals (T. Jones, 1998).

Some of the other traits associated with successful programs are strong administrator leadership, whole-staff training, and behavior management practice based on conflict resolution theories. Administrator leadership is central to being able to overcome any attitudinal or structural resistance to a new school program such as peer mediation (Cohen, 2001). Daunic et al. (2000) described the pressure on many school administrators to develop both antiviolence programs and constant academic improvements in their schools. Administrators need to be committed and responsible to the ideas behind conflict resolution and peer mediation programs by investigating the effort and resources necessary to creating a truly effective program. In general, the comprehensive efforts suggested for making programs most successful are highly dependent on strong administrator leadership (Cohen, 2001; Girard, 1995; P. Jones, 1998; Lupton-Smith et al., 1996; Pilchard, 2000; Schrumpf, Crawford, and Bodine, 1997; Singh, 1995).

In a schoolwide program with more comprehensive goals, teacher training becomes nearly as important as student training: "Without sufficient training to address teachers' own behavior, there is the danger that the adults' words will not match their actions" (Girard, 1995, p. 2). Because modeling is such a powerful teaching tool, it is very important that teachers do model positive conflict negotiation and mediation skills (Bodine, Crawford, and Schrumpf, 1994; Deutsch and Raider, 2000; Singh, 1995). Coleman and Deutsch (2000) have explained that training all school staff

> can help institutionalize the changes through adult modeling of the attitudes and behaviors desired for the students; demonstrates the value of such approaches; and encourages the development of new language, norms, and expectations around conflict and conflict management throughout the school community. (p. 2)

In their "systems approach" they have also encouraged broader community training and recruiting parents, caregivers, clergy, local police, and other community members to take part in planning school efforts.

Teacher training can help overcome any skepticism and resistance that teachers may experience when faced with a new and demanding project (Bell et al., 2000). Singh (1995) quotes Cameron and Depuis (1991) that "it takes students (an estimated) two years to accept peer mediation as a dispute resolution process and teachers five years" (p. 509). Although teacher "buy-in" is not always easy to achieve (P. Jones, 1998), it is crucial to the success of a program for logistical as well as pedagogical reasons.

Johnson and Johnson (1995) have written extensively on the importance of establishing a cooperative context in which to learn and practice conflict resolution. They contrast a cooperative learning environment, in which students have a stake in maintaining a positive relationship with others, with a competitive environment, in which students strive to outdo their opponents. In Johnson and Johnson's Teaching Students to Be Peacemakers Program (TSP), trainers instruct teachers, administrators, and students on how to establish a cooperative environment (Fitch and Marshall, 1999). Johnson and Johnson (1995) have also looked at more academic applications of conflict resolution such as creative controversy, an assignment in which pairs of students take turns exploring and debating an issue from different perspectives. In addition to giving students rich experience in skills fundamental to mediation and negotiation such as perspective taking, creative controversy has also resulted in increases in student achievement, critical thinking, higher-level reasoning, and intrinsic motivation (Johnson and Johnson, 1979).

Research has begun to look at what kind of teacher training is most efficient and effective. According to Kmitta et al. (2000), training is most effective when it is voluntary and when it gives at least as much time to teaching teachers how to mediate their own conflicts as to teaching teachers how to train students in mediation.

Although the importance of schoolwide teacher training is well documented, small cadre programs are often coordinated by an individual person who may or may not have gone through training himself or herself. School counselors have the flexibility to train and monitor student mediators during the school day, and many tend to integrate proactive, student-centered, skill-building interventions such as peer mediation into their overall guidance plans (Humphries, 1999; Thompson, 1996). For these reasons, school counselors are often asked to implement programs or will initiate them on their own.

If a school seeks to promote mediation and negotiation skills among students, not only does it need to train teachers in these skills, but also to replace school and classroom behavior management practices based on punishment with practices that reflect principles of conflict resolution. Crawford and Bodine (2001) emphasized the difference between external and internal methods of controlling behavior. External methods are coercive and inflict punishment on students who are caught behaving in an undesirable way. Internal methods encourage responsible behavior in students by encouraging them to evaluate the logical consequences of their behavior. This presupposes a cooperative context in which all students have something to gain by participating positively in a group (Bodine, Crawford, and Schrumpf, 1994). A basic assumption of the Teaching Students to Be Peacemakers Program is that the "norms, values, and culture of a school should promote and support the use of the negotiation and mediation procedures" (Johnson and Johnson, 2001, p. 6). This implies that the same dispute resolution procedures are used when teachers and students have conflicts as when conflicts arise between students.

Paul Jones (1998, p. 179) recommends that teachers and administrators replace "discipline based on rewards and punishments with teaching values." Punishment-based discipline gives children the message that they can do whatever they like as long as they are not caught. If school rules are based on values, however, following the rules means doing one's part because he or she cares about others and maintaining relationships with them.

In 2000 CREnet organized a research symposium sponsored by the United States Department of Education. Educators, practitioners, and researchers were invited to come together to examine the existing research, to identify current research needs, and to develop a publication that would make this information accessible to the field (Jones and Kmitta, 2000). The result was a collection of chapters titled *Does It Work? The Case for Conflict Resolution Education in Our Nation's Schools*. It is obvious from the title that the collection advocates for conflict resolution education and concludes that it does, indeed, "work." It emphasizes comprehensive programming and devotes a whole chapter to institutionalization of programming. In the conclusion of the document Kmitta observes: "Throughout this volume, educators, researchers, and practitioners emphasize the futility of research if we cannot find a way to make conflict resolution education a more permanent component of the educational institution" (p. 146). In other words, the research can show what a successful conflict resolution program looks like. It can also describe the preconditions for a successful program: time, money, support, enthusiasm, ongoing, quality training, and long-term commitment. As long as these preconditions are not available to most schools on a consistent basis, putting research into practice is difficult if not entirely unrealistic.

The *Does It Work?* collection is significant because it looks to the experienced voices of practitioners without compromising the vision of well-considered, well-funded research projects. It does not solve the dilemma of how to make comprehensive programs accessible to more schools but at least it recognizes the issue. More research could be done, however, to look at what small-scale programs are able to achieve and how they could be implemented to maximize their success and to increase their longevity in schools that are not yet prepared to implement comprehensive programs.

METHOD

Participant Recruitment

The original proposal for this study involved interviewing six middle school counselors who had been coordinators of their schools' peer mediation programs for at least two years. Because the study is a qualitative one, descriptive and exploratory in nature, it was important to find participants who were able and willing to give detailed information about their schools' programs and about their own experiences with and perspectives on peer mediation programs. Diversity in schools represented as well as diversity in participant background were also priorities in selection. In order to recruit a diverse group of participants, the search was focused on middle schools in a three-county area of North Carolina, each county having a very distinct school system facing different challenges and having access to different resources.

As it turned out, recruitment was difficult. In the two smaller counties, all middle schools were called to find out if they currently had a peer mediation program. In one county, one program that had existed had been abandoned and two out of three existing programs were brand new. In another county, three out of the four programs listed on the county's Web site no longer existed, although a new unlisted program had just begun. A senior guidance director in the largest county gave the researcher a list of counselors who included peer mediation in their yearly developmental guidance programs. From this list it appeared that nine middle schools in the county had current programs. Upon contacting each counselor, it turned out that four of the programs no longer existed and one program was coordinated by a social studies teacher. That left four programs in the county coordinated by middle school counselors. Two counselors felt too overwhelmed in the last months of the school year to participate in the study.

This left a total of four participants in the three-county area who had been coordinating programs for at least two years. Although she had only been coordinating her program for one year, an additional counselor was interviewed to add another perspective. This recruitment process was informative in and of itself as it demonstrated how quickly programs seem to come in and out of existence.

The five counselors who became the study sample were a relatively diverse group. Although all five were women, they differed in age, experience, ethnic background, as well as school and program conditions.

Participants and Their Programs

Dana

Dana is an Anglo-American woman in her mid-thirties. She has been a school counselor for six years and has been at her current school for four years. She has coordinated two peer mediation programs for a total of five and a half years. Dana was exposed to conflict resolution education through a national conference sponsored by SPIDR and CREnet. She has also attended several training workshops.

Dana's school, Preston Middle School, is located in a small university town, which is well known for the quality of its schools. Her school of 804 students has a student-teacher ratio of 13.2 to 1, three school counselors, and 15 percent of students enrolled in the Free and Reduced Lunch program. The student body is roughly 66 percent Anglo American, 17 percent African American, 14 percent Asian American, and 2 percent Latino.

Dana's program is four years old. Several years before Dana began at Preston, the school district required that conflict resolution be taught in its schools. Preston started a peer mediation program, but it did not work well and was abandoned. When Dana came to the school, she worked hard to sell the program to the teachers and administration. Today the principal and teachers are generally very supportive. There are 13 trained staff members on the mediation team, including Dana. Thirty student mediators represent the school each year and mediate roughly 50 conflicts during that time. Mediators are selected by peer and teacher recommendation and once selected are allowed to continue as mediators throughout the rest of their years at the school. Each year, there is one full day of training (six hours) and minicourses designed for more intensive practice of specific skills. The program offers basic training for new mediators and advanced training for returning mediators. Mediators fundraise each year for special events. One year they attended the National Peacemakers Conference in Arizona. In 2001 they visited a mediation team in Washington, DC, to compare notes and learn from other mediators. This year the team from DC is coming to visit them. Dana says the program's main objectives are to "teach kids to actively listen and to help others come up with their own answers." The program is evaluated by evidence that it is commonly used but not always by the same students. If the same referrals are made over and over again, that would be a sign that mediation was not working. In addition to this, Dana surveys her returning mediators each year to find out what they think is effective or not effective about the program.

Adele

Adele is an African-American woman in her mid-thirties. She has been a school counselor for nine years and has been at Kingsbridge Middle School for seven years. When the peer mediation program began at her school six years ago, the school had designated drop-out prevention money for a staff member to act as a program coordinator. The next year that position was cut and Adele took over the program. She had been involved with a program at her first job as an elementary school counselor, but did not have any formal training in conflict resolution education or mediation.

Kingsbridge is an International Baccalaureate magnet school in a midsize city. The school of 412 students has a student-teacher ratio of 11.8 to 1 and has only one school counselor. Twenty-eight percent of students receive free or reduced lunch. The student body is roughly 71 percent African American, 25 percent Anglo American, 2 percent Asian American, and 2 percent Latino.

Adele's program has a total of 30 mediators each year. New mediators are trained when former mediators leave the school or choose to stop mediating. Each year Adele makes an announcement that anyone interested in becoming a mediator should pick up an application form in her office. She interviews all students who hand in applications. She screens applicants for interest and responsibility level and tries to select a diverse group of students. Mediators receive one day of training from veteran high school mediators. Adele has no one to help her with the program, which often means asking her students to take on more responsibility. Students mediate about 30 conflicts a year. Their biggest complaint is that they do not have more cases to mediate. Adele says that though the principal and faculty are extremely supportive, they are not very involved with the program. She is not sure that the principal really understands what the program is all about even though the principal likes the idea of having it. The teachers at Kingsbridge are very supportive, but they do not have to make any sacrifices for the program, especially since there are so few mediations that happen each year. Adele's main objectives for the program have been keeping it going, and giving her students the opportunity to develop and practice their leadership skills. The program is evaluated based on what students have to say about it: If they say it works, then it does. If they leave a session and the conflict is solved, that is success.

Sue

Sue is an Anglo-American woman in her early 50s. She has been a school counselor for 20 years and has worked at Erhart Middle School for 18 years. She has been working with the peer mediation program at her school for almost ten years and has been coordinating it for the past four or five years. She began her career as an advancement counselor working with at-risk students in the early 1980s.

Erhart Middle School is located in a wealthy suburban town near a large city. Some of its students are bussed in from housing projects in the city. It has approximately 1,000 students, one counselor for each grade level, and a student-teacher ratio of 14 to 1. The student body is 67 percent Anglo American, 22 percent African American, 6 percent Latino, and 5 percent Asian American; 27 percent of students receive free or reduced lunch.

In the early 1990s her school system began pushing conflict resolution and peer mediation programs throughout the district. They offered a three-day training, which Sue attended. A year or two later, the principal created a position which would allow one staff member three periods a day to devote to a peer mediation program in the school. Although the rest of the faculty was not formally trained, they did receive substantial staff development about the program and about conflict resolution in general. Over the years they have been very supportive. Twenty students participate in the program as mediators each year, and in that time they mediate roughly 90 conflicts. New mediators are generally recruited from the sixth grade. Each year new and returning mediators receive a full day of training (six hours) and then practice skills during the half hour after lunch, student ER time (enrichment and remediation). Sue coordinates the program with help from the school resource officer and the ISS (In-School Suspension) teacher. Sue says the main objective of the program is "to have the kids solve their own conflicts . . . instead of going to ISS." She evaluates the program's success by monitoring how many students are using the program and what kinds of conflicts are happening in the school. They look to see that fewer students are getting into the serious conflicts that can turn into disciplinary issues.

Libby

Libby is a 30-year-old Anglo-American woman. She began her career as a school counselor at Lansing Middle School three and a half years ago. Before that, during her internship, she worked closely with a middle school counselor in the same county who coordinated a peer mediation program. She learned a lot from that experience and thought her school could benefit significantly from such a program.

Lansing Middle is located in an inner-city neighborhood. It has about 900 students and three counselors. The student-teacher ratio is 13.2 to 1, and 65 percent of its students receive free and reduced lunch. The student body is roughly 57 percent Anglo American, 29 percent African American, 13 percent Asian American, and 1 percent Latino.

Libby started the program at Lansing three years ago. Each year she has worked hard to win the support and enthusiasm of the school's administrators and teachers, and each year she has, indeed, won over more of the school faculty. More teachers refer more conflicts each year. When she began the program, she trained 12 sixth graders to be mediators for the sixth grade. The next year she kept on the mediators from the previous year who were now seventh graders and trained 12 new sixth graders. This past year was the first year of the program during which mediators were trained in all three grades. To become mediators, students have to submit two referrals from peers and two referrals from teachers, fill out an application, have parent permission, and maintain an average of C or above. Students also have to go through Libby's classroom guidance session on conflict resolution. Once selected, students go through a two-day (12-hour) training session and then practice skills. Libby monitors their mediations until they have mastered the process and the basic skills (eye contact, communication, listening, etc.). She says her students mediate roughly three conflicts a week. Her program's main objectives are to teach leadership skills and conflict resolution skills to the mediators and to help students establish positive relationships with peers throughout the school. In addition to evaluating mediator skills, she sends out a yearly evaluation form to the staff to get their feedback on the program.

Cathy

Cathy is an Anglo-American woman in her mid-twenties, who has been a school counselor for two years at Staunton Middle School. This was her first year coordinating a peer mediation program and she had no prior experience or training in mediation.

Staunton is in a rural area, but is not far from two midsize cities as well as a small town, which serves as the county seat. It has 712 students, a student-teacher ratio of 14 to 1, and two school counselors. Twenty-seven percent of students receive free or reduced lunch. The student body is approximately 69 percent Anglo American, 28 percent African American, 2 percent Latino, and 1 percent Asian American.

Cathy was excited about starting a peer mediation program this year. Although she had read about peer mediation programs, she did not have prior experience with mediation herself. The school had had a program in the past that was largely supported by the county dispute settlement center. Cathy turned to the dispute settlement center again when looking to rekindle the project. She could not come up with all the money that the center had originally asked for, but had been awarded a few hundred dollars in school system grant money. The center agreed to work with the school for this amount of money. The center's school coordinator trained 12 students once a week for one hour from August till December. In January, the students were supposed to begin mediating, but the whole schedule for the school changed, and the "acceleration" time on Fridays during which the students were going to mediate was eliminated. It took a while for teachers to agree to have students taken out of their classes for mediation, but there was no other way for students to mediate. This year Cathy's students did 20 mediations. She said that the program's main objectives were to: introduce students to options for solving problems, teach communication skills, generate alternatives to fighting, and give mediators a solid foundation from which to understand the purpose of mediation and conflict resolution. This year the struggle to keep the program going was so overwhelming that Cathy and her co-worker did not have time to follow any evaluation procedure.

Instrument

A questionnaire was designed to elicit general background information regarding each school's demographics, the age and size of the program, funding, program goals and design, student and staff training, evaluation procedures, and participant/counselor background (see Appendix A). In addition to this, a semistructured interview (see Appendix B) was designed to provoke counselors' practical ideas and opinions regarding traits of programs that are highly recommended in the professional literature. First, it asked participants to comment on five potential benefits of peer mediation programs commonly found in the research, namely, peer mediation's ability to contribute to

1. the prevention of school violence,
2. the reduction of bullying and teasing,
3. improvement of student self-esteem,
4. improvement in academic achievement, and
5. improvement in school and classroom atmosphere.

Second, it asked participants to estimate the importance of each of five traits that have been described as central to a successful program in the research, namely:

1. strong administrator leadership,
2. teacher/staff/administrator training,
3. behavior management systems in accordance with conflict resolution theory,
4. schoolwide conflict resolution curriculum, and
5. practice opportunities for all students.

Procedure

Data Collection

Counselors were contacted via telephone and e-mail to establish their appropriateness for the study, their willingness to participate in it, and finally a date for an interview. At the beginning of the interview with each participant, the informed consent form was reviewed (see Appendix C). In particular, the general premise of the study, procedure, confidentiality, and follow-up contact information were explained. Aware that in the final section of the interview they would be asked to compare their own programs to what might be considered an "ideal program," the researcher explained that the purpose of the interview was to find out what was most important to a program in her experience, and that what was happening in the program was more important for the study than what was not happening. Once the participant signed the consent form, the tape recorder was turned on and the remainder of the meeting was recorded.

Before beginning with the semistructured interview, the participant completed the questionnaire, orally or in writing. After this was completed, the interview began. As previously explained, the interview was designed to provoke counselors to discuss their experiences and opinions in relation to common findings in the professional literature first, regarding benefits of programs, and second, regarding traits important to successful programs.

Data Analysis

Each interview was partially transcribed. Names of participants and their schools were changed to protect confidentiality and anonymity. The main themes of each interview were summarized based on the tape recording and transcriptions. These were then sent electronically to each participant in order to verify that they had been understood accurately. At the same time, each interview was analyzed and coded with particular attention to (1) how each supported, modified, or negated common findings in the literature, and (2) how each differed from or agreed with the other interviews. The coding process began with participants' responses to the specific questions contained on the interview instrument, which was fairly specific (e.g., to what extent do you think peer mediation programs contribute to the prevention of school violence?). Similar responses to questions were written up in general terms and more detailed or unique responses were highlighted as quotations or paraphrases. After the interviews had been coded in light of the original questions, they were analyzed again for themes that were stressed very strongly by a participant or stressed by more than one participant.

Audit Process

To confirm that the results of the study were credible and not due to researcher bias, an auditor was asked to review the informed consent forms that each participant had signed, the questionnaires that the participants had filled out, and the recorded interview material on tape and as transcriptions. The auditor determined that the results did come from the data and that any inferences made were logical and not constructions of researcher bias (see Appendix D).

RESULTS

Benefits of Peer Mediation Programs

Questions 1 and 2 of the survey asked the counselors (a) to what extent they believed that peer mediation programs were effective strategies for preventing school violence, decreasing bullying and teasing, improving school and classroom atmosphere, improving individual students' academic performance, and improving student self-esteem, and (b) to what extent they believed their programs accomplished these goals.

Cathy did not discuss each individual item but rather all five together. She felt strongly that peer mediation programs should be able to make a positive impact on all of these points and explained that it was her conviction about this that inspired her to initiate a program for her school. Because of the difficulties she had acquiring the support she needed to implement the program in a more successful way, her mediators did very few mediations this year. For this reason, she did not think that her program could lay claim to having had much of an impact on anything besides the lives of the mediators who went through the training. The four other participants' responses are presented as follows.

Prevents School Violence and Decreases Bullying and Teasing

Dana, Adele, Sue, and Libby agreed that peer mediation programs had a positive impact on both preventing school violence and decreasing bullying and teasing. Each of them emphasized that peer mediation taught kids to "talk, not fight," and that this kept bullying and teasing from escalating into something more violent. Libby said that most of her school's referrals came from bullying and teasing issues and that she felt peer mediation was an effective strategy for addressing these issues. She said she was not sure if this particular opportunity, which helped some kids, had a schoolwide impact. That was her one reservation about saying that programs, including her own, could prevent school violence.

Sue and Dana made distinctions between the majority of the students who go through mediation and exceptionally aggressive students. Sue said, "Most of the mediation sessions I don't really consider violent. Most of them are hurt feelings and things like that. . . . If a student is your really aggressive-type child, I don't know if it affects that, but it does help basic fighting." Dana explained that peer mediation can be a good way to deal with bullies: "You can teach them too, to talk, not fight." But she also made the point that the success of this strategy depends on the bullier: "Usually bullies are dealing with deeper self-esteem issues or problems at home. The aggression that comes from more personal issues aren't really addressed by peer mediation."

Adele emphasized that bullying and teasing are "just natural in a middle school environment." She said she would be worried about her students if they didn't tease one another. At the same time, though, people's feelings do get hurt, and if you play around with someone on the wrong day fights often ensue. "That's where peer mediation comes in and prevents what could happen if there wasn't a place to deal with these things."

Improves School and Classroom Atmosphere

Three of the four counselors felt strongly that their programs did contribute to the improvement of school and classroom atmosphere. Dana explained that "if you teach people to work out their conflicts productively, that's going to make things better in the classroom." She believed that her program did, indeed, benefit the school in this way. Libby also made a strong statement: "I definitely think [our program] has improved school and classroom atmosphere." She went on to explain what a large role race and diversity issues seemed to play in students' lives at school. She believes her peer mediation program has helped many students learn to respect one another's differences.

Adele described peer mediation as a strategy for lowering the general stress level of the atmosphere in the classroom and in the school in general. "Students know they can depend on something to help them get through a situation they're dealing with at school; there's support for them. And I think that makes them feel their atmosphere is safer . . . kids have a lot of stress . . . it's just not the stress we have, like bills and car problems, that kind of thing. They have stress and if we can alleviate some of their stress, it is always going to improve classroom atmosphere."

Improves Individual Students' Academic Performance

Libby and Sue did not see any correlation between peer mediation programs and student academic performance. Dana and Adele spoke solely about mediators. They explained that their mediators were inspired to work harder in school because they had to get decent grades to stay in the program. Although both counselors described the importance of keeping a diversity of students on the mediation team, "not just straight-A students," their programs also insist on mediators being responsible about making up any work they miss in the classroom and have consequences for grades slipping below C. In Dana's program, students are on probation from mediation for Ds and are dismissed from the program for Fs. In Adele's and Libby's programs, students must maintain at least a C average.

Improves Student Self-Esteem

All counselors stressed that the program did not improve student self-esteem on a schoolwide basis, but did have a very positive effect on the mediators' self-esteem. Dana discussed the powerful effects of being selected to be a mediator in the first place: "It is an honor to say that you were picked by your teachers and fellow classmates . . . to know 'I was chosen for my skills and my honesty.'" She also described how mediators begin to use their new skills in their own conflicts with friends and at home. She said that she hears funny stories from parents about how her students will communicate with them in new ways. Sometimes their efforts are successful and sometimes they are not. "But when it does work, it affects their self-esteem."

Adele's emphasis was on the social aspect of peer mediation and on being a role model to other students: "Because they are part of something that is obviously going to boost their self-esteem." In addition, having the opportunity to show their leadership skills and be recognized by their peers improves the way mediators feel about themselves.

Similarly, Sue described the experience of being a peer mediator as one that "enhances [mediators'] self-esteem because they take ownership of problems" happening at their school. They have a role that is valued and a skill to contribute. This makes them feel different about who they are at school.

Most Significant Result of Program

When asked about the most significant result of their programs, three of the participants focused on how the program helped mediators. Adele and Sue focused on the leadership skills that the mediators develop and how it helped students blossom, even those who were not otherwise excelling in school. "If we don't do anything else but touch the lives of a few mediators, that is worthwhile," Sue explained. Because of the logistical difficulties her program faced this year, Cathy did not think that her program was able to influence the whole student body. "Hopefully the kids learned some new strategies for solving conflicts for themselves personally . . . I don't think enough kids in the student body saw this as an option for resolving their conflicts. So I think it was more of a personal gain for the mediators than for the other students or teachers."

Dana was the only participant who focused on a more general schoolwide achievement her program has made: creating opportunities for kids to help kids. This in itself represents a shift of focus in schools that is empowering and productive for students as well as teachers.

Wish List: Changes to Program

Questions 4 and 5 asked what the counselors would change about their programs if they could and what they would need to be able to make those changes. All of the counselors wished for more time to be able to give to one aspect of the program or another. Dana has wanted to implement a schoolwide conflict resolution curriculum for years. When asked what she would need to finally be able to do so, she explained: "Time, and that is the piece that always falls through." Sue would like someone to keep records on the program. Ever since her program lost their paid coordinator, no one has had enough time to document the activities of the program. She emphasized that it was lack of money that kept the school from being able to hire someone to focus solely or primarily on the program. Cathy wished to be able to spend more time working consistently with the mediators throughout the year. "We have to drop everything that we're doing to do what the administrators think is important, or the county. There are different things that we have to do for different people, so it is hard to be consistent with the program when all these things factor in." In order to have more time on a more consistent basis Cathy felt that she would need far greater administrator support.

Adele wished for either more time to give to the program or an assistant to help her. "To have more time to do it would mean to cut out some of my duties . . . other duties like testing coordinator, or records, or SAP (Student Assistance Program), or 504s, or registration, or five-year plans, . . . or any of that, you know . . . I could go on and on. Or give me an assistant. Or give me someone else to help. But you know they all have just as much. But, hey, that's education. You do what you can, with what you have." She suggested that inadequate funding was what kept everyone in public education overburdened and this is what would have to change for her to be able to focus more time on the program.

Libby's main desire was to have more faculty involvement with the program. In particular she thought that it would be nice if the seventh-and eighth-grade counselors took responsibility for following up with the seventh- and eighth-grade mediators. As it stands, Libby trains the sixth-grade mediators and does all the work with the experienced mediators as well. "I would need administrator support to encourage people to get involved. We do have a budget for guidance. So we'll have a budget next year for peer mediation. So things are getting better."

Cathy also mentioned a desire to have more training for students, teachers, and counselors, and more resources overall (books, videos, pamphlets, etc.). To have this, she thought she would need more administrator support and money.

Important Traits for Successful Programs

Questions 6 and 7 asked counselors to evaluate the importance of each of five traits to the success of peer mediation programs generally, and to explain how those traits described their own program.

Teacher and Administrator Training

Three of the counselors, Adele, Dana, and Sue, felt that it was important for teachers to be aware of the peer mediation programs at their schools and to have a clear understanding of what they are about. These three did not think that faculty training was necessary to providing this awareness and understanding. Libby felt that training was very important to the success of a program, but if training wasn't possible, it was essential to have teacher awareness and understanding. Cathy felt that teacher and administrator training was essential to a successful program.

Dana stressed the importance of staff "buy in" and described the work she had done to get it. She explained that just before she'd come to her school, the district had said, "Oh, here! Do conflict resolution training with your kids!" The teachers did not know what to do. They started a peer mediation program and it was not working. Dana explained: "Nobody was buying into it. I had started a program in Maryland. I brought the program here. Peer mediation is just a part of conflict resolution. It doesn't work if people don't buy into it. So before I came in and said that we were going to have this program, I did a lot of talking and a lot hype to get people to buy into the idea. Once the staff bought into it, we started the program." In her school, there are 13 trained staff members on the peer mediation team. Not all teachers in the school have been trained, but all teachers, new and returning, are introduced to the program at the beginning of each school year. As some staff leave the mediation team and others join, the number of staff at the school who have been trained grows.

Sue's program has been around the longest of any of the programs in this study. It enjoys support from an administrator who believes it should be an integral part of the school's mission to give students the skills they need to solve conflicts. When the program began nine years ago, teachers learned about it through staff development meetings at the start of the school year. This introduction is no longer made on a yearly basis, which means that while most teachers are very supportive of the program, newer teachers might not even know that it exists. When discussing this, Sue said: "There has been so much turnover, it is probably time to do that [introduction] again."

When asked how important teacher and administrator training was, Adele also stressed that awareness was more important than training, however, her responses over the course of the interview seemed to indicate that she thought that the whole school should share basic principles of conflict resolution. "Teachers must be aware of the program and what it is all about. I mean, how can you be in education if you're not [aware of peer mediation and conflict resolution]. There should be principles that people use in classrooms and all, but I don't really know if that happens."

Libby does a review of her program each year for the teachers at her school. Not only does she explain how it works, but she teaches listening skills and does a workshop on diversity training, which includes material from a conflict resolution curriculum. When she began her program three years ago, she had to work very hard to get support from teachers. "Because they hadn't seen the validity in it, what's good in it, I had to show them," she said. "Some teachers are at about one hundred percent now and there are some that don't really care. But it's getting better."

Cathy had made several requests of the principal to allot a small amount of time and money to include a teacher workshop on conflict resolution and peer mediation on a staff development workday. Although the principal agreed to it, she never followed through. Cathy had hoped that training would help generate support for the peer mediation program, but also help to generate a broader interest in teaching conflict resolution throughout the school.

Opportunities for All Students to Practice As Mediators

Dana, Adele, and Libby felt that it was somewhat important to make the experience of being a mediator available to all students, but it did not seem to be a priority to any of them. Dana said that if it were possible to train all students, then it would be important to give them practice opportunities, but this is not how her program is set up. Adele did not feel that all students would benefit from going through training and practicing as a mediator. "Some students who have a lot of parent involvement might not really need [the skills and experience] as much as others." At Libby's school, all sixth graders are introduced to conflict resolution and are given opportunities to practice mediation and negotiation skills in a quarter-long class. Although she thinks that all students should have conflict resolution training, she does not think that all students need to have the experience of being a mediator.

Sue said that it is very important to have all students in school practice mediation. "I wish we could do it," she said. As at Libby's school, students at her school do get a few opportunities to practice in the context of the violence prevention program, Second Step, but these classroom opportunities are few and do not receive the legitimacy and importance that school mediation does.

Cathy thought that it was very important to allow all students to have the opportunity to serve their school as mediators.

Conflict Resolution Curriculum

All participants agreed on the importance of having a comprehensive conflict resolution curriculum to accompany a peer mediation program. Dana said that it was important, but very difficult to realize this because it demands so much time. Although it has been a wish of hers to implement such a program for many years, "that is always the piece that doesn't get done." In contrast to this, the peer mediation program can exist because it is "doable." Lansing Middle School and Erhart Middle School are in the same school system and both have violence prevention curricula in place. Libby's school uses the Get Real about Violence curriculum and Sue's school uses Second Step. Libby said that a conflict resolution curriculum is essential to the success of a peer mediation program and that her school "sort of" offers this. By this, she meant that Lansing uses a violence prevention program which includes some themes akin to conflict resolution. Sue did not distinguish between Erhart's violence prevention curriculum and a curriculum more specific to conflict resolution.

Administrator Leadership

When asked about the importance of administrator leadership to the success of a peer mediation program, Dana quickly said: "Administrator support [is important], but not necessarily leadership. Having a strong coordinator is what's important." In her case, her administration was relatively supportive, but did not have the expertise and knowledge that Dana already had when she started working at the school as a counselor. Dana had a clear idea of what it took to establish a successful peer mediation program and was proactive about getting support from the whole school staff before implementing the program. "The key is having a coordinator and having support. You have to ask [the staff]: Do you want to do this? If you want to, I will plan it, but I'm not going to do it alone."

All of the other counselors felt that it was very important or essential to have strong administrator leadership in implementing a program. Sue's administrators have been strong advocates of the program from the very beginning. Early on, that meant allotting budget monies for a paid coordinator. Now, that means referring many students to the peer mediation program and supporting projects in general that encourage students to develop good problem-solving skills.

Adele has appreciated her principal's leadership and support during the time she has worked on the program, but said: "She doesn't know what goes on. She just likes the fact that we have it." Her principal's willingness to advocate for the program has helped maintain teacher cooperation and readiness to let students out of class.

Libby has had to work to get her administration to buy in to the program, but each year that has gotten better. "It is easier for them to refer [student issues] to peer mediation than to deal with it themselves. So I don't know if it is out of love of the program, but to get [work] off of their backs. So they're learning to appreciate it." Her work would have been easier if the administrators had taken more interest and responsibility in advocating for the program from the beginning.

Based on her own rough experience this past year, Christie explained: "I think administrator leadership can make or break you. If you don't have the support from the head honcho for anything you're doing, it's hard. If you have their backing then the teachers will accept it." She was continually frustrated that the principal did not follow through on things she said she would do to support the program and that the principal was only supportive of the program insofar as it didn't conflict with what she needed from the counselors on any given day.

Behavior Management in Accordance with Conflict Resolution Theory

Four of the participants said that creating behavior management practices consistent with conflict resolution ideas was very important. The same four also felt that their schools had done this more or less implicitly. Cathy was the only one who felt that her school leaned toward more authoritarian ways of confronting students. She thought that it was important for teachers and administrators to model constructive problem solving and good communication even when they might be angry or frustrated with students.

Other Themes

Following is a brief summary of additional points that participants emphasized in their interviews.

Different schools/different programs. Dana was the only participant who had coordinated more than one program. She was also the only one who had received training by any of the national organizations. She said several times throughout the interview that just as no two schools are alike, no two peer mediation programs can be alike. A program has to be designed in light of a particular school's resources, structure, and needs.

Diversity of mediators. All participants stressed the importance of recruiting the most diverse group of mediators possible. Dana, Cathy, and Libby suggested that this creates more trust and credibility in the program throughout the school and encourages more students to use the program.

Diminishing district support. Sue, Dana, and Adele all mentioned that their programs had been pushed during the mid-1990s and now received less support from their county system. Sue received training that was offered by her school district. The district also came into Erhart to introduce the program to teachers. The principal allotted half of a teacher's position for the coordination of the original peer mediation program at the school. Almost ten years later, teachers no longer receive this introduction from the county and the paid position was eliminated five or six years ago. Dana's school system required Preston Middle School to implement a conflict resolution program in the mid-1990s. Her school tried a peer mediation program, which was abandoned after a short time. When she started the new program four years ago, she was given a budget, which has since been taken away. Adele's program was put into place as part of the county school system's dropout prevention program. This too was discontinued after a few years. It has been up to her alone to keep the program going ever since.

PR/student and teacher buy in. Dana, Sue, and Libby coordinate high-profile peer mediation programs. Sue and her mediators have trained mediators at other middle schools. Libby's mediators have been highlighted on UNC-TV's "Making a Difference." Dana and her mediators attended the National Peacemaking Conference in Arizona and meet each year with a peer delegation of mediators from a school in Washington, DC. All of these events have helped win the programs legitimacy among their schools' staff and student bodies.

Although Sue's school system and the principal at Erhart did a lot to advertise the program before it started, Adele and Libby described the work that they had to do to win "buy in" among their colleagues. They both described this as a process that they initially had to invest a great deal in. As the programs become more established, some of the more resistant faculty come to recognize their benefits when they finally have occasion to experience mediation themselves.

Dana and Sue also work to keep their programs well advertised within the student body. Dana's students wear T-shirts that say "Talking Works" and "Talk and Mediators Listen." Sue's students put together an advertisement for the program that is played on the school television network periodically.

Continuity. Libby and Cathy discussed the problem of turnover at their schools. Libby said that the school counselors at Lansing did not have much respect when she first began working there because they had had a different counselor every year in every grade level for five years. She had to win the trust and respect of the teachers and administrators, which took time. Cathy and the other school counselor at Staunton were planning to leave their jobs at the end of this school year. She described what she was doing to wrap up her program so that the counselors coming in could continue with it if they wanted to. She was concerned that it would be difficult for them: "We'd have a lot to work with if we were going to be here next year. If [the new counselors] choose to do it, they'll be starting from scratch just like we did. That makes it really hard. You have to restart and restart. Never get anywhere."

Expectations and program maturity. Libby's story illustrated the importance of having a long-term perspective. She started her program with 12 mediators in one grade and now has mediators in each grade. She started the program with very little teacher and administrator support, and now feels that most teachers and administrators support the program. Next year she will have a budget. Although she still wished for more help with the program, she also recognized what the program has accomplished so far. Cathy was very discouraged with her first year implementing and coordinating the program at Staunton, but she also recognized that her disappointment might have something to do with lack of experience: "Maybe if someone with more experience had taken this on, they would have had more realistic ideas about what was going to happen. We were all gung ho and thought that it would be great. Maybe if we had had more experience, we would have had more realistic expectations."

DISCUSSION

In the world of conflict resolution education, the question of the 1990s was, "Does it work?" The resounding answer was affirmative but conditional: comprehensive programs with plenty of administrator commitment and teacher training consistently have positive results. But the new concern is how to create successful programs that are feasible in most schools. Although violence prevention continues to be important, high-stakes testing and accountability issues are the new priorities on the national education agenda. School counselors, who might have been asked to be peer mediation coordinators ten years ago, are becoming testing coordinators today. State budget crises are hitting school budgets and cutting dispute settlement centers. Federal cuts threaten school counselor positions that had been created in the 1990s. The current configuration of issues in education makes the competing demands of comprehensiveness and feasibility in peer mediation programs all the more difficult to reconcile.

Although the professional literature tends to push comprehensive programs and criticize what they characterize as "ad hoc," "fix-it" programs that tend to be smaller and less theoretically grounded, these latter programs are designed to operate within the parameters of individual schools' immediate resources. This is certainly a primary reason why they are so widespread, if also perhaps why they can be short-lived. Whatever can be learned about how counselor coordinators are negotiating the tension between ideal conditions for a program and their school's resources might help keep conflict resolution education within the grasp of more schools rather than becoming a passing fad.

Considerations

By analyzing the ways that coordinator perceptions confirm or contradict the research findings about what makes programs successful, this study has generated some general and some specific considerations for anyone starting a new program or maintaining an existing one.

Establishing Goals: How Comprehensive?

Before getting into particular details of program design, it is important to note the discrepancy between the comprehensive programs recommended by the literature and the actual programs that the study participants have coordinated. Comprehensive programs would include developmentally appropriate conflict resolution education at each grade level, teacher and administrator training, a schoolwide peer mediation program, and discipline strategies consistent with principles of conflict resolution. Although there was certainly a range of comprehensibility in the programs represented by this study, none of them could be described as comprehensive programs. Two schools had violence prevention curricula that included a few lessons about conflict resolution, but none of the schools made an explicit effort to integrate thorough conflict resolution curricula into their programming. In the best-case scenarios, teachers and administrators received a lot of education about peer mediation, but it was only at Preston Middle School that a significant number of staff had been trained. All of the programs were cadre programs rather than schoolwide programs.

When evaluating the most significant result of their programs, four of the five coordinators focused on the benefits that the program brought to student mediators rather than to the whole school. Only Dana mentioned a more abstract and general result: "Kids helping kids." This is not to say that the coordinators did not see their programs benefitting the whole school. In fact, with the exception of Cathy, all coordinators thought that their programs improved school and classroom atmosphere and increased nonviolent and productive problem solving within the student body. Dana, Libby, and Sue all described scenarios in which teachers went through mediation with students and became strong advocates of the program. Libby also felt strongly that her program was "crucial, not just for conflict resolution, but for the diversity . . . having understanding and respect for other people." These are significant achievements and they provide important learning opportunities for students and teachers who have contact with the program.

At the same time, long-term advocates of conflict resolution education would argue that some of the most powerful potentialities of conflict resolution education can be overlooked or undervalued when programs do not attempt to change the whole structure of a school. Conflict resolution is an effective strategy for violence prevention because it is proactive and based on clearly defined skills or competencies, but its goals are far greater than preventing physical violence.

Problem-solving strategies such as mediation and negotiation are especially useful for addressing issues of psychological violence that are so common, yet often minimized or dismissed in competitive, punishing school environments (Schrumpf et al., 1997).

Psychological struggles that take place in schools may have consequences that turn out to be as tragic and disastrous as some of the horrific incidences of school violence that have attracted nationwide attention. To illustrate this point, statistics about school violence have actually decreased almost every year since 1994 (Annual Report on School Safety, U.S. Department of Education, 2000). This is certainly a trend deserving of celebration; however, other disturbing facts underscore that students and teachers experience plenty of painful and unresolved conflicts during the school day. First, despite the drop in violent crime, students do not perceive schools as being safer. A poll done by the Justice Policy Institute and the Children's Law Center indicated that seven out of ten Americans believed a shooting was likely to happen in their schools and 62 percent believed that juvenile crime was on the increase. From 1998 to 1999, the percentage of students who felt that their classrooms were safe dropped from 40 to 33 percent. Second, after progress was made in the 1970s and 1980s to reduce high school dropout rates, they continued to be very stable during the 1990s (Department of Education, National Center for Education Statistics). When this finding was released to the media on November 15, 2001, U.S. Secretary of Education Rod Paige commented: "Despite the growing investment in education at all levels, student achievement has lagged . . . the study released today is another indicator that we have not made enough progress in recent years to improve access to quality education and that comprehensive change is needed." Third, it is increasingly difficult to keep new teachers in the field of public education. Today between 30 and 60 percent of new teachers leave the field within the first three years depending on how much training they began their career with (Darling-Hammond, 2000). Classroom management is consistently among the top complaints of teachers today. For many reasons it seems that schools fail to provide the conditions for an increasing number of students and teachers to thrive personally, academically, or professionally.

Can conflict resolution education really hope to make this kind of impact on the day-to-day functioning of the school as it is experienced by all students and teachers? Researchers in the field certainly believe that it can and that it should work toward total school reform, but these broad and far-reaching goals *would* demand a more comprehensive program in terms of extent of training and number of students and faculty involved. Is this what anyone with ambitions for starting a program needs to aspire to?

Long-Term versus Short-Term Goals:
Institutionalization and Maturation

The importance of having a long-term perspective on any project cannot be underestimated, particularly in schools where staff and student turnover is fast and widespread. If there are goals that are worth establishing then they must be backed up by a vision of how they can be achieved over time under varying conditions. Peer mediation programs can be quick to come and go when they rest solely on one person's efforts and do not seek to draw in the participation and enthusiasm of other educators.

Lupton-Smith et al. (1996) described the value of limited peer mediation programs as well as the importance that they develop and mature into more comprehensive programs over time. This seems like a sensible and positive approach to building a program: beginning with what resources are available and working toward a more expanded program while exploring or developing new resources to support it.

Dana, who was the only coordinator who had received training from CREnet, had a good sense of what she needed from the school to make her school's program worthwhile as well as how she would like to see the program develop in the future. She said several times that given the resources, she would institute a full conflict resolution curriculum for each grade level at her school, but there had been school crises that had taken priority over this project as long as she had been at Preston.

Conflict Resolution in the Classroom versus Peer Mediation

All of the participants in the study agreed that having a schoolwide conflict resolution curriculum would be very important to the success of a peer mediation program. The literature also emphasizes the importance of developmentally appropriate conflict resolution curricula that students learn from throughout their whole school experience. If there were a question of putting into place a conflict resolution curriculum or a peer mediation program, it would seem that a conflict resolution curriculum could have a greater impact on the whole school environment because it tends to be more thorough and engages students and teachers in learning and practicing skills together. Peer mediation can be an important extension of such a program whether as a schoolwide program or a cadre program, but neither is a good substitute for one. The problem, of course, is that asking teachers to implement another program with their students is not realistic in most schools. Doing so would require time, money, and schoolwide enthusiasm that few public schools have to spare. Peer mediation, on the other hand, "is doable." It can have powerful effects on the lives of mediators and on other teachers and students.

Cadre Programs versus Schoolwide Programs

It may be desirable to offer peer mediation as a schoolwide program so that all students learn and practice skills themselves, however, this would be highly impractical in many schools without drastic redistribution of time and funding. In addition, cadre programs may be able to have a significant impact on school environments. A small program must be highly creative and consistently visible to be capable of influencing a whole school environment. The administration and faculty must invest in creating a school culture that values mediation skills and fosters respect for student mediators. Finally, mediators must be both diverse and well liked by their peers. Each of the study participants mentioned the importance of selecting mediators who represented different aspects of the student body. This seems essential for building trust and interest in the program throughout the student body.

Becoming Informed

When beginning a program, be aware of other practitioner experiences and research findings. Although it may not be possible or necessary to follow all the recommendations that the professional literature make about how to design a successful program, being familiar with well-researched best practices can give those starting programs a sense of what to expect from their first year with the program and how to solve problems more effectively as they arise. It can also provide a sense of how a program might develop in the future and how to set goals that are realistic and "doable."

National associations are important resources for connecting with other practitioners and for keeping abreast of research recommendations. The Association for Conflict Resolution (ACR) is an excellent source of information as are organizations such as Educators for Social Responsibility (ESR), School Mediation Associates (SMA), the Colorado School Mediation Project (CSMP), the Community Board Program, and the National Center for Conflict Resolution Education (NCCRE). Most of these programs have Web sites and are useful for locating books, videos, and curricular material as well as for finding out about training, grants, and conferences.

Resource Assessment, Planning, and Support

In this study, it was Dana who reiterated several times: "You have to design a program to fit the school you are at. Otherwise it won't work." Schools have vastly different resources at their disposal and vastly different needs that they attempt to address. Doing a formal or informal assessment of needs and resources can help anyone designing a program to focus their initial efforts more efficiently and proactively.

Adele brought up the fact that some students have more to gain from going through intensive mediation training than others. Likewise, in schools where there is more strife and less harmony, a peer mediation or conflict resolution training program might be a higher priority than in more peaceful schools.

School mission and philosophy, population, extent of student and teacher turnover, number of student and support staff, type of schedule, extent of administrator and teacher interest, are just some of the variables that need to be considered in how a program is designed and implemented.

The study largely confirmed the importance of administrator leadership to program success. Surely, the more enthusiastic and informed support that can be stirred throughout the administration and faculty, the better. Administrators have the power to allot time and money for the program and, if they have good rapport with teachers, can do a lot to win teacher support for the program. At the same time, Libby's story in particular also suggests that much can be done with minimal administrator support and that administrators can become more supportive over time as they see the program making important contributions to the school.

In this study it was clear that the schools in which the teachers had the most exposure to and awareness of conflict resolution and peer mediation were also the schools that enjoyed the most support and the least resistance to the program. As Adele emphasized, everyone in public education is overwhelmed. Teachers are often resistant to new projects that might demand extra time or work on their part or that might take students out of their classes. Pushing innovations on teachers before they are convinced that they are worth the time and effort can breed resentment and mistrust of new ideas and projects. Therefore, it is important to assess teacher knowledge and interest in a peer mediation program well before initiating the program and doing whatever possible to draw them in. Dana and Libby emphasized how much work they put into building hype around the program and educating teachers about its structure and goals. Creating a place for, or even requiring, staff involvement from the beginning, as Dana did, removes some of the burden from the coordinator, takes a step toward institutionalizing the program by making it viable even if she were to leave, and adds legitimacy and potency to the program as more adults model the many skills fundamental to mediation and conflict resolution.

Libby's story highlighted findings by Singh (1995) and Paul Jones (1998) that winning support from teachers and administrators takes time and effort. Be prepared for a certain amount of resistance to the project and to create a forum for faculty feedback. Soliciting the opinions and experiences of teachers and administrators on a regular basis gives them an opportunity to voice concerns or complaints that should be addressed, but also gives coordinators opportunities to recognize the support they are gaining even if small and gradual.

The most immediate way to build support for a program may be to train the whole faculty. The teachers at Erhart Middle School received some significant staff development on conflict resolution in the mid-1990s, but no follow-up training has been done. Libby offers a staff development workshop on listening skills and diversity at the beginning of each year. This is the most systematic and extensive training offered to teachers in the schools represented in this study. Several of the participants discussed turning points with teachers who became excited about mediation after working through a conflict referred to the program by a student. The literature recommends that conflict resolution curricula be developmentally appropriate and this is surely important for teachers who are learning new skills as well. They need to learn how to mediate themselves, not simply how to teach students to mediate. If teachers experience success in working through issues that they have with one another or with students through conflict resolution strategies, they will be much more apt to recognize the value in sharing these skills with their students.

When asked to estimate the importance of administrator leadership to peer mediation programs, Dana asserted, "It is not essential if you have a strong coordinator." Her program certainly does. Although the other counselors seemed less willing to assert their own leadership per se, they all mentioned the importance of having a strong and committed coordinator. Indeed, none of these programs would exist without the women who are working hard to keep them going today. Coordinators' convictions that these programs are valuable and worthwhile and their motivation to keep them going despite all that they are required to do can take a program a long way even in difficult circumstances.

Local organizations are a great source of support within a school. Many states still have county dispute settlement centers and many of these have staff who work exclusively on school programs. Although the program at Cathy's school suffered from a lack of internal support, the training that the local center offered the students in the program was excellent. Even when such a center might not be able to work with a school on an ongoing basis, it can often be a valuable source of materials and information.

Juvenile justice programs, teen court, and boys and girls clubs sometimes have grant monies for projects that involve young people in community service or violence prevention efforts. Linking school and community efforts reinforces both and can often be another source of support in the form of money or volunteer time.

Other schools that have active peer mediation programs can be a source of inspiration and ideas for coordinators beginning programs and for students once they are mediating. Dana's staff mediators and student mediators have made contacts nationally and internationally and are better able to evaluate their own work and recognize its importance. Libby and Sue's students have trained other students, which boosts their personal sense of accomplishment and has been important for the schools who received their training. From the other side, Adele's students have been trained by experienced high school students and went through training with students from another middle school in their county.

Limitations

This study has generated ideas about how to conceive of peer mediation programs that can be effective, realistic, and sustainable. The qualitative data resulting from the interviews provided a more complex understanding of the dynamics of each school, their program, and their evolution over time than quantitative data could. The data, however, are limited by the small sample size, the short-term nature of the study, and the self-selection that occurred in recruiting study participants. All of the counselors who agreed to participate in the study were strong advocates for their programs and believed that their investment in the programs were important and worthwhile. Interviews with counselors who had experienced less success or who were less motivated by and committed to conflict resolution education may have generated significantly different results.

Recommendations for Future Research

Researchers have tended to be dismissive of programs that are not based on theoretical work. At the same time, many realize that practitioners are constantly struggling to do as much as they can with the few resources that they have. Designing and executing programs based on solid research is often not as big a priority as getting a feasible program in place. As research professionals look at comprehensiveness and institutionalization of programming as ultimate goals and best practices, it is also important to look at what is actually happening in most schools. More research needs to be done on cadre programs and how they can be designed to have the most impact on the larger school environment. In addition, more work could be done to give practitioners guidelines on building more stable and mature programs over time. Finally, more research could be done in the spirit of this study, which focuses on what kind of programming exists despite the theory. Although often such a project confirms the hypotheses of professional research, looking at the field from the practitioner's perspective can open new avenues for inquiry and build a better understanding of what can be achieved with limited resources.

APPENDIX A:
QUESTIONNAIRE—MIDDLE SCHOOL
PEER MEDIATION PROGRAMS
CURRENTLY COORDINATED
BY SCHOOL COUNSELORS

Please provide the following descriptive information about your school.
Name of school: _____
County: _____
Estimated total population of students in your school: _____
Estimated percent of students in Free and Reduced Lunch Program:_____
Estimated percent of students   African-American: _____
                                    Asian-American: _____
                                    Euro-American: _____
                                    Latino: _____
                                    Other: _____
Number of school counselors: _____

Please provide the following descriptive information about your peer mediation program.
How long has the program been in existence? _____
How many students participate each year as mediators? _____
How many conflicts are mediated each year? _____
How are students referred for mediation? (Circle those that apply)

        Self-referral   Teacher Referral
        Administrator Referral   Parent Referral

Does your program have its own budget?_____
If so, how much? _____
When do students mediate? (Circle those that apply)

        Any time needed   During activity periods
        After school   Other _____

How long is student training? (Number and length of sessions): _____
How many staff members are actively involved in the program? _____
Have teachers and administrators also received mediation and/or conflict resolution training in your school? _____ If so, to what extent? (Number and length of sessions): _____How many teachers/administrators?

On a scale of 1 to 10, how supportive of peer mediation is your principal?_____
On a scale of 1 to 10, how supportive of peer mediation are most teachers?_____

Is there a conflict resolution education curriculum taught on a schoolwide basis in your school? _____

Are your school's behavior expectations and behavior management system consistent with conflict resolution theory? _____

What are your program's main objectives?

_____

_____

_____

How is your program evaluated?

_____

_____

_____

And finally . . . about your background:
How long have you been a school counselor? _____
How long have you worked as a school counselor at this school? _____
How long have you been coordinating the peer mediation program?_____
What prior experience in conflict resolution education or peer mediation have you had? _____

APPENDIX B:
INTERVIEW INSTRUMENT—THE REAL AND THE IDEAL
IN MIDDLE SCHOOL PEER MEDIATION PROGRAMS

1. In your opinion, how effective is peer mediation as a strategy:

   To prevent school violence?
   To decrease bullying and teasing?
   To improve school and classroom atmosphere?
   To improve individual students' academic performance?
   To improve student self-esteem?

2. Do you feel your program accomplishes some of these things?
3. What do you feel is the most significant result of your program?
4. What would you change about your program if you could?
5. What would you need to make those changes?
6. How would you rank the importance of the following five traits to a successful peer mediation program? Please fill in the blank next to each trait with either: N (not important), S (somewhat important), V (very important), or E (essential).

   _____teacher and administrator training

   _____a comprehensive K-12 conflict resolution curriculum

   _____practice opportunities for all students

   _____school behavior management systems based on conflict resolution theory

   _____strong administrator leadership

7. Place a check next to each of the same traits if they apply to your program:

   _____teacher and administrator training

   _____a comprehensive K-12 conflict resolution curriculum

   _____practice opportunities for all students

   _____school behavior management systems based on conflict resolution theory

   _____strong administrator leadership

APPENDIX C:
NORTH CAROLINA STATE UNIVERSITY
INFORMED CONSENT FORM

Title of Study: The Ideal and the Real in Middle School Peer Mediation Programs

Principal Investigator: Maura Dillon **Faculty Sponsor:** Dr. Stanley B. Baker

You are invited to participate in a research study. The purpose of this study is to generate a list of practical concerns for school counselors advocating for or co-ordinating peer mediation programs in middle schools. By comparing the experiences and expertise of schools counselors currently running programs to the recommendations made in the professional literature, I hope to assemble some useful information about what is working in middle schools now and what some of the obstacles to more successful programs might be.

INFORMATION
Participation in the study would involve filling out a questionnaire regarding your school's demographics, your peer mediation program structure, and your professional background in conflict resolution education (20-30 minutes) and one recorded interview (45-60 minutes) and a brief follow-up interview (15-20 minutes).

RISKS AND CONFIDENTIALITY
The potential risk of the study is that the principal investigator will have access to the data. This information will be analyzed and your identity disguised. **All information collected for this study will be kept strictly confidential. Data will be stored securely and be made available only to persons conducting the study unless you specifically give permission in writing to do otherwise. No reference will be made in oral or written reports which could link you to the study.**

BENEFITS
By participating in this study, you will contribute to a better understanding of the characteristics that are most essential to organizing and maintaining successful peer mediation programs in middle schools.

PARTICIPATION
Your participation in this study is voluntary; you may decline to participate without penalty. If you decide to participate, you may withdraw from the study

at any time. If you withdraw from the study before data collection is completed your data will be returned to you or destroyed.

CONSENT

I have read and understand the above information. I have received a copy of this form. I agree to participate in this study.

Participant's signature_____**Date:** _____

Investigator's signature_____**Date:** _____

APPENDIX D:
LETTER OF ATTESTATION

October 10, 2002

To Whom it May Concern:

I have been the designated auditor for the thesis of _____, master's student in the Department of Counselor Education at _____University.

My role as auditor has been to ensure that the results of this study are dependable, credible, and confirmable, and not based on researcher bias.

My primary responsibilities as auditor have been to: (1) review and verify the data gathered from the research participants, and (2) to attest to having done so.

The audit process consisted of the following:

- Reviewing auditor expectations with the researcher
- Familiarizing myself with the study by reading Chapters 1 and 3 of the thesis
- Reviewing informed consent forms signed by each participant and written questionnaires
- Reading interview transcriptions and listening to some recorded interview material
- Examining researcher's interpretations and categories in Chapter 4 for their appropriateness

Upon completing this process I attest that the findings in this study are dependable and confirmable. No inconsistencies, illogical inference, or research bias were found during the course of this process; therefore, the research findings are also credible.

Sincerely,

_____

NOTE

1. In 1994, NAME merged with the National Institute for Dispute Resolution (NIDR) to become the Conflict Resolution in Education Network, or CREnet. In September 2001, CREnet merged with the Academy of Family Mediators (AFM) and the Society for Professionals in Dispute Resolution (SPIDR) to become the Association for Conflict Resolution (ACR).

REFERENCES

Baker, M., French, V., Trujillo, M., and Wing, L. (2000). Impact on diverse populations: How CRE has not addressed the needs of diverse populations. In T. S. Jones and D. Kmitta (Eds.), *Does it work?: The case for conflict resolution education in our nation's schools* (pp. 61-78). Washington, DC: Conflict Resolution Education Network.

Bell, S. K., Coleman, J. K., Anderson, A., and Whelan, J. P. (2000). The effectiveness of peer mediation in a low-SES rural elementary school. *Psychology in the Schools, 37,* 505-516.

Benson, A. J. and Benson, J. M. (1993). Peer mediation: Conflict resolution in schools. *Journal of School Psychology, 31,* 427-430.

Bodine, R. J. and Crawford, D. K. (1998). *The handbook of conflict resolution education.* San Francisco: Jossey-Bass Publishers.

Bodine, R. J., Crawford, D. K., and Schrumpf, F. (1994). *Creating the peaceable school: A comprehensive program for teaching conflict resolution.* Champaign, IL: Research Press.

Carruthers, W. L., Carruthers, B. J. B., Day-Vines, N. L., Bostick, D., and Watson, D. C. (1996). Conflict resolution as curriculum: A definition, description, and process for integration in core curricula. *The School Counselor, 43,* 345-373.

Carruthers, W. L., Sweeney, B., Kmitta, D., and Harris, G. (1996). Conflict resolution: An examination of the research literature and a model for program evaluation. *The School Counselor, 44,* 5-18.

Casella, R. (2000). The benefits of peer mediation in the context of urban conflict and program status. *Urban Education, 35,* 324-356.

Cohen, R. (2001). CREnet fact sheet: Implementing a peer mediation program. Conflict Resolution Education Network. Retrieved June 11, 2001. Available online: <http://www.crenet.org/Research/peer.htm>.

Coleman, P. and Deutsch, M. (2000). Cooperation, conflict resolution, and school violence: A systems approach. *Choices Briefs, 5,* 1-6.

Conflict Resolution Education Network (1996). Recommended standards for school-based peer mediation programs. Retrieved August 6, 2002. Available online: <http://www.acresolution.org/research.nsf/key-print/PMStandards1996?OpenDocument>.

Crary, D. R. (1992). Community benefits from mediation: A test of the "peace virus" hypothesis. *Mediation Quarterly, 9,* 241-252.

Crawford, D. K. and Bodine, R. J. (2001). Conflict resolution education: Preparing youth for the future. *Juvenile Justice Journal, 8,* 1-9.

Darling-Hammond, L. (2000). "Solving the dilemmas of teacher supply, demand, and standards." National Commission on Teaching and America's Future. Retrieved January 12, 2002. Available online: <http://www.tc.columbia.edu/nctaf/publications/solving.html>.

Daunic, A. P., Smith, S. W., Robinson, T. R., Landry, K. L., and Miller, M. D. (2000). Schoolwide conflict resolution and peer mediation programs: Experiences in three middle schools. *Intervention in School and Clinic, 36,* 94-101.

Deutsch, M. (1994). Constructive conflict resolution: Principles, training, and research. *Journal of Social Issues, 50,* 13-32.

Deutsch, M. and Raider, E. (2000). Foreword. In T. S. Jones and D. Kmitta (Eds.), *Does it work?: The case for conflict resolution education in our nation's schools* (pp. vii-ix). Washington, DC: Conflict Resolution Education Network.

Elliot, D. S., Hamburg, B. A., and Williams, K. R. (1998). *Violence in American schools: A new perspective.* Cambridge, UK: Cambridge University Press.

Fingerhut, L. A. (1992). Firearm and nonfirearm homicide among persons 15 through 19 years of age. *Journal of the American Medical Association, 267,* 3048-3053.

Fitch, T. and Marshall, J. L. (1999). *The teaching students to be peacemakers program: Program overview and review of the literature.* Washington, DC: ERIC Clearinghouse on Teaching and Teacher Education (ED 436 517).

Fitzell, S. G. (1997). *Free the children: Conflict education for strong, peaceful minds.* Philadelphia: New Society Publishers.

Gentry, D. and Benenson, W. (1993). School-to-home transfer of conflict management skills among school-age children. *Families in Society: Journal of Contemporary Human Services, 4,* 67-73.

Gerber, S. (1999). Does peer mediation really work? *Professional School Counseling, 2,* 169-171.

Girard, K. L. (1995). *Preparing teachers for conflict resolution in schools.* Washington DC: ERIC Clearinghouse on Teaching and Teacher Education (ED 387 456).

Humphries, T. L. (1999). Improving peer mediation programs: Student experiences and suggestions. *Professional School Counseling, 3,* 13-21.

Johnson, D. W. and Johnson, R. (1979). Conflict in the classroom: Controversy and learning. *Review of Educational Research, 49,* 51-61.

Johnson, D. W. and Johnson, R. T. (1995). Why violence prevention programs don't work—and what does. *Educational Leadership, 52,* 63-68.

Johnson, D. W. and Johnson, R. T. (1996). Conflict resolution and peer mediation programs in elementary and secondary schools: A review of the research. *Review of Educational Research, 66,* 459-506.

Johnson, D. W. and Johnson, R. T. (2001). Teaching students to be peacemakers: A meta-analysis. Paper presented at the annual meeting of the American Educational Research Association, April. Seattle, WA. ED 460 178.

Johnson, D. W., Johnson, R., Dudley, B., Ward, M., and Magnuson, D. (1995). Impact of peer mediation training on the management of school and home conflicts. *American Educational Research Journal, 32,* 829-844.

Jones, P. L. (1998). Values education, violence prevention, and peer mediation: The triad against violence in our schools. *Educational Horizons, 76,* 177-181.

Jones, T. S. (1998). The Comprehensive Peer Mediation Evaluation Project: Insights and directions for curriculum integration. Retrieved August 8, 2002. Available online: <http://www.ncip.org/articles/Integration.html>.

Jones, T. S., Johnson, D., and Lieber, C. M. (2000). Impact of CRE on school and classroom climate. In T. S. Jones and D. Kmitta (Eds.), *Does it work?: The case for conflict resolution education in our nation's schools* (pp. 85-102). Washington, DC: Conflict Resolution Education Network.

Jones, T. S. and Kmitta, D. (Eds.) (2000). *Does it work?: The case for conflict resolution in our nation's schools.* Washington, DC: Conflict Resolution Education Network.

Kmitta, D., Chappell, C., Brown, J., and Wiley, P. (2000). Does it work? Shared insights and future directions. In T. S. Jones and D. Kmitta (Eds.), *Does it work?: The case for conflict resolution education in our nation's schools* (pp. 139-148). Washington, DC: Conflict Resolution Education Network.

Lane, P. and McWhirter, J. J. (1992). A peer mediation model: Conflict resolution for elementary and middle school children. *Elementary School Guidance and Counseling, 27,* 15-23.

Lupton-Smith, H. S., Carruthers, W. L., Flythe, R., Goettee, E., and Modest, K. H. (1996). Conflict resolution as peer mediation: Programs for elementary, middle, and high school students. *The School Counselor, 43,* 374-391.

National Center for Education Statistics (2001). *Dropout Rates in the United States:* 2000. Available: <http://nces.ed.gov/pubs2002/droppub_2001/>.

Pilchard, H. E. (2000). Conflict resolution in the United States. In T. S. Jones and D. Kmitta (Eds.), *Does it work?: The case for conflict resolution education in our nation's schools* (pp. 1-14). Washington, DC: Conflict Resolution Education Network.

Sandy, S. V., Bailey, S., and Sloane-Akwara, V. (2000). Impact on students: Conflict resolution education's proven benefits for students. In T. S. Jones and D. Kmitta (Eds.), *Does it work?: The case for conflict resolution education in our nation's schools* (pp. 15-32). Washington, DC: Conflict Resolution Education Network.

Schrumpf, F., Crawford, D. K., and Bodine, R. J. (1997). *Peer mediation: Conflict resolution in schools program guide.* Champaign, IL: Research Press.

Singh, D. (1995). Pathways to peer mediation. Paper presented at the annual meeting of the Australian Guidance and Counseling Association. Hobart, Tasmania, September. ED 404 593.

Stop the Violence (1994). *Scholastic Update,* January, pp. 2-6.

Thompson, S. M. (1996). Peer mediation: A peaceful solution. *School Counselor,* *44,* 151-155.

U.S. Department of Education (2000). *Annual Report on School Safety.* Available: <http://www.ed.gov/PressReleases/10-2000/102600.html>.

Webster, D. (1993). The unconvincing case for school-based conflict resolution programs for adolescents. *Health Affairs, 12,* 126-140.

Chapter 7

Because No One Ever Asked: Understanding Youth Gangs As a Primary Step in Violence Prevention

Laura Kallus

Gangs offer something of value to our youths. Much like other social groups, gangs fulfill significant needs for many young people. Only by understanding these needs and acknowledging the intrinsic value of young people within their communities can any genuine efforts to curb the gang violence that spills over into our schools begin. Understanding and valuing youths are among the most fundamental and the least expensive building blocks that exist in the prevention of youth violence. This begins with asking the right questions, listening to what our youths are saying, then developing appropriate strategies for meeting their needs at various stages of their development. Engaging high-risk youths early in the process is a strategy that is often overlooked.

A common reaction within a community with an emerging gang problem is denial. This allows the underlying causes of gang formation to remain untended and generally allows the youth gang culture to take root and develop. Only when the level of violence or destructiveness reaches a point of intolerance within a community does the public become outraged. The pressure is then placed on law enforcement to solve the gang problem. Far too often, suppression tactics and zero-tolerance policies designed to target youth gangs are born out of hysteria, and fail. They fail because suppression does little to alleviate the root causes of gang formation. It can only offer a Band-Aid approach in dealing with a very complex issue. Suppression should only be viewed as a last resort to a community-based strategy that combines understanding, prevention, and intervention.

In many cases, by the time a community begins to take action the youth gang culture has already become established on neighborhood streets and in school hallways. The gang has become a viable source of love, discipline, protection, and excitement for young people. It is critical to understand not only what the gang offers our youths but also why certain young people choose the gang to fulfill their needs over other social groups. This chapter combines the real voices of gang members from a Washington, DC, community with current research in the field of youth violence and delinquency. The case studies employed in this chapter were taken from tape-recorded life history interviews of gang members conducted primarily between 1999 and 2002. Gang members shared the experiences in their families, schools, and communities that were influential in their trajectory from children to gang members. Many of the reasons they cited for joining gangs point to specific risk factors in their homes, schools, and communities that research has linked to destructive behavior such as violence, delinquency, and substance abuse (Bellamy et al., 1997; Hawkins and Catalano, 1992; U.S. Department of Health and Human Services, 2001). Although researchers have categorized risk factors for youth violence into five domains, this chapter highlights two, the family and school environment.

RISK FACTORS

Many theories have been developed to explain the occurrence and perpetuation of youth gangs throughout history (Bursik and Grasmick, 1995; Kent and Felkenes, 1998; Vigil, 1988). The social development model identifies risk factors that interfere with the healthy development and socialization of individuals (Bellamy et al., 1997). Research shows that the risk factors for gang membership are the same as those for violence in general. However, once children join a gang the chances are greater that they will engage in more delinquent and more violent acts than other at-risk, nongang youth (Battin-Pearson et al., 1998; Thornberry et al., 1995; Esbensen, Huizinga, and Weiher, 1995). Therefore, it is important to understand the risk factors that predict violence and delinquency in early childhood as well as late adolescence. Hawkins et al. (2000) reviewed long-term studies of violence predictors and identified risk factors that statistically correlate to youth violence. Current research arranges the factors into the following domains that impact a child's development: individual, family, school, peer groups, and community factors.

During childhood the majority of risk factors are found in the individual and family domains as children learn to respond to their immediate surroundings. Individual factors that predict violence include childhood aggressiveness, early involvement in violent and antisocial behavior, and favorable attitudes toward deviant behavior. Risk factors in the family domain include parents who engage in criminal behavior, physical abuse and neglect, sexual abuse, poor family management strategies, and exposure to marital and family conflict (Hawkins et al., 2000). The family plays the most vital role in the child's development until puberty when peer groups assume greater importance.

Once a child enters school, various risk factors predict later violence and delinquency. Research indicates that early academic failure, low bonding to school, and truancy increase later risk of violence and delinquency. Additional factors such as frequent changing of schools and attending schools with high delinquency rates also compound these risks (Bellamy et al., 1997; Hawkins et al., 2000). Having delinquent siblings, associating with antisocial peers, and membership in a gang are also strong predictors of violence for adolescents. Within the community, certain factors have been shown to predict youth crime and violence. These include poverty, community disorganization, easy access to drugs and weapons, and exposure to violence and racial prejudice (Hawkins et al., 2000).

The predictive powers of certain risk factors in specific domains vary according to youths' developmental stages. For example, risk factors that predict violence at ages six to 11 are different than those that predict violence at ages 15 to 25. In addition, risk factors commonly exist in clusters and youths with multiple risk factors are much more likely to engage in violent or delinquent behavior than others (Hawkins et al., 2000). As the risk factors that contribute to youth violence and delinquency change as children transition through key developmental stages, so too must strategies for prevention and intervention.

FROM VIOLENT HOMES TO VIOLENT STREETS

During childhood, the family is the primary social realm for learning positive, appropriate behavior. Unfortunately, many young people are growing up in family environments wrought with violence, neglect, and substance abuse. Other risk factors that increase chances of violence and delinquency in youths, such as poverty, low education levels, and community disorganization also influence parenting skills. Explaining why they joined the gang, "problems at home" is a common response. Discussions of problems at home generally yield descriptions of domestic violence, child abuse, neglect, and parental alcohol/drug abuse. By adolescence, many gang members have been witnesses and victims of consistent violence in their homes.

A 21-year-old gang member, Carlitos, thoughtfully considered the effects of such exposure to violence in childhood: "I think the major thing about this gang problem is some parents, not all parents but some parents, they beat their kids and that's how the kids start to get violent." What this young man realizes is that children learn by example and early exposure to aggression and family conflict increases the risk for crime and violence in later adolescence (Bellamy et al., 1997; Hawkins et al., 2000). Although most gang members do not make such direct associations, they discuss violence in their childhood as problems from which to escape. For many of them, exposure to domestic violence and child abuse caused great anxiety and feelings of helplessness. Gino's situation is a typical example:

> You know my stepdad used to beat on my mom. When we were *chavelitos* (children) and shit he used to hit on her. I mean it used to be a terror when you are a little kid. It's not like now that if I see my stepdad hit my mom, it would be all over. But before we used to be scared. We used to live on the third floor and downstairs on the second floor there used to be a *chiviada*— a gambling place, you know. He used to go and then come drunk upstairs talking all this bullshit. All this crazy shit. We were *chavelitos;* we couldn't do shit but to run.

Another gang member, Elmer, realized as he got older that drugs and alcohol played a role in the violence his father inflicted against his mother. When asked if he has a good relationship with his father, he replied:

Not really, I didn't because he was beating up on my mom. He used to go home at five in the morning, wake her up. Beat her up for no reason. And one night she went to my room and said, "Oh, stop your dad from hitting me!" He was in the living room. And then I told him to stop. He was like, "Oh, what you going to do about it? You a man now? You going to fight me?" He was talking crap. He was really drunk. I was about almost eighteen. Then I didn't want to take it so far, but I did. You know, now I regret it, but it's too late. I don't like people hitting on a woman like that . . . I didn't know back then about that [cocaine], but now I know. I used to see him, but I didn't know. Now I know . . . actually, I wasn't closer to my mom, to either one. But it was like . . . imagine someone beating on your mom? All right then. I wasn't close to her, but that doesn't mean I didn't feel something for her.

When children are young, they are helpless in the face of violence. They are scared and angry. They often fantasize about the day they can fight back and protect themselves and those they love. Like Elmer, as they get older and physically stronger, they often will challenge their victimizers and end up on the streets with nowhere to go. Others emotionally detach from those that hurt them and fail to protect them.

One gang-affiliated young woman, Chinita, describes the reasons she ran away from home:

CHINITA: Like when I was like thirteen I had run away from home the first time because every time I used to get in trouble my mom used to hit me and stuff. And like I got tired of it.

LAURA: What grade were you in?

CHINITA: Seventh grade.

LAURA: Where did you go?

CHINITA: To my boyfriend's house.

Chinita's boyfriend was the leader of a local gang. She was 12 years old when she fell in love with him. She lived with him for almost two years before she left: "I had left him because he was cheating on me and that wasn't the first time. And he hit me for no reason so I was like, 'This is the last time he does this, I'm not going to take this no more.' So I just left." A couple of weeks after they broke up he was shot by members of a rival gang as he was at a bar celebrating his 22nd birthday. Chinita was 14 years old.

After Chinita's boyfriend was murdered, his best friend Cristopher took his place as the gang leader. He remembers one way the gang offered protection from an abusive father:

> I never get along with my father. . . . He used to beat my mom, you know. And I didn't like that stuff and I used to fight with my dad too. I used to fight him too when I seen my mom fighting with him. When I was real skinny and tiny he used to grab me from my throat and put me down on the floor like nothing—like a piece of trash. But later on when he seen that I hang around with those guys [the gang], he was like, he didn't talk to me. He was scared of me. Like he didn't do nothing to me. He kind of respect me and Mom some more—it's not respect, it's like leaving alone my mom, you know. He was scared too. I think he still is.

So-So, another 15-year-old gang member with a documented history of abuse, neglect, and early delinquency, sought solace and guidance in the streets at a very early age:

> I got problems with my mom because of my sister's father because he used to be drinking and hitting on me. My mom used to let him. And that's when I started hanging out [in the streets]. . . . That's why I changed. I started changing and hanging out when I was like eight or nine.

Other gang members recall that So-So used to be poor, always dirty, and running the streets. The gang began to look out for him. So-So agreed: "At first, the grown-ups used to take advantage of me. They used to give me stuff [drugs] to hold . . . but they still took care of me, buy me shoes and clothes and everything." Too young to work and with no one to care for him, So-So began selling drugs when he was ten years old: "That's when I started getting smart and selling by myself . . . street-smart." Early on, So-So emotionally and physically disassociated himself from those who failed to protect him and failed to provide for his basic needs. When he refers to becoming "street-smart" he is describing a variety of learned basic survival skills. So-So has been continuously in and out of foster homes, residential placements, and detention facilities. Although known to the courts and the community as a drug dealer and gang member, So-So is highly intelligent and resilient. Like many gang members who may lack formal education, by early adolescence So-So already exhibited the type of savvy business sense and interpersonal skills that are valued in the business world. He cultivated them to his advantage. So-So adapted to his environment and not only survived but also managed to earn enough money to buy clothes and eat.

The gang provided the kind of support and affection that So-So needed at such an early age. A sanctuary where he felt protected and respected, the gang offered him a sense of control over his life at a time when so many things were beyond his control. So-So was not a violent young man. He simply needed to take care of himself. "I used to be real, real dirty because I had just come out [from a foster home] and I had no clothes, no money, nothing." He discusses why he began selling drugs with the gang at age ten:

SO-SO: Because when I was little I knew a rack of people that used to be selling big, big drugs. They used to be tight as shit with me, so I used to see them—how they sell and stuff and that's when I started getting into it myself.

LAURA: What made you want to do it?

SO-SO: I used to be real, real poor. And I just liked money since I was little.

LAURA: You wanted nice things?

SO-SO: Yeah, I used to be just wanting to have the money because when you be having the money, people be respecting you. They be like "Damn, he's tight."

LAURA: Did your mom try to keep you off the street?

SO-SO: Nah, she didn't used to say nothing.

By the age of thirteen, So-So was battling an addiction to crack cocaine. He began to owe money to his suppliers in the gang. One of them, a member of the same gang, put a gun to his head because So-So owed him $500. So-So's addiction and debt deepened until he was arrested again at age 15. Six months in the juvenile detention facility helped So-So recover from his addiction: "I am glad that I got locked up because I would still be doing that shit. I couldn't stop by myself. I was stuck to that stuff." Fortunately, some gang members forgave his debt and others let him pay it back little by little because they loved So-So, and they understood the nature of addiction.

For many youths in urban environments (and increasingly in suburban and rural environments as well) gangs are a normalized part of their social landscape. Gang members, discussing their earliest memories, revealed how many gang youths had family members who were also involved in gangs. This early exposure influenced the belief that gangs were just a normal part of everyday life and impacted their eventual decision to join (Kallus, 1999). Gino, when asked about his earliest impressions of gangs, laughed and replied:

> Cool as shit! My brother was from La Raza . . . I used to go, "You motherfucker, you in the gang. I want to be in the gang, too, man!" But I was too small, you know . . . when we moved to the ghetto he was in the gang. All his friends used to come pick him up. I was always like, "Damn, I want to be like that!"

In various communities with a chronic gang problem, parents and even grandparents have a history of gang affiliation. This not only normalizes gang culture and influences a youth's desire to join a gang, it can also become a matter of basic survival (Valdez, 1997; Vigil, 1988). However, if early role models in the family domain engage in violent or antisocial behavior, the risk that their children will learn the same behavior increases if their communities are also violent. In the neighborhood where these youths are living, opportunities for economic and social mobility are limited. Drugs, crime, and gangs provide attractive economic opportunities for adults in the community as well as for youths. Adults are visible participants in the drug trade, both as addicts and suppliers. They can also be seen on the street corners gambling, drinking, and using drugs as they socialize. The impact of these early experiences had profound effects on these young people. For example, Gino relates:

> The way we grow up was wrong. I am the first one to admit I know God ain't just drop me here to be going through this. I guess

our childhood is over. 'Cause ain't nothing funny and everything
I love like my mom, sister . . . but I think this world is polluted.

The gang members in this chapter grew up in turbulent family environments wrought with substance abuse, violence, and neglect. Witnessing violence against their mothers seemed to affect the gang members more than their own experiences of abuse. In any event, research shows that children and adolescents react diversely to domestic violence exposure and child abuse (Atnafou, 1995; Dobbin and Gatowski, 1996). Children who witness family violence often suffer from academic performance problems that stem from preoccupation, inability to concentrate, increased conflict with teachers, and sporadic school attendance. In comparison to girls, boys often fight more with peers, rebel in school, and exhibit more destructive and disobedient behavior (Dobbin and Gatowski, 1996). Girls usually react with increased dependency and clingyness, secrecy, and depression. As they reach adolescence youths may exhibit behavior problems such as running away from home, aggression, hostility, depression, and withdrawal. Abused and neglected children have the increased likelihood of committing violent crimes and being arrested as juveniles and adults (Dobbin and Gatowski, 1996).

SCHOOL

Although many gang members in Washington, DC, reported the presence of gangs in the communities for as long as they could remember, it was not until they entered school when the decision to identify with a gang became important. This marks a distinct developmental stage in adolescent identity formation when the influence of the peer group supercedes the family. If a child is a member of an ethnic minority or is a recent immigrant, other factors such as language barriers and discrimination can influence his or her decision to bond with a peer group that offers protection, solidarity, and companionship (Fernández-Kelly and Schauffler, 1994; Kallus, 1999; Vigil, 1988). An immigrant from El Salvador, Gino, shares his experience entering elementary school:

I didn't know nothing. I didn't know what the hell was going on. You don't know nothing. I was just so mad, scared! Scared and all that shit. You don't know nobody. You don't know what the hell they're talking about.

So-So agreed with Gino. He recalls a particularly frustrating memory: "I remember one day when I had to use the bathroom real bad and I didn't know how to say it [in English]. And I just did it on myself. And then after that, from that time on, I just got real mad." Unable to speak English and being victimized by other children marked their earliest memories of school in the United States. Years earlier, they had moved into a predominately African-American community with little experience with diversity. Their minority status and inability to speak English alienated them from the other students. They experienced discrimination. Carlitos explains, "A lot of kids from different races, they want to fight you only because they think this is their country." Cristopher agreed:

> Black people, they picked on Spanish people because we don't know how to defend ourselves. So if I was alone there, they would pick on me 'cause I didn't have no friend, you know . . . so I start having friends, bad friends like the ones who are gangsters.

Gino was kicked out of one elementary school for skipping classes and negatively influencing his friends. After he was transferred to another school, his peer group became a protective factor.

> I was in fifth grade. I went to this all-black school then and there was discrimination because there was like five Spanish guys and four Spanish girls. So we had to make a little gang, you know, to watch our ass and shit. So we made a little gang and carried little sticks. We sharpened them like shanks—like when you in jail and stuff. After that, they kicked me out of there 'cause I never went to school.

Factors such as language barriers and racial or ethnic discrimination further contribute to the risk factors these youths struggled with at home. They had to adapt to violence and aggression within their family and school environments. For protection and companionship, many banded together into peer groups based on ethnicity and neighborhood boundaries. Like most peer groups, the bonds between these youths were strong and long-lasting. For many of them, delinquent behavior such as skipping school, drinking, and doing drugs began in junior high school. A 19-year-old gang member, Jose Lopez, remembers:

> When I was like eleven, I was hanging out. I used to go to a middle school. It was for bad people, only bad people go there. It's a school just for bad people that had gotten kicked out of school. And I had got kicked out of my school 'cause they found me with a gun. . . . I took it out on this dude. We had got in a fight, a Spanish dude. We started fighting and then I got mad and I took out the gun. I got locked up and they put me in that school. And then I started hanging out with wrong people. Started breaking into houses and stuff, started smoking weed and drinking Old English.

For various youths, like Jose Lopez, So-So, and Gino, delinquent behavior precluded gang membership and was influenced by older role models that were gang affiliated. For others, drug use, truancy, and crime began after they joined a gang. In all cases, such activity and behavior intensified after gang membership. Although they began to identify with and emulate older gang members in their families and communities at an early age, many reported being initiated into the gang around age 14. Other studies of gang members report that initiation into the gang most often occurred in junior high school when the youths were around 13 or 14 years old (Decker and Van Winkle, 1996; Cruz and Peña, 1998; Vigil, 1988). This demonstrates a critical stage in these young people's development. The influence of peer groups becomes stronger than the family's influence as youths move toward establishing their own identity and gradual independence.

As youths transition into adolescence, three factors in the peer domain considerably affect later violent or delinquent behavior. These include weak social ties to healthy peer groups that engage in conventional social activities, identification with a delinquent peer group, and gang membership (U.S. Department of Health and Human Services, 2001). Often, these factors are related as young people who feel rejected by the popular group seek acceptance among antisocial or delinquent peers. Such associations can introduce young people to behaviors and activities to which the youngsters may not have been exposed. Carlitos, a gang member who graduated from high school, remembers his school experiences as positive but acknowledges the negative influence of his friends:

> Sometimes when I started to go to school it was really nice. But then I started to hang with my friends, started to get high, and that's when I got in trouble. . . . I used to get good grades when I came here [to the United States] but when I started to join the gang and I turned seventeen years old, my grades went down. . . . Sometimes you like to do things that are wrong—and you know they are wrong. But when you start to hang with your friends and they tell you to get high, smoke, drink, and that's when your life is messed up.

Regardless of the consequences, having a reputation as a gang member carries certain privileges, especially for youths who feel marginalized or rejected by the mainstream. The gang offers them protection from groups who bully them. Gang members feel powerful because they have friends who would do anything for them:

LAURA: What is it that makes you want to get in [the gang]?

KARTOON: You got protection.

CASCABEL: Yeah, you got friends.

KARTOON: And nobody touch you.

CASCABEL: Yeah, but you still got to be watching your back.

KARTOON: That's the only bad part about it.

LAURA: What's all the good things about it?

KARTOON: You chill with all your friends, go to parties, you got a rack of girls, drink.

The need for protection is another recurring theme for young people who struggle with violence in their homes, schools, and communities—the places that should serve as sanctuaries. For young people who must navigate neighborhoods where crime and violence are common and access to drugs and firearms is easily accessible, protection is perceived as necessary for survival (Decker and Van Winkle,

1996; Kallus, 1999; Vigil, 1988). When asked how easy it is to get a gun, one neighborhood youth replied, "You could just buy it! Like if I had two hundred fifty dollars I could get a nine millimeter by tomorrow."

Gang members often talk of gaining respect as a perk for joining. Many of them have felt devalued and helpless throughout their lives. Their idea of respect, in essence, is the ability to instill fear. People are afraid of them. Even teachers may feel threatened by them. Younger kids now look up to them. Gang members no longer feel like victims. When discussing the issue, Kartoon explained, "You know how you get respect? You don't be scared of nobody." Cascabel added, "You always be there for your friends, you know. If you got to fight and if you don't back down. If you always there, you know, and they don't see you scared." Many gang members were attracted to the excitement and adventure that the gang offers. Kartoon said, "They want to experience it. Actually for me, I want to experience everything. . . . Everybody be saying it's fun, you know, I want to experience it." Kartoon's uncle and cousin were early founders of the local gang.

When gang members discuss the attraction of joining, they talk about having fun, being protected, and having a reputation that commands respect, as well as popularity with girls. All of these are significant, healthy desires of adolescents. They often joined for reasons other than violence and criminal behavior. For example, Elmer explains his attraction to gang life:

> At first I thought it was really cool 'cause you get the girls, you hang around, drink. It was fun at first but . . . now, if I think about it, if I could go back and if I could change it, I would change it. 'Cause it's a lot of trouble. You get into fights . . . looking at it, all of my idea of being in a gang was to have fun not to have violence.

Even though problem behaviors emerged as early as elementary school, the traditional response even at that early stage was to transfer the youths to other schools. There was no intervention or outreach to these young people until they became involved in the juvenile justice or child welfare system. Even then, strategies for helping them cope with the stressors in their lives were nonexistent. Many were placed in foster homes, shelter houses, and other residential facilities where they were further victimized. They often ran away and came back home to the streets. Throughout the years, they fell further and further behind academically. Frustrated schools either kicked them out or passed them on to the next grade. Gino remembers:

> They just passed me! I don't know how. They didn't like me, the teachers. I never went to school or did no homework and I passed the grade. They didn't like me. Probably they didn't like me or they didn't care. So they passed me to the sixth grade. Then from sixth grade they just didn't care, you know. So fuck it. So they passed me to seventh . . . it was from fifth to eighth grade. I didn't get no certificate for passing. I didn't graduate from elementary; they just passed me on.

Gino never made it to high school. He spent two years in seventh grade then dropped out of school. Gino was attracted to the economic pull of the gang's drug-selling activities. His problems at home had intensified and he found himself on the streets before he was 16 years old.

> So I said, "What the hell, I'm in the street. I ain't doing shit. I ain't worth shit. Let me change my life around." . . . So I started selling that crazy shit [cocaine]. Then I got more into the gangs because then I had money, clothes. I became a member of La Raza. I was *the man* then . . . nice clothes, nice perfume, Versace and shit. I was totally different than before asking for dollars. You know, I was a drunky begging for a dollar. I couldn't handle it. Then with nine hundred dollars in my pocket—it changed me around!

Eventually he moved back into his mother's house. "I was paying the whole apartment then. I was like 'take it, Mom.' She didn't know. She was like, 'What the fuck? Are you stealing? Robbing?' I said, 'Just take it.' I was paying my rent, my brother's rent, and my other brother's rent." Gino also sent a great deal of money to support his extended family in El Salvador. When his brothers got deported because of their criminal activities, Gino supported them, too. With a level head for business, Gino eventually made enough money to provide small business loans to family members in El Salvador. By this time, he was 19 years old with two children of his own. His decision to sell drugs gave him not only material gain but also a sense of confidence and self-worth. He viewed his trajectory from abused, troubled child to the financial provider for his extended family as a success. Never graduating from junior high school, Gino used his survival skills to become a young capitalist. For many youths such as Gino and So-So, these survival skills—or as the youths say "street smarts"—are vital adaptations to the realities of a harsh environment.

Another young gang member, Romero, was also passed when he got to be too old for junior high. Also a victim of abandonment and neglect, Romero entered the juvenile justice system at an early age and has been institutionalized almost consistently since he was 15 years old. At one point, when the judge was going to release him to a residential home, Romero begged her to let him stay in the detention facility so that he could finish out his school year in one place. Today, at age 19, he can barely read and write. He never received his diploma or GED. His frustration is immense. He will be released to the community with no education and no vocational skills, although he had asked the courts repeatedly to provide him with the opportunity to learn. He had wanted to become a carpenter.

DISCUSSION

The school environment has had to adapt to the influence of gangs. Often schools are the front lines where gang formation, recruitment, and conflict take place. Very little training is provided to equip our educators, counselors, and youth workers with the tools to effectively deal with gang members and their influence in our schools. Primarily, school administrations are responsible for providing the larger student body with an environment that is safe and conducive to learning. To achieve this, many schools have adopted policies that lack the flexibility and creativity needed for working with gang members and other high-risk youths. The traditional response to antisocial behavior at school has been to suspend or expel youths.

Currently, public schools that receive federal funding are required to implement zero-tolerance policies for weapon offenses. Originally designed under the Gun-Free Schools Act (GFSA) of 1994, zero-tolerance policies mandate a one-year mandatory expulsion for bringing a weapon to school. Although the act allows school districts to judge such expulsions on a case-by-case basis, many school districts have broadened its scope to include a wide array of behaviors that mandate out-of-school suspensions or expulsions regardless of circumstances (Gordon, Della Piana, and Keleher, 2000). Such policies tie the hands of administrations and prevent creative strategies for addressing problem behaviors to emerge.

Depending on the severity of the behavior, youths may be barred from attending school for varying periods of time. Because parents work, suspended youths are often left home unsupervised. If the behavior is severe, youths may be required to attend an alternative school during the time they are suspended from their regular school. Edgar, an 18-year-old gang member, explains the unintended effect of such suspensions:

> When you get suspended they send you to another school—more harder. Everybody who gets suspended go to there so they can pass the grades. The school is strict. I went for a week then left. When I used to get suspended I used to be chilling and making skipping parties at my house! If they kick you out then you be having fun! When you get back, all your grades are going to be fucked. They need to do something so the person can understand and be better. 'Cause if a person be in the streets they gonna be drinking, smoking, doing skipping parties. . . .

Not only does suspension allow youths to be at home and unsupervised, it also lures other students from school. Skipping parties take place during the day when parents are at work. Young people from the same social group or gang will skip school to attend. At these parties alcohol consumption, drug use, and sex commonly occur.

For young people who are already resistant to attending school, suspension is not a punishment. It may have the unintended consequence of promoting delinquent behavior because it allows these youths to remain at home or on the streets unsupervised. It may also entice other students to join them in unsupervised delinquent activities. In other instances, youths may be expelled from their regular school and forced to transfer to another. If little is done to assist young people with the underlying causes of their behavior, it will likely continue and intensify. Disruptive behavior and academic failure may begin as early as elementary school and create a spiraling effect. The result of this is youths such as Gino who were passed on to the next grade levels because they were too old to remain in their current placements. Predictably, Gino dropped out of school and returned to the streets.

Schools need to intervene early with youths and continue to work with them until they graduate high school. School-based strategies should be flexible and well-grounded in research. Many strategies have been proven effective in working with delinquent youths at various educational stages (Sherman et al., 1998; Wasserman, Miller, and Cothern, 2000). Alternatives to suspension and expulsion that are creative, flexible, and intensive need to be employed. Teachers and school counselors must be educated about gangs in their schools and provided training to respond effectively. The time must be taken to understand what youths are going through. As Edgar noted, "They need to have patience. And they need to talk to you."

The gang members in this chapter have raised some key issues that school administrations should consider. School strategies should include an emphasis on training for the early detection of child abuse, neglect, and other family conflict, which have been proven to affect children's ability to thrive and increases their risk for later violent and delinquent behavior. Although some intervention in this area may be beyond the scope of a school's capabilities, administrations can provide the necessary linkages to community resources that will assist families in crisis. School personnel can be trained on early detection and educated on the local resources available in the community.

In addition, school personnel must also be aware of peer dynamics that may isolate or persecute some groups of young people. Recent immigrants who do not speak the predominant language or members of a cultural or racial minority may be particularly vulnerable to isolation and discrimination by the larger social groups. Efforts must be made to foster inclusion and appreciation of diversity within the school culture. Similarly, diversity and sensitivity training is beneficial for school staff who may not be aware of hidden biases or perceptions that may impact their disciplining practices. They are also in a position to provide outreach and support to marginalized youths.

Finally, the practice of social promotion should be reexamined. Students who are promoted to the next grade level based on anything other than their academic achievement are at increased risk of dropping out of school. Truancy, academic failure, and problem behaviors tend to intensify. Too many young people are entering, and sometimes graduating, high school without basic academic skills. Suspensions, expulsions, and transferring youths to other schools further exacerbate the problems. There is also the perception that teachers or administrations no longer want to deal with these youths and are shifting the responsibility onto someone else. Gang members and other high-risk youths can be extremely challenging to work with; however, the price that is paid for giving up is immeasurable.

CONCLUSION

The first step in the prevention of gang and youth violence begins with understanding. Understanding comes from engaging youths in dialogue and listening to what they are saying. All youths and their experiences are unique. There is not one easy or simple solution that will apply to all of them. Gang members and other high-risk youths must be involved in the problem-solving process. As their voices in this chapter show, they are acutely aware of their needs. They seek ways to adjust and survive. While conducting fieldwork with gang members in Washington, DC, it became obvious that these youths are intelligent, resilient young people that want understanding. The following excerpt from my notes illustrates this point:

> After two hours of deeply personal questions, I was incredulous of the genuine show of trust that the gang leader exhibited toward me—a total stranger. It defied everything I had assumed about the difficulties of conducting fieldwork with gang members. I had no money to pay them, no guarantee that their stories would ever appear in print, no funding for programs, no clout with the courts . . . no incentives to offer. I had to ask, "Why are you helping me with this research?"
>
> Cristopher looked me in the eye and said simply, *"Because no one ever asked."*

As if all we had to do to learn was simply to ask. As if all people want to tell their stories if only someone out there in the world thought it was important. These kids, and countless others, are living and dying on our streets. Very few people value their stories, or in essence, value their lives. To many of us they are only statistics. To some of us they are monsters who show little regard for life and decency and hard work. To others, they are our lost sons and daughters who slipped from our grasp, our students who fell through the cracks.

What we fail to realize over and over again is that these were once children who dreamed, whose lives were supposed to mean something, who wanted what we all wanted—to be valued and respected. Many of these children were failed by those they needed the most, those who were supposed to protect them, cherish them, and teach them how to make their way in this world. They learned from what they saw around them and they found ways to survive. They learned to fight, to hustle, to laugh, and to play. They also learned how to build walls around their hearts so things would not hurt as bad. By the time they enter our detention facilities, our programs, or our classrooms they are hardened, detached, and angry.

The gang provides a great deal that appeals to youths from various backgrounds. It provides structure, rules and discipline, passionate commitment, and loyalty. For youths who may feel that their lives lack meaning or importance, the gang offers them something to live and die for. Gangs are valuable to youths because they fulfill needs. Until communities take responsibility for fulfilling those needs in other ways, the gang will be there for the youths that need it.

REFERENCES

Atnafou, R. (1995). Children as witnesses to community violence: A call for more understanding of the problem and its treatment. *Options* (Newsletter of the Adolescent Violence Resource Center), 2, 7-11.

Battin-Pearson, S.R., Thornberry, T.P., Hawkins, J.D., and Krohn, M.D. (1998). Gang membership, delinquent peers, and delinquent behavior. *Juvenile Justice Bulletin* (October). Office of Juvenile Justice and Delinquency Prevention. Washington, DC: U.S. Department of Justice.

Bellamy, N.D., Hayes, J.G., Sorensen, S.L., Delory, M., Chow, D., and Walsh, E.M. (1997). *Youth violence prevention: A resource manual for preventing violence in public housing and community settings.* U.S. Department of Housing and Urban Development, Office of Crime Prevention and Security, in collaboration with the Centers for Disease Control. Bethesda, MD: SPARTA Consulting Corporation.

Bursik, R.J. and Grasmick, H.G. (1995). The effect of neighborhood dynamics on gang behavior. In M. Klein, C. Maxson, and J. Miller (Eds.), *The modern gang reader* (pp. 114-124). Los Angeles, CA: Roxbury Publishing Company.

Cruz, J.M. and Peña, N.P. (1998). *Solidaridad y violencia en las pandillas del gran San Salvador: Mas allá de las vida loca.* San Salvador, El Salvador: UCA Editores.

Decker, S. and Van Winkle, B. (1996). *Life in the gang.* Cambridge, UK: Cambridge University Press.

Dobbin, S.A. and Gatowski, S.I. (1996). *Juvenile violence: A guide to research.* Reno, NV: National Council of Juvenile and Family Court Judges.

Esbensen, F., Huizinga, D., and Weiher, A. (1995). Gang and nongang youth: Differences in explanatory factors. In M. Klein, C. Maxson, and J. Miller (Eds.), *The modern gang reader* (pp. 192-201). Los Angeles, CA: Roxbury Publishing Company.

Fernández-Kelly, M. and Schauffler, R. (1994). Divided fates: Immigrant children in a restructured economy. *International Migration Review,* 28:662-689.

Gordon, R., Della Piana, L., and Keleher, T. (2000). *Facing the consequences: An examination of racial discrimination in U.S. public schools.* Oakland, CA: The Applied Research Center.

Hawkins, J. D. and Catalano, R.F. Jr. (1992). *Communities that care.* San Francisco: Jossey-Bass.

Hawkins, J.D., Herrenkohl, T.I., Farrington, D.P., Brewer, D., Catalano, R.F., Harachi, T.W., and Cothern, L. (2000). Predictors of youth violence. *Juvenile Justice Bulletin* (April). Office of Juvenile Justice and Delinquency Prevention. Washington, DC: U.S. Department of Justice.

Kallus, L. (1999). La Mara: Gangs, identity and life for Salvadoran youth in Washington DC. In J. Lipson and L.A. McSpadden (Eds.), *Negotiating power and place at the margins: Selected papers on refugee and immigrants,* Volume VII (pp. 198-231). Arlington, VA: American Anthropological Association.

Kent, D.R. and Felkenes, G.T. (1998). *Cultural explanations for Vietnamese youth involvement in street gangs.* Westminster, CA: Westminster Police Department, Office of Research and Planning.

Sherman, L.W., Gottfredson, D.C., MacKenzie, D.L., Eck, J., Rueter, P., and Bushway, S.D. (1998). Preventing crime: What works, what doesn't, what's promising. *National Institute of Justice: Research in Brief* (July). Office of Justice Programs. Washington, DC: U.S. Department of Justice.

Thornberry, T.B., Krohn, M.D., Lizotte, A.J., and Chard-Wierschem, D. (1995). The role of juvenile gangs in facilitating delinquent behavior. In M. Klein, C. Maxson, and J. Miller (Eds.), *The modern gang reader* (pp. 174-185). Los Angeles, CA: Roxbury Publishing Company.

U.S. Department of Health and Human Services. (2001). *Youth violence: A report of the Surgeon General.* Rockville, MD: U.S. Department of Health and Human Services, Centers for Disease Control and Prevention, National Center for Injury Prevention and Control; Substance Abuse and Mental Health Services Administration, Center for Mental Health Services; and National Institutes of Health, National Institute of Mental Health.

Valdez, A. (1997). *Gangs: A guide to understanding street gangs.* San Clemente, CA: LawTech Publishing Co., Ltd.

Vigil, J.D. (1988). *Barrio gangs: Street life and identity in Southern California.* Austin, TX: University of Texas Press.

Wasserman, G.A., Miller, L.S., and Cothern, L. (2000). Prevention of serious and violent juvenile offending. *Juvenile Justice Bulletin* (April). Office of Juvenile Justice and Delinquency Prevention. Washington, DC: U.S. Department of Justice.

Chapter 8

Weapons in Schools

David C. May

INTRODUCTION

To put it bluntly, I think students bring weapons to school to save their own lives. They have a constant fear of being attacked, whether for money, for drugs, or for some other reason. They feel they need to bring a weapon with them to school. ("Students speak out," 1988)

The preceding words were written by a 15-year-old student for *The Washington Post* on the subject of why other students felt the need to bring weapons into the school environment. The youth wrote that response in December of 1988, almost ten years prior to the shootings at Columbine High School which triggered the present concern for school safety. Nevertheless, though over fourteen years have passed since that response, some suggest the words still ring true today.

A "weapon" is any instrument used to attack another person (National School Safety Center, 1993). Although most citizens in the United States think of a firearm (or gun) when they hear the word weapon, there are a wide variety of weapons available to youths. Other weapons commonly found among adolescents include (but are not limited to) knives of various types, billy clubs, metal knuckles, straight razors, and box cutters. These other weapons cannot be ignored. Knives and other weapons play an important role in violent crime, particularly nonlethal violent crime, both at school and away from school. The U.S. Departments of Treasury and Justice (1999) report that for those offenders 17 and under who commit nonlethal crimes of violence, 5 percent use firearms, 6.9 percent use knives,

8 percent use other weapons, and 80 percent use no weapon at all. Simon (1996) reviews a number of studies which indicate that while most youth homicides can be attributed to firearms, knife assaults are more likely to result in nonfatal injury, and woundings from stabbings outnumber firearm-related injuries in some jurisdictions by over 300 percent. In addition, Louis Harris and Associates (1999) report that knives, razors, scissors, penknives, switchblades, pepper spray, and box cutters all outrank guns as the type of weapon that students tend to carry.

The presence of firearms and other weapons at school also influences the quality of education offered in public schools. Using data collected from the 50 states and their six territories, Gray and Sinclair (2000) report that 3,523 students were expelled under the Gun-Free Schools Act for the 1998-1999 academic year for bringing a firearm to school, a 4 percent reduction from the previous year. Three out of five expulsions (59 percent) were for bringing a handgun to school, while approximately one in eight (12 percent) was for bringing a rifle or shotgun to school, and approximately one in three (29 percent) was for some other type of firearm or "destructive device" (e.g., bombs, grenades, or starter pistols).

Recently, the general public appears to have developed the perception that the prevalence of weapons in and around schools has increased dramatically. Incidents such as those in Littleton, Colorado, Pearl, Mississippi, and Santee, California, have led many to believe that our schools are inundated with weapons and are no longer safe places for children to learn. This perception, however, directly contradicts empirical evidence to the contrary (Kaufman et al., 2001) and perceptions of students, teachers, and law enforcement officials nationwide that violence and weapons in public schools have decreased (Louis Harris and Associates, 1999).

In addition, during the 1998-1999 school year, which included the Columbine shootings, the National School Safety Center reported that there were 26 school-associated violent deaths—a 40 percent decline from the previous year. Furthermore, this number has continued to decline, so that in the 2001-2002 school year, there were only five deaths on school grounds (National School Safety Center, 2002). Since there are approximately 50 million students in America's schools, the odds of dying a violent death in a school in the United

States that year were one in ten million, making schools one of the safest places that children can be.

Crime among school-aged children (including weapons offenses) must be viewed in a context of crime among young people in the larger society as schools often are a microcosm of the larger area in which they are located. Thus, if crime among juveniles is decreasing in the larger society, it should be decreasing at school as well. This appears to be the case, as arrests of juveniles for murder fell 2 percent from 2000, and were 47.3 percent lower than 1997 and 62 percent lower than 1992. Juvenile robbery arrests also decreased 3.5 percent in 2001 and were down approximately 30 percent from 1992 (Federal Bureau of Investigation, 2002).

Despite the decline in violent crime among juveniles (those under age 18) (Federal Bureau of Investigation, 2002), violence still remains a problem. Homicide remains the third leading cause of death among youths, following motor vehicle crashes and other unintentional injuries (Grunbaum et al., 2002). In 2001, there were an estimated 1,402 murder victims who were under the age of 18.[1] Two in three (934) were male. Of the 1,402 murder victims under 18, 612 (43.7 percent) were killed with a firearm, 102 (7.2 percent) with a knife or cutting instrument, 58 (4.1 percent) with a blunt object, and 322 (22.9 percent) with personal weapons (hands, fists, feet, pushing someone to his or her death, etc.). Firearms were largely responsible for adolescent deaths, as three in four adolescents (aged 13 to 19) murdered in 2001 (75.8 percent) were killed with firearms (Federal Bureau of Investigation, 2002).

These numbers have caused many parents and other concerned citizens to feel that children today are more at risk than in previous years. This perception that violence is on the rise is particularly acute when parents are asked about the safety of schools in the United States. Brooks, Schiraldi, and Ziedenberg (2000) review a number of polls conducted in the late 1990s, including one that finds three in four (71 percent) Americans thought it was likely that a school shooting could happen in their community and three in five (60 percent) respondents reported school violence as an issue that "worried them a great deal." In addition, they review two polls conducted by Gallup for *USA Today* which indicate that respondents were 49 percent more likely to be fearful of schools in 1999 than in 1998.

Despite the fact that schools are one of the safest places for children, and crime among youth has been falling since the mid-1990s, parents are correct: schools are not without crime. In 1999, students ages 12 through 18 were victims of about 2.5 million total crimes at school, 186,000 of which were considered serious violent crimes (e.g., rape, sexual assault, robbery, and aggravated assault). Louis Harris and Associates (1999) suggest that these numbers may be even higher, as one in four public school students admitted that they had been the victim of a violent act in or around school. Nevertheless, the proportion of students in grades nine through twelve threatened or injured with a weapon on school property has not changed significantly in the past decade, as each year, about 7 to 8 percent of students reported being threatened or injured with a weapon on school property in the past year (Kaufman et al., 2001; Grunbaum et al., 2002).

Due to the emphasis given to school safety as a result of the perceived "upsurge" in school violence, many public schools now have the same appearance as prisons. Administrators feel that by reducing weapons in school, they can reduce the violence perpetrated with those weapons on school grounds. Sheley (2000) interviewed 48 school administrators from areas throughout the country and found that almost all (96 percent) had incorporated automatic suspension as punishment for weapons violations, and two in three (66 percent) had designated their school as a "gun-free zone" and had begun to use dress codes (63 percent). Sheley suggests that weapons in school are viewed by most school administrators, teachers, and parents as one of the most problematic aspects in a school setting and a major contributor to the violence in schools.

INCIDENCE AND PREVALENCE OF WEAPONS IN SCHOOLS

The incidence and prevalence of weapons at school and weapons at locations other than schools have been examined by numerous researchers using a wide variety of samples. With this wide variety of samples have come an equally wide variety of estimates as to the incidence and prevalence of weapons among adolescents, both at school and away from school. As is the case in many research efforts, measurement issues permeate the literature regarding weapons in schools. Measurement problems in the research concerning weapons in schools are fourfold:

1. Some researchers ask youths about lifetime possession of weapons while others ask about a shorter time period (usually 30 days, six months, or a year).
2. Some researchers ask youths about weapon ownership, not possession. Youths can and often do carry weapons they do not own; thus, an honest answer that they do not own the weapon would not count them as weapon possessors, although they may regularly carry that weapon.
3. Some researchers ask about possession and ownership of "weapons" while others ask about possession and use of "firearms" or "guns." Weapons is a much broader category.
4. Most important, some researchers ask youths whether they carry a gun/weapon but do not specify "to school"; others specify "to school" but do not specify "into the school building."

The combination of these four problems makes it difficult to compare one study with another without knowing how the researcher addresses each of the four measurement issues. As such, a somewhat detailed discussion of each of the studies reviewed for this chapter is provided as follows. A number of studies have used data collected from students throughout the United States to assess prevalence and incidence of weapon possession both at and away from school. These studies will be reviewed first, followed by a review of studies using smaller local or regional samples.

Grunbaum et al. (2002) and Kaufman et al. (2001) reported that among 13,601 students in grades nine through twelve in the United States, approximately one in five students (17.4 percent) had carried a weapon and one in 20 (5.7 percent) had carried a gun in the previous 30 days. In addition, 6.4 percent had carried a weapon on school property in that same time period. These numbers were lower than in 1993, when 22 percent carried a weapon anywhere and 12 percent carried a weapon at school. In a study of 15,877 middle and high school students from throughout the United States, the Josephson Institute of Ethics (2001) determined that one in five (21 percent) high school boys and one in seven (15 percent) middle school males took a weapon to school at least once in the past year. Using responses from 1,000 students from throughout the United States, Louis Harris and Associates (1999) determined that one in eight students had carried a weapon to school and one in 50 had fired a gun or used a knife on school grounds in the previous 30 days. Using data from 10,904 high school students collected through the 1995 Youth Risk Behavior Survey, Simon, Crosby, and Dahlberg (1999) determined that one in five adolescents had carried a weapon within the previous days and approximately one in ten (9.6 percent) carried a weapon on school grounds during that time period. Further, Forrest et al. (2000) examined data collected from 6,450 students in grades seven through twelve between 1994 and 1996 as part of the National Longitudinal Survey of Adolescent Health. In their sample, approximately one in ten students reported carrying a weapon on school property in the last 30 days. Among those who reported carrying weapons to school, two in three (65.7 percent) reported carrying a knife, while almost one in five (18.7 percent) reported carrying a gun to school. Finally, in a study discussed in detail next, Sheley and Wright (1995) determined that one in two (50 percent) incarcerated youths and one in eight (12 percent) inner-city high school students in various parts of the United States carried a gun outside the home all the time or most of the time in the one or two years preceding their confinement or the interview. Approximately 50 percent of the inmate sample carried a gun most or all of the time while 3 percent of the students reported carrying a gun to school all or most of the time (Sheley and Wright, 1995).

In summary, the studies that use data collected from national or seminational samples of adolescents indicate that about 10 percent of students had carried a weapon to school in the previous 30 days. Much smaller proportions (less than 3 percent) had carried a gun to school in the previous 30 days.

In addition to these studies using data from samples of students throughout the country, a number of studies have been conducted using smaller, regional samples as well. Using data collected in 1996 from 6,169 students in grades six through twelve from 21 schools in Kentucky, Wilcox-Rountree and Clayton (2001) determined that 4 percent of the students they surveyed had taken a weapon to school in the previous 30 days, while 2 percent of the students said they had taken a gun to school in the previous 30 days. Wilcox-Rountree (2000) examined data collected from 4,008 public high school students in grades six through twelve in three counties in Kentucky in 1996. She determined that 4.6 percent of her sample had brought a weapon to school in the past 30 days. When asked specifically about firearms, 1.4 percent (Urban County), 1.7 percent (Western County), and approximately 3 percent (Eastern County) responded that they had brought a firearm to school in the previous 30 days (Wilcox-Rountree, 2000). Using data collected in 1997 from a sample of 1,139 students in grades nine through eleven, Nofziger (2001) determined that 15 percent had carried a weapon on school property in the previous 30 days, and a slightly larger number (15.2 percent) had carried a weapon in the past 30 days. May (1999) analyzed results from a sample of 8,338 public school students in grades ten through twelve in Mississippi and determined that eight percent of the sample had carried a gun to school in their lifetime. Malek, Chang, and Davis (1998) analyzed results from data collected from 567 seventh graders in Louisiana and Massachusetts in 1991. They determined that one in three (34 percent) of the respondents in their study carried a weapon at least once in the past 30 days.

Webster, Gainer, and Champion (1993) used data from a sample of 294 black junior high students in Washington, DC, collected in 1991. Students were asked if they had "ever carried a gun with you for protection or to use in case you get into a fight?" and if they had "ever carried a knife with you for protection or to use in case you get into a fight?" (Webster, Gainer, and Champion, 1993, p. 1605). Nearly half of the males and just over one-third of the females had carried a knife for protection; one in four males and less than one in 20 females had carried a gun for protection. Sheley (1994b) determined that 12 percent of his sample of inner-city youths carried a gun routinely, and 23 percent carried a gun occasionally. Orpinas, Murray, and Kelder (1999) found that, among their sample of 8,865 sixth, seventh, and eighth graders in Texas, one in ten students had carried a handgun and one in four students had carried a weapon other than a handgun in the past 30 days. Simon et al. (1998) determined that, among their sample of 2,200 high school seniors in California, one in five (21.8 percent) boys and one in twenty (5.3 percent) girls reported carrying a gun in their lifetime. Bailey, Flewelling, and Rosenbaum (1997) determined that among a sample of 1,503 seventh and eighth graders in Illinois,

15 percent had brought a weapon to school in the previous month. In contrast, Callahan, Rivara, and Farrow (1993), using a sample of 89 incarcerated male youths in Washington State, determined that three in five detainees (59 percent) reported owning a handgun, and almost half (46 percent) had carried a gun to school. Limber and Pagliocca (2000), in a study discussed in detail as follows, determined that three in four (74.3 percent) incarcerated adolescent males had carried a handgun at some time in their lives, and almost half (43.6 percent) had carried a rifle or shotgun. In addition, Limber and Pagliocca (2000) also examined how often the males in their sample carried a knife or gun before they were incarcerated. Most carried a knife no more than a few times a year while most carried a gun a few times a month. Finally, 17.4 percent of the respondents stated they carried a gun to school now and then, while 6.5 percent reported carrying a gun to school most of the time, and 2.9 percent stated they carried a gun to school all the time. One in three (30.2 percent) carried a weapon other than a gun to school occasionally, 10.8 percent carried a weapon other than a gun to school most of the time, and 8.6 percent carried a weapon other than a gun to school all the time. The weapon other than a firearm carried to school most often was a pocketknife (20.1 percent), followed by brass knuckles (7.9 percent), switchblades (4.3 percent), straight razors (3.6 percent), and hunting knives (2.9 percent) (Limber and Pagliocca, 2000).

Hawkins et al. (2002) interviewed 1,465 students in an affluent (median household income of $68,790) community south of San Francisco. One in four males (26.4 percent) and almost one in ten (8.2 percent) females had carried a weapon "for protection or in case of a fight" during their lifetime. Three in five (59.2 percent) of those who carried weapons carried a knife or blade while approximately one in five (22.5 and 18.3 percent, respectively) reported carrying a gun or a weapon other than a gun or knife for protection as well. In sum, while the findings from the local and regional studies are more diverse, they provide more specific data not provided by the national studies. With the exception of the study done by Callahan and Rivara, it appears that between one in 50 and one in 15 students take guns to school in a 30-day period, while between one in 20 and one in ten students take weapons other than firearms to school in a 30-day period. Finally, the weapon of choice at school is generally some type of knife.

DEMOGRAPHIC AND CONTEXTUAL PREDICTORS
OF WEAPONS OFFENDERS

Despite the variation in prevalence and incidence of youth weapon possession both at school and away from school, a number of demographic and contextual predictors of weapons possession are identified in the literature. The vast majority of the researchers agree that males are more likely than their female counterparts to carry weapons, both at school and away from school (Bailey, Flewelling, and Rosenbaum, 1997; Callahan and Rivara, 1992; Durant et al., 1997; Grunbaum et al., 2002; Hawkins et al., 2002; Kaufman et al., 2001; Lizotte and Sheppard, 2001; Louis Harris and Associates, 1999; May, 1999; Simon et al., 1998; Wilcox-Rountree and Clayton, 2001), although some researchers have found nonsignificant gender differences in some contexts (Wilcox-Rountree, 2000). In addition, some researchers suggest that, among those youths who carry weapons, females are more likely to carry weapons to school than males (Simon, Crosby and Dahlberg, 1999) and blacks are more likely than whites to choose firearms as their weapon of choice for defensive possession (May, 2001).

The relationship between race and weapons possession is more ambiguous. Several researchers find no significant racial differences in weapons possession either at school or away from school (Kaufman et al., 2001; Simon et al., 1998; Wilcox-Rountree, 2000); others report that nonwhites are more likely than their Caucasian counterparts to carry weapons (Forrest et al., 2000; May, 1999; Simon et al., 1999; Wilcox-Rountree and Clayton, 2001). Other researchers have determined that the interaction between race and gender is also important in predicting weapons possession. Grunbaum et al. (2002) determined that black female students (8.6 percent) were significantly more likely than white female students (5.1 percent) to have carried a weapon, while white male students (31.3 percent) were significantly more likely than black male students (22.4 percent) to have done so.

The relationship between socioeconomic status and weapon possession is also ambiguous. Some researchers report that those of lower socioeconomic status are more likely to carry weapons to school (Wilcox-Rountree and Clayton, 2001) and in general (Simon et al., 1998), but one study suggests that those with higher socioeconomic status are more likely to carry weapons to school (May, 1999). Nevertheless, most research efforts (see Wilcox-Rountree and Clayton, 2001, for review) report that, after controlling for other demographic and contextual variables, socioeconomic status has little impact on weapon possession at school.

One of the clearest predictors of weapons possession both at school and away from school is gang membership, as practically all studies find that gang members are more likely than nongang members to carry and own weapons (Bjerregaard and Lizotte, 1995; Lizotte and Shepherd, 2001).

In addition, most researchers have determined that those who carry weapons, both at school and away from school, are more likely to engage in other deviant behaviors as well (Bailey, Flewelling, and Rosenbaum, 1997; Callahan and Rivara, 1992; Durant et al., 1997; Lizotte et al., 1994; May, 2001; Sheley and Wright, 1995; Simon et al., 1998, 1999; Webster, Gainer, and Champion, 1993; Wilcox-Rountree, 2000).

Some researchers also report that youths who had been previously victimized or threatened with victimization are more likely to carry weapons both to school (Simon et al., 1999; Wilcox-Rountree and Clayton, 2001) and away from school (Simon et al., 1999; Webster, Gainer, and Champion, 1993), although others find no relationship between victimization (either threatened or actual) and weapons possession (May, 2001; Wilcox-Rountree, 2000).

The relationship between age and weapons possession is also somewhat ambiguous. Some researchers suggest older youth are more likely than their younger counterparts to carry weapons to school (May, 1999) and away from school (Kaufman et al., 2001) while other researchers argue that the relationship between age and weapons possession is curvilinear, reaching its peak in grades nine and ten and then declining in grades eleven and twelve (Forrest et al., 2000; Wilcox-Rountree and Clayton, 2001; Wilcox-Rountree, 2000).

Finally, as mentioned previously, the vast majority of these studies indicate that protection is the primary reason youths carry weapons to school (see May, 2001, for review). Despite the fact that so many youths state that protection is the reason for their weapons possession, the relationship between fear of criminal victimization and weapons possession does not appear to support that argument, as most studies determine that fearful youths are no more likely to carry weapons than nonfearful youths (May, 2001; Wilcox-Rountree, 2000), although there are some exceptions (Durant et al., 1997).

In summary, the aforementioned studies show that those who carry weapons to school are significantly more likely to be male, gang members, involved in other delinquent activities, and carrying the weapon for protection. None of the demographic variables have an unambiguous relationship with weapons possession and thus appear to be dependent on either the contextual and structural factors of the sample under study or the measurement strategies of the researcher conducting the study.

WHERE DO JUVENILES OBTAIN THEIR WEAPONS?

Despite the ideological debate over the impact of guns in school shootings, one common area of concern has emerged: how do adolescents come to possess a firearm? Some of the school shooters alluded to earlier obtained their weapons from locked gun cabinets in their homes (most recently, Andy Williams in Santee, California, and Elizabeth Bush in Williamsport, Pennsylvania), however, many adolescents who possess firearms and other weapons obtain them from other sources. In fact, a substantial number of youths report they could easily get guns if they wanted to (Josephson Institute of Ethics, 2001; Kissell, 1993; Larson, 1994; Louis Harris and Associates, 1999; Page and Hammermeister, 1997; Sheley and Wright, 1995). This fact makes the question of adolescent weapon possession even more pertinent. Is it difficult for adolescents to obtain firearms and other weapons? Where do they obtain them?

Although a limited number of studies have focused on sources from which adolescents obtain firearms (May and Jarjoura, 2001), no studies exist that examine where students obtain knives, mace, clubs, and other weapons, the weapons most commonly found on adolescents in schools (Louis Harris and Associates, 1999). Anecdotal evidence suggests, however, that youths who carry these weapons buy them from retail outlets that sell those weapons legally or, in cases where the law forbids juveniles from owning those weapons (e.g., mace, some clubs in some jurisdictions), they obtain them from acquaintances or relatives. The studies that examine sources of firearms among adult criminals and youths are reviewed as follows.

Wright and Rossi (1986) were the first researchers to examine where criminals obtained their firearms. Using self-report data from a sample of 1,874 incarcerated male adults, they sought to estimate the prevalence of gun use and the means through which the respondents had obtained their most recent firearm. Three in four of the respondents admitted that they owned firearms. Of those that had owned a gun, the vast majority (87 percent) owned a handgun, the firearm most regularly used in firearm-related crimes (Federal Bureau of Investigation, 2002). Despite this fact, only 15 percent had applied for a permit to carry their handgun and only one in four of the handgun owners had registered any of their guns with police (Wright and Rossi, 1986).

Wright and Rossi then examined the means and sources from which the convicted offenders obtained their handguns. They determined that while one in three (309 of the 970) of the felons purchased their most recent handgun, only one in three (35 percent) handgun *purchasers* obtained their handgun from a source that would be concerned about the legality of the transaction (e.g., gun shop, pawnshop, hardware or department store). Two in three handgun purchasers (64 percent) purchased their handgun from either family or friends or from some "street source" (e.g., fence, off the street, drug dealer, or black market). In addition, one in three (32 percent) of the handgun owners stole their most recent handgun, while the remainder rented or borrowed (8.7 percent), traded for (7.5 percent), or received as a gift (8.0 percent) their most recent handgun. Consequently, the vast majority of the offenders (831 out of 939) obtained their most recent handgun from sources that would not be covered by any legislation that exists, either in 1986 or 2002. Furthermore, even among respondents who owned long guns, only one-third had obtained their most recent long gun from a retail outlet; two in three had not. Thus, Wright and Rossi (1986) argued that "regulations imposed at the point of retail sale miss the overwhelming majority of all criminal handgun transactions" (p. 185). A decade later, Harlow (2001) uncovered similar findings from interviews with state and federal prisoners.

A decade after the groundbreaking study by Wright and Rossi, Sheley and Wright (1995) extended the examination of firearm acquisition among convicted offenders to the realm of juveniles. Sheley and Wright (1995) provide a more detailed analysis of weapon use and acquisition among adolescents, using data collected in self-report surveys administered to 835 male inmates in six correctional facilities located in California, Illinois, Louisiana, and New Jersey and 758 male students in ten inner-city high schools in the United States. Their findings are discussed in detail in this chapter.

Sheley and Wright (1995) assessed how respondents would go about obtaining a firearm if they wanted one. Among the incarcerated youths, the most popular method of obtaining a firearm was "off the street" (54 percent). Almost one in two (45 percent) stated that they would borrow one from a family member or friend. Approximately one in three responded that they would "get one from a drug dealer," "get one from a junkie," or "buy one from a family member or friend." Less than one in five (17 percent) stated that they would steal one from a house or an apartment, while a slightly smaller number (14 percent) said they would steal one from a person or car. Thus, street sources and informal purchases and trades with family, friends, and acquaintances were the primary means through which the inmates would obtain their firearms (Sheley and Wright, 1995).

On the other hand, the most popular method of obtaining a firearm among the students was to borrow one from a family member or friend (53 percent). About one in three students stated that they would "get one off the street." Approximately equal numbers (one in four) would get one from a drug dealer, get one from a junkie, or buy one from a gun shop. Thus, among students, family members and friends were even more important sources of firearms than among the incarcerated youths; interestingly, students were also twice as likely (28 percent versus 12 percent) to state that they would "buy one from a gun shop" (Sheley and Wright, 1995). Thus, Sheley and Wright (1995) determined that not only do most incarcerated youths own guns immediately prior to their incarceration, both incarcerated youths and students can easily obtain these guns through illegal means.

May and Jarjoura (2001) partially replicated the Sheley and Wright study by interviewing 318 incarcerated adolescent males in Indiana in the summer of 1999. Their findings reveal a number of similarities to those of Sheley and Wright as just over 40 percent of the sample indicated that if they needed a gun, they would borrow a gun from a friend or relative. The proportion in their study reporting they would steal a gun from a car or house (14 percent) was also similar to results reported by Sheley and Wright. Several differences were found as well. Youths in the May and Jarjoura study were somewhat less likely to report stealing or buying a gun from a drug dealer or drug addict (about one in five compared with one in three in the Sheley and Wright study). A much smaller percentage reported getting the gun "off the street" (8.5 percent compared with over 50 percent in the earlier study). May and Jarjoura also determined that one in four (26 percent) stated that they would buy a gun legally, although it is unclear what the youths mean by "legally," as the majority of the sample could not purchase a firearm legally.[2]

Limber and Pagliocca (2000) interviewed 140 male youths in 1997 incarcerated in a secure juvenile justice facility in South Carolina. Sixty-nine had referrals for weapons offenses; 71 did not. Six of the youths had a school weapons charge as one of their most recent offenses, while 50 had a nonschool weapons charge as one of their most recent offenses. Finally, 84 had no current weapons offense. The boys were asked how and where they obtained their most recent firearm. Approximately two in five reported obtaining handguns most frequently from friends and from illegal means (e.g., a fence, "on the street," stolen from someone's home, or a "junkie"). Youths also reported obtaining handguns from family members (13.2 percent) or from a store or pawnshop (7.0 percent) (Limber and Pagliocca, 2000).

Approximately one in three youths stated that they obtained rifles (31.3 percent) and shotguns (32.9 percent) through illegal means, with the most common source being a drug dealer or junkie, while the same proportion of the sample said they obtained shotguns from friends. A slightly smaller proportion stated they obtained rifles from friends (26.6 percent) or family members (21.9 percent), while one in four (23.3 percent) indicated they obtained shotguns from family. One in twenty (5.5 percent) stated they obtained their shotgun from a pawnshop while approximately one in six (15.6 percent) stated they obtained their rifles from that same source (Limber and Pagliocca, 2000).

Table 8.1 compares the results across the studies. The findings from the studies indicate the following: Those youths who want firearms will not obtain them in legal transactions that can be deterred by

TABLE 8.1. Comparison of Sources of Firearms by Study

Authors	Rank-Ordered Method of Obtaining Firearm
Sheley and Wright (1995) student sample	1. Borrow from family or friend 2. Get one off the street 3. Buy one from family or friend 4. Get one from a drug dealer 5. Get one from a junkie 6. Buy one from a gun shop
Sheley and Wright (1995) inmate sample	1. Off the street 2. Family or friend 3. Get one from a drug dealer 4. Get one from a junkie 5. Buy from family member or friend
May and Jarjoura (2001) inmate sample	1. Borrow from friend or relative 2. Steal or buy one from a drug dealer 3. Steal or buy one from a drug addict 4. Buy it legally 5. Steal from a car or house
Limber and Pagliocca (2000) inmate sample	1. From friends 2. Illegal means (fence, on the street, etc.) 3. Family members 4. Pawnshop or store

regulation and enforcement. Youths who want firearms will go to illegal sources on the street or family or friends.

WHAT WEAPONS DO JUVENILES PREFER?

The groundbreaking study by Sheley and Wright (1995) reviewed earlier was the first to ask incarcerated juveniles about their firearm preferences. Sheley and Wright (1995) determined that 83 percent of the inmate sample owned a firearm at the time they were incarcerated. Among these youths, the most commonly owned firearm was a revolver (72 percent had owned one at one point in their lives, and 58 percent owned a revolver at the time of their incarceration). Two-thirds of the sample had owned automatic and semiautomatic handguns[3] at some point, with 55 percent owning an automatic or semiautomatic handgun at the time of their incarceration. About one-half of the youth owned a sawed-off shotgun, and 39 percent owned a regular shotgun at the time of their incarceration. Finally, about one-third of the incarcerated boys owned an assault weapon (i.e., military-style automatic or semiautomatic rifle) at the time of their incarceration.

Among the students, the results were almost as startling. Sheley and Wright (1995) and Sheley (1994b) determined that 22 percent of the student sample owned a firearm at the time they were interviewed. Among these youths, the most commonly owned firearm at the time of the study was an automatic or semiautomatic handgun (18 percent owned one at the time of their interview) followed by a revolver (15 percent). About equal numbers (14 percent) had owned a sawed-off shotgun, an unmodified shotgun, and a military-style weapon at some point in their lives; 6 percent presently owned a military-style rifle.

May and Jarjoura (2001) determined that the overwhelming majority (74.5 percent) of the youths in their sample who had used a gun in a crime used an automatic or semiautomatic pistol in the last gun crime they committed prior to their incarceration. As respondents were allowed to respond with more than one type of firearm, revolvers (30.3 percent) were the second most popular gun type used in crime, followed by shotguns (20.6 percent), automatic rifles (10.9 percent), and assault rifles (9.1 percent). These results are somewhat unexpected based on the findings from Sheley and Wright (1995). In the earlier study, the youths were about as likely to own revolvers as automatic or semiautomatic pistols at the time of their incarceration. As Sheley and Wright report, handguns are much more popular among the gun criminals than long guns (shotguns and rifles).

Limber and Pagliocca (2000) asked the incarcerated adolescent males in their sample which weapons they had ever possessed. Four in five (80.7 percent) had owned or possessed a handgun, while two in three (63.6 percent) had owned or possessed a rifle or shotgun.

Thus, once again, using four diverse samples, the aforementioned studies arrive at the same results. Juveniles who carry guns prefer handguns (either semiautomatics or revolvers), followed by sawed-off or unmodified shotguns, and, finally, rifles. As mentioned earlier, however, the weapon most preferred by youths is not a firearm; when weapons are carried to school, knives (whether switchblade, hunting, or folding) are the weapon most youths admit to taking to school. Thus, among firearms, the handgun is the weapon of choice to carry to school; among *all weapons,* the knife is the preferred weapon by those youths who carry weapons whether at school or away from school.

PROTECTION OR AGGRESSION: THEORETICAL PREDICTORS OF WEAPONS POSSESSION

A number of motives have been suggested to explain why juveniles carry weapons to school. These include: for protection from crime both en route and at school, as a status symbol, and because they want to hurt someone (Louis Harris and Associates, 1999). Understanding the motivation of young people is important so that programs can be designed to combat weapons at school. This is made more complex, however, because the reasons for carrying weapons to school are so diverse. As O'Donnell (1995) suggests, if self-protection is the primary reason for carrying weapons to school, the number of weapons in school can be reduced by measures that make students feel more secure in the school environment. These include (but are not limited to) metal detectors, random locker searches, and transparent book bags. On the other hand, increased security measures such as these are unlikely to deter those youths who carry weapons to school as just another criminal act for those involved in a web of delinquent and criminal activities.

As mentioned earlier, the most common reason offered for weapon carrying among youths is protection, assumably from crime and from other youths who possess weapons. Although protection is an often-cited reason for weapon possession among adolescents, few studies attempt to examine the etiology of weapon possession specifically for protection. Webster, Gainer, and Champion (1993) used data from a sample of 294 black junior high students in Washington, DC, collected in 1991. Students were asked if they had "ever carried a gun with you for protection or to use in case you get into a fight?" (p. 1605). They were also asked another question worded in the exact same manner with the only exception being that the word "knife" was substituted for "gun." Approximately half of the males and one in three females had carried a knife for protection; one in four males and less than one in twenty females had carried a gun for protection. Among both males and females, those who had been threatened or attacked with a knife or gun were more likely to carry knives for protection than their counterparts. Males who had been threatened with a gun or knife were more likely to carry guns. As such a small number of females (six in the sample) had carried firearms, no models were estimated for that group (Webster, Gainer, and Champion, 1993). DuRant et al. (1997), using data collected from a sample of 3,054 public high school students in Boston, examined the relationship between weapon possession at school ("During the past 30 days, on how many days did you carry a weapon such as a gun, knife, or club?") and fear of school crime ("During the past 30 days, how many days did you not go to school because you felt you would be unsafe at school or on your way to or from school?") (p. 362). After controlling for a number of other variables previously demonstrating a statistically significant association with weapon possession, they determined that students who had not attended school on six or more days in the previous month because of fear were over five times more likely to carry weapons to school (DuRant et al., 1997).

May (2001) assessed the relationship between fear of crime and weapons possession, and determined that the relationship between fear of crime and weapons possession (whether guns or other weapons) is not statistically significant. May (2001) uncovered a strong relationship between perceived neighborhood incivility and weapons possession, however, finding that those youths who perceive their neighborhoods as criminogenic are more likely to carry weapons for protection than their counterparts who do not, as do Simon et al. (1998). They suggest that the reason for the disagreement between the studies is due to the measurement of fear of crime and weapon possession used in previous research efforts.

This finding, coupled with research reviewed earlier, suggests that self-help theory may offer a viable explanation for weapon possession at school, at least among some youths. Simon (1996) suggests that self-help theory, a derivative of social control theory, can be used to explain weapon carrying among those who offer this as an explanation for their behavior. Based on social control theory, those who exhibit a weaker bond to society will be more likely to engage in violent forms of delinquency. Social control theorists suggest that only those individuals who have strong social bonds and attachments to society and social institutions (such as the family and school) are able to refrain from delinquent acts because these agencies express disapproval when individuals violate the norms of society. According to Hirschi (1969), there are four elements of the individual's bond to society: attachment, commitment, involvement, and beliefs. The more committed an adolescent is to the rules of society, and the stronger the attachment between the adolescent and society, the less likely the juvenile will be to engage in delinquency, such as weapons carrying.

Black (1983) argues that, following self-help theory, some individuals engage in behaviors to protect themselves or their interests when they feel that societal institutions are not protecting them well enough. Thus, following Black (1983), self-help theory would suggest that some individuals are motivated to engage in aggressive actions (weapons possession) as a response to real or perceived vulnerability to criminal victimization because they feel that societal institutions (namely law enforcement and school officials) do not offer them adequate protection from this criminal victimization.

Tests of the relationship between attachment to social institutions and weapons possession generally indicate that those attached to school and family are less likely to carry weapons (Bailey, Flewelling, and Rosenbaum, 1997; Durant et al., 1997; May, 1999; Wilcox-Rountree and Clayton, 2001). However, some determine that the relationship between attachment and weapon possession may be dependent on other demographic factors (Wilcox-Rountree, 2000).

Nevertheless, not all adolescents who carry weapons to school do so out of a heightened sense of vulnerability. Harris (1993, p. 15), in an analysis of data collected from 2,508 public and private school students across the United States, determined that those youths who had carried a gun to school in the past 30 days were twice as likely *not* to be worried "about being in danger of being attacked physically" as their counterparts who had not carried a gun in the past 30 days. As mentioned earlier, numerous studies suggest that those individuals who carry weapons, both at school and away from school, are more likely to engage in other forms of delinquency as well. Nevertheless, the nature of this relationship is not clear. Lizotte et al. (1994) suggest that weapons possession does not necessarily cause subsequent violent, firearm, and drug crime; youths who carry weapons (for protection or not) might just find it more convenient to commit crime. May (2001) concurs and argues that youths who carry weapons may be taking precautions to protect themselves from danger yet often place themselves at risk of greater danger of both criminal victimization and criminal participation.

Thus, there appears to be another explanation for weapons possession among youths. This explanation suggests that weapons possession is just another type of a series of criminal and delinquent behaviors in which some youths engage. Furthermore, youths who do carry weapons are not alone; they often associate with peers who engage in weapons possession and other delinquent behaviors. Youths who possess weapons often do so to impress friends or be accepted by peers (Louis Harris and Associates, 1999). They are more likely to have friends who possess and approve of weapons, be a member of a delinquent gang, use drugs, and engage in violent behaviors (Bailey, Flewelling, and Rosenbaum, 1997; Callahan and Rivara, 1992; Forrest et al., 2000; Sheley, 1994a,b; Sheley and Wright, 1995; Webster, Gainer, and Champion, 1993). Thus, it appears although self-help theory might explain weapon possession among some youths, differential association theory offers a valid explanation why other youths carry weapons.

DIFFERENTIAL ASSOCIATION THEORY

Differential association theory proposes that youths whose friends have values and beliefs that encourage breaking the law are most likely to engage in criminal and delinquent behavior, including weapons possession at school. Sutherland (1947) argued that people engage in deviant activity because of "an excess of definitions favorable to violation of law over definitions unfavorable to violation of law" (p. 6). Individuals learn to engage in criminal behavior through interactions with others (commonly referred to as peer groups or cliques) whose values and beliefs encourage breaking the law. This is the principle of differential association. Williams and McShane (1999) reviewed numerous studies testing differential association and concluded that association with peers who are criminal or delinquent is one of the strongest predictors of involvement in delinquency.

May (2001) has conducted two studies which tested the relationship between differential association and weapons possession. In one study, he determined that those youth who had friends with attitudes favorable to delinquency were more likely to carry both firearms and weapons other than firearms in general (May, 2001). In the other study, he determined that, even after controlling for all the demographic and contextual variables mentioned previously, differential association was second only to gang membership in predicting who carried weapons to school (May, 1999). In addition, Lizotte and Sheppard (2001) determined that those who have peers who own guns for protection are much more likely to own guns for protection than those who do not, even among gun owners. Furthermore, several researchers determined that those youths who perceive that a number of other youths carry weapons to school are more likely to carry weapons to school themselves (Bailey, Flewelling, and Rosenbaum, 1997; Simon, Crosby, and Dahlberg, 1999) as are those whose peers carry weapons (Wilcox-Rountree and Clayton, 2001).

It appears that weapon possession at school is based largely on two theoretical perspectives. The self-help/social control perspective suggests that some youths, who have weak bonds to social institutions such as family, schools, and religious organizations, perceive that these and other societal institutions do not offer them the protection from criminal victimization they feel they deserve. This fact, combined with their lack of concern for the rules (brought about by their weak attachment to these societal institutions), makes them more likely than their counterparts to bring weapons to school. The second (and somewhat complementary) theoretical perspective argues that some youths perceive that others are bringing weapons to school and have friends (often fellow gang members) that own weapons and often carry them to school. As such, they perceive that they should bring weapons to school as well and are thus more likely to engage in weapon possession at school than their counterparts who do not have these same definitions favorable to weapon possession at school.

PROGRAMS AND POLICIES
TO COMBAT WEAPONS IN SCHOOLS

As the National School Safety Center (1993) suggests, there is no magic formula to ensure that weapons are not found at school. Nevertheless, a wide variety of programs and strategies are available to reduce the prevalence and incidence of weapons at school. Several of these are discussed next.

One of the most effective methods for reducing the number of students who bring weapons to school is the creation of a "positive reporting climate" (National School Safety Center, 1993). In schools with positive reporting climates, students are encouraged to alert teachers and administrators when other students bring weapons to school. Schools can ease this process by providing staff and students a toll-free, anonymous hotline where they can report weapons offenses and other criminal activity. Hiring school resource officers who are trained in law enforcement and work well with young people can also contribute to this positive reporting climate, as can training teachers to emphasize that students who report illegal behavior of other students are not "rats," but are actually doing themselves and other students a favor by reporting the criminal behavior (National School Safety Center, 1993). A positive reporting climate is important to reduce weapon possession and other violent crime at school; in three of four school shootings examined by the Secret Service, the attacker told a friend, schoolmate, or sibling about his idea for a possible attack before actually attacking (U.S. Secret Service and U.S. Department of Education, 2002). It is quite possible that a positive reporting climate could have prevented some of those deaths.

Another popular response used by schools to prevent students from bringing weapons to school is the use of metal detectors, either stationary or portable (and sometimes both). Use of stationary metal detectors screens out weapons holders as they enter school; mobile metal detectors allow school security officers to expand school security to the parking lots and routes that lead to school property (Kenney and Watson, 1998). As the National School Safety Center (1993) suggests, use of metal detectors has both pros and cons. Metal detectors send a strong message to students that the school recognizes the serious nature of weapon possession at school and is seriously trying to solve that problem. Critics argue, however, that metal detectors create unrealistic expectations that one metal detector will completely cure the problem of weapons at school. Furthermore, metal detector programs are labor-intensive and expensive. Perhaps most important, however, is the constitutional question raised by the use of metal detectors: Does a metal detector search meet the reasonable expectation standard of the Fourth Amendment which courts have ruled is required by the Constitution?

Although Constitutional challenges to the legality of searches with metal detectors in schools are rare, they do exist. Only one lower-level New York court has ruled on this matter (*People v. Dukes,* 1990), and in that case the court upheld a metal detector search of a student at a New York City high school which was conducted according to guidelines established by the board of education in 1989. The court determined that the district had demonstrated a need for conducting such searches and had created detailed procedures for conducting searches; as such, the search was Constitutional.

Along with metal detectors, other popular intervention strategies also are considered intrusive by individual rights advocates. These methods include sweeps and locker searches, restrictions on book bags (e.g., allowing only clear plastic or mesh book bags), or even bans of book bags altogether. In fact, some schools provide two sets of textbooks for students, one for home and one for school. Furthermore, other schools have removed lockers based on the same premise (National School Safety Center, 1993).

Although the issue of right to privacy among public school students remains murky at best, most researchers and legal scholars suggest that the courts will uphold metal-detector and locker searches for weapons when the presence of a knife or gun has been reported. In addition, a federal court decision by Judge Robert Doumar (*DesRoches by Des-Roches v. Caprio* [1998]) provides additional clarification of this issue. According to Judge Doumar,

1. When school employees want to find property, they can search more than one student as long as they have reasonable suspicion that student has the property.
2. Schools should ask students for their consent prior to search.
3. Unless school employees have reason to suspect a student who does not consent to a search, they should not search that student (Dowling-Sendor, 1998), although there is less agreement when the issue is a locker search.

Thus, those schools that choose to use metal detectors, random sweeps, and locker and book bag searches to maintain security must understand the various legal issues surrounding their use and be careful to train their personnel to abide by those rules.

In an extensive review of school-based crime prevention programs, Gottfredson (1997) determined that there were three types of programs schools can effectively use to reduce crime and delinquency. The first type of program are "programs aimed at building school capacity to initiate and sustain innovation." These programs are designed to change decision-making processes or authority structures within schools by using teams of staff and (sometimes) parents, students, and community members to plan and carry out activities to improve the school (Gottfredson, 1997). One such program was developed by Kenney and Watson (1998) who developed a program to empower students to improve safety in schools by using problem-solving techniques to reduce crime, disorder, and fear on the school campus. Using this method, students use a four-step method commonly used in problem-oriented policing interventions to identify problems, analyze possible solutions, formulate and implement a strategy, and evaluate the outcomes of the intervention. Students and teachers work together to identify the greatest problems at school and develop strategies to reduce them. When compared with a control school, the experimental school had reduced fear of crime and actual criminal incidents. Although this program did not focus on weapons reduction exclusively, the tenets of this program can be used by school administrators to effectively reduce weapons in school as well as fear of crime and actual criminal incidents.

Gottfredson (1997) also determined that other programs are effective in combating school-related violence. In her review, programs that clarify and communicate norms about behaviors by establishing school rules and programs that improve consistency of rule enforcement were determined to effectively reduce school violence. The National School Safety Center (1993) suggests that schools should have clear policies with regard to weapons violations, including zero-tolerance suspension and expulsion policies for possession of firearms at school. Some districts also use expulsion for weapon possession, although critics of these policies argue that they are not an effective long-term solution because they remove students from school and put them and their weapons on the street with little potential for conformist behavior. An alternative to expulsion would be to develop alternative placement programs for youth who are found to have weapons at school (National School Safety Center, 1993).

Gottfredson (1997) also reports that programs which communicate norms through schoolwide campaigns or ceremonies also work to reduce crime and delinquency. Programs of this genre include activities such as posters, newsletters, and ceremonies during which students declare their intention to remain drug, alcohol, or violence free. Some well-known interventions in this category include schoolwide campaigns against bullying; Red Ribbon Week, sponsored through the Department of Education's Safe and Drug-Free Schools and Communities program; and student letter-writing campaigns to reduce violence and weapons in schools.

Finally, Gottfredson (1997) suggests programs that focus on comprehensive instructional strategies which teach a wide range of social competency skills (e.g., developing problem-solving, self-control, stress-management, decision-making, and communication skills) delivered over a long period of time also work in reducing crime and delinquency. Examples of these programs include the Communities in School program and Goldstein and Glick's (1987) Aggression Replacement Training program which uses structured learning, moral education, and anger management training to reduce weapons possession at school.

Another popular program to reduce weapons in school uses law enforcement officers or other security personnel to serve as deterrents for students who bring weapons to school. The National School Safety Center (1993) suggests that use of security personnel and law enforcement officers can effectively reduce weapons possession at school by meeting the following criteria: They (1) are trained in current law enforcement practices; (2) use the principles of community policing; and (3) communicate regularly with teachers, administrators, and students about their role in school safety to establish a positive reporting climate.

CONCLUSION AND POLICY IMPLICATIONS

One of the more interesting findings from the literature reviewed in this chapter concerns the lack of relationship between demographic and contextual variables when it comes to choice of firearm. One explanation for this finding is that guns and other weapons are a prevalent part of society and are readily available for juveniles. Those youths who desire to have a gun or other weapon may have so many sources from which to choose that there are no clear patterns of acquisition; when youths want firearms or weapons, they may simply go to the source most readily available, which in some cases could be a friend or relative, but in other cases might be a drug dealer or drug addict.

The implications of the previously reviewed literature concerning weapons in schools are numerous. First, most of the guns used by the juvenile offenders in the commission of a crime and by youths who take weapons to school are obtained illegally, either through family or friends, theft from the "street," or purchase from some other illegal source. Thus, existing gun laws, as presently enforced, will have little impact on this phenomenon. Second, guns are a prevalent part of the adolescent community; even when youths are not engaged in illegal activity or committing property crimes, many have guns with them. Third, the lethality of guns is an important determinant of choice of gun to be carried, as the firearm of choice is a semiautomatic handgun, a weapon that is both easy to conceal and extremely lethal.

The results of this research have important policy implications, primarily in the area of firearms. The primary focus of efforts to reduce gun violence among adolescents should focus on the removal of illegal firearms from the adolescent population at large. Lizotte and Sheppard (2001) report that there is sizable turnover in adolescent male illegal gun ownership; furthermore, youth who carry weapons are more likely to be involved in other forms of violent delinquency than their counterparts. As such, confiscating a single gun may stop several boys from possessing that gun over a period of time. This, in turn, could decrease gun possession among a large group of boys, and avert many serious crimes. The results of this study indicate, however, that introducing more gun legislation may not be the most effective mechanism to achieve this goal. There are a number of potentially effective strategies. First, targeted deterrence efforts, such as Operation Ceasefire in Boston (U.S. Department of Justice, 2000) that combine the efforts of school and court officials, law enforcement officers, and juvenile probation officers and share information and monitor students who have criminal records or who fail to complete aftercare programs successfully, should be replicated throughout the country. Second, criminal justice officials should use tracing and ballistic imaging to uncover and punish those who provide weapons to juveniles and strengthen criminal penalties for those who transfer handguns to juveniles (Sheley and Wright, 1995). Despite the rhetoric of both gun-control advocates and opponents that the black market in firearms is a major source of firearm problems among juveniles, law enforcement officials rarely give it the attention given to prostitution and narcotics. As such, local law enforcement officials, school administrators, and school resource officers should work together to trace the source of illegal weapons brought to school, particularly firearms. School officials should demand information about weapons sources from those students who are caught bringing weapons to school, perhaps using the idea of a lesser punishment for the offender if they reveal the source of the weapon. This increased attention given to "black market" sources of weapons and firearms may not reduce adolescent weapon possession immediately; nevertheless, if we could reduce the number of these dealers over time, it could potentially reduce firearm availability among adolescents in the future. Third, enforcement efforts should concentrate on the activities that surround the exchange of stolen weapons, not just the sources. We need to examine ways for law enforcement agencies to interrupt these methods of weapons transfer. In addition, efforts should be made to publicize the treatment of illegal weapons dealers who deal firearms and other illegal weapons to kids. Although the general public may overlook illegal weapons transfers to adults, few think children should have illegal weapons, particularly guns. This negative public reaction and the stigma that it brings to individuals who may run otherwise legitimate businesses, along with the positive reaction it would give to law enforcement and prosecutors and judges who punish these offenders may combine to reduce the problem of weapons among youths.

Finally, as May (2001) suggests, those youths who carry firearms regularly are likely to be involved in a web of activities that threaten both their own safety and the safety of others. We cannot be sure whether the ownership causes or is caused by the dangers of criminal activity. As May (2001) suggests, any attempt to disarm adolescents without offering alternative means of protection might drive those youths into gangs for self-protection, which defeats the purpose of disarmament in the first place. As Sheley and Wright (1995) suggest, there are simply too many youths with firearms to think that the cause and cure lies within the individual gun carriers; the problem is much larger than that.

In conclusion, steps need to be taken to reduce the demand for guns and other weapons. Limber and Pagliocca (2000) offer an innovative approach to reducing weapons possession and weapon-related violence. They asked an open-ended question to the incarcerated young males in their sample which gave them the opportunity to identify steps that could be used to keep kids from carrying and using weapons. Interestingly, only 16 percent indicated that nothing could be done, while only 5.7 percent "didn't know" what could be done. The most common suggestions were as follows:

- Prevention and early intervention initiatives (e.g., mentoring, violence prevention programs) (28.6 percent).
- Stricter regulation of firearms and weapons to make them more difficult to obtain (20.7 percent).
- More parental involvement and supervision (13.0 percent).
- Stricter punishments for weapons violations (7.1 percent).
- Increased surveillance at school (5.0 percent).

These young males believe that stringent punishments for those youths who carry and use guns are not an effective strategy for reducing gun use. They agree that convincing juveniles not to own, carry, and use guns and other weapons involves convincing them that they can survive in their neighborhoods and schools without being armed. Until we can do that, we will have little success in curbing the problem of weapons in school among adolescents.

NOTES

1. The FBI does not receive data from all jurisdictions. As such, they provide estimates for those jurisdictions from which they do not receive data. In addition, the statistics cited are statistics about the victim. These individuals were victims of both adults and adolescents.

2. Respondents were asked, "If I needed to get a gun, I would get one by . . ." "Buy it legally" was one of the item response options. The Gun Control Act of 1968 made it illegal for federal firearms dealers to sell handguns to persons under 21, and the Youth Handgun Safety Act of 1994 generally prohibited possession of handguns by anyone under 18. Although there is no age restriction on transfers from non-

licensed dealers (e.g., individuals who own guns) of rifles and shotguns, licensed dealers may only sell long guns to individuals over 18 (U.S. Departments of Treasury and Justice, 1999). Thus, it is probable that many of the youths who gave this response were unclear on the legality of firearms purchases and possession for adolescents.

3. Sheley and Wright (1995) offered the juveniles a list of firearms and asked them which they had owned and possessed. The types listed by Sheley and Wright were (1) hunting and target rifles; (2) military-style automatic or semiautomatic rifles; (3) regular shotguns; (4) sawed-off shotguns; (5) revolvers (also called regular handguns); (6) automatic or semiautomatic handguns; (7) derringers or single-shot handguns; (8) homemade guns (also called zip guns). Sheley and Wright categorized semiautomatic and automatic handguns in the same category. As Sheley and Wright note, most police authorities and criminologists find that juveniles are unable to make the technical distinction between the two and most juveniles who say they own automatic weapons actually own semiautomatic firearms (p. 39).

REFERENCES

Bailey, S. L., Flewelling, R. L., and Rosenbaum, D. P. (1997). Characteristics of students who bring weapons to school. *Journal of Adolescent Health, 20,* 261-270.

Bjerregaard, B. and Lizotte, A. J. (1995). Gun ownership and gang membership. *The Journal of Criminal Law and Criminology, 86*(1), 37-58.

Black, D. (1983). Crime as social control. *American Sociological Review, 48,* 34-45.

Brooks, K., Schiraldi, V., and Ziedenberg, J. (2000). *School house hype: Two years later.* Washington, DC: Justice Policy Institute. Available online at <http://www.cjcj.org.pubs/schoolhouse/ssh2.html>.

Callahan, C. M. and Rivara, F. P. (1992). Urban high school youth and handguns: A school-based survey. *Journal of the American Medical Association, 267*(22), 3038-3042.

Callahan, C. M., Rivara, F. P., and Farrow, J. A. (1993). Youth in detention and handguns. *Journal of Adolescent Health, 14,* 350-355.

Dowling-Sendor, B. (1998). Before you search that locker. *The American School Board Journal, 185,* 24-25.

DuRant, R. H., Kahn, J., Beckford, P. H., and Woods, E. R. (1997). The association of weapon carrying and fighting on school property and other health risk and problem behaviors among high school students. *Archives of Pediatric Adolescent Medicine, 151,* 360-366.

Federal Bureau of Investigation (2002). *Crime in the United States—2001.* Washington, DC: Government Printing Office.

Forrest, K. Y. Z., Zychowski, A. K., Stuhldreher, W. L., and Ryan, W. J. (2000). Weapon-carrying in school: Prevalence and association with other violent behaviors. *American Journal of Health Studies, 16*(3), 133-140.

Goldstein, A. P. and Glick, B. (1987). *Aggression replacement training: A comprehensive intervention for aggressive youth.* Ottawa, Ontario, Canada: Research Press.

Gottfredson, D. (1997). School-based crime prevention. In Sherman, L. W., Gottfredson, D., MacKenzie, D., Eck, J., Reuter, P., and Bushway, S. (Eds.), *Preventing crime: What works, what doesn't, and what's promising* (Chapter 5). University of Maryland: Department of Criminology and Criminal Justice, NCJ 165366. Available online at <http://www.cjcentral.com/sherrman/sherman.htm>.

Gray, K. and Sinclair, B. (2000). *Report on state implementation of the Gun-Free Schools Act: School year 1998-99.* Rockville, MD: Westat. (Prepared for U.S. Department of Education). Available online at <http://www.ed.gov/offices/OESE/SDFS/GFSA/gfsa9899.doc>.

Grunbaum, J. A., Kann, L., Kinchen, S. A., Williams, B., Ross, J. G., Lowry, R., and Kolbe, L. (2002). *Youth risk behavior surveillance—United States, 2001.* Atlanta, GA: Centers for Disease Control and Prevention. Available online at <http://www.cdc.gov/mmwr/preview/mmwrhtml/ss5104a1.htm>.

Harlow, C. W. (2001). *Firearm use by offenders.* Washington, DC: U.S. Department of Justice, Bureau of Justice Statistics (NCJ 189369).

Harris, L. (1993). *A survey of experiences, perceptions, and apprehensions about guns among young people in America.* Washington, DC: L.H. Research, Inc., Study 930019.

Hawkins, S. R., Campanaro, A., Pitts, T. B., and Steiner, H. (2002). Weapons in an affluent suburban school. *Journal of School Violence, 1*(1), 53-65.

Hirschi, T. (1969). *Causes of delinquency.* Berkeley, CA: University of California Press.

Josephson Institute of Ethics (2001). *2000 report card: Report #1 The ethics of American youth: Violence and substance abuse data and commentary.* Marina Del Ray, CA: Josephson Institute of Ethics. Available online at <http://www.josephsoninstitute.org>.

Kaufman, P., Chen, X., Choy, S. P., Peter, K., Ruddy, S., Miller, A. K., Fleury, J. K., Chandler, K. A., Plany, M. G., and Rand, M. R. (2001). *Indicators of school crime and safety: 2001.* Washington, DC: U.S. Departments of Education and Justice, NCES 2002-113/NCJ-190075. Available online at <http://nces.ed.gov/pubs2002/crime 2001/>.

Kenney, D. J. and Watson, S. T. (1998). *Crime in the schools: Reducing fear and disorder with student problem solving.* Washington, DC: Police Executive Research Forum.

Kissell, K. P. (1993). Guns on the rise in rural schools. *The Morning Call,* March 21.

Larson, E. (1994). *Lethal passage: How the travels of a single handgun expose the roots of America's gun crisis.* New York: Crown Publishers.

Limber, S. P. and Pagliocca, P. M. (2000). *Firearm possession and use among youth: Reanalysis of findings from a survey of incarcerated youth.* Electronic publication available online at <http://www.scdps.org/ojp/Reanalysis %20final %20report.pdf>.

Lizotte, A. J. and Sheppard, D. (2001). *Gun use by male juveniles: Research and prevention*. Washington, DC: U.S. Department of Justice, Office of Juvenile Justice and Delinquency Prevention (NCJ 188992).

Lizotte, A. J., Tesoriero, J. M., Thornberry, T. P., and Krohn, M. D. (1994). Patterns of adolescent firearms ownership and use. *Justice Quarterly, 11*(1), 51-73.

Louis Harris and Associates (1999). *The Metropolitan Life survey of the American teacher, 1999: Violence in America's public schools—five years later*. New York: Louis Harris and Associates.

Malek, M. K., Chang, B. H., and Davis, T. (1998). Fighting and weapon-carrying among seventh-grade students in Massachusetts and Louisiana. *Journal of Adolescent Health, 2*, 94-102.

May, D. C. (1999). Scared kids, unattached kids, or peer pressure: Why do students carry firearms to school? *Youth and Society, 31*(1), 100-127.

May, D. C. (2001). *Adolescent fear of crime, perceptions of risk, and defensive/protective behaviors: An alternative explanation of violent delinquency*. Lewiston, NY: Edwin Mellen Press.

May, D. C. and Jarjoura, R. G. (2001). Gun possession among adolescent male offenders: Where do they get their guns? Unpublished paper presented at the annual meetings of the North Central Sociological Association, April 7, 2001, Louisville, KY.

National School Safety Center (1993). *Weapons in schools: NSSC resource paper*. Malibu, CA: National School Safety Center.

National School Safety Center (2002). *School associated violent deaths*. Westlake Village, CA: National School Safety Center In-House Report. Available online at <http://www.nssc.org/savd.pdf>.

Nofziger, S. (2001). *Bullies, fights, and guns: Testing self-control theory with juveniles*. New York: LFB Scholarly Publishing LLC.

O'Donnell, C. R. (1995). Firearm deaths among children and youth. *American Psychologist, 50*(9), 771-775.

Orpinas, P., Murray, N., and Kelder, S. (1999). Parental influences on students' aggressive behaviors and weapon carrying. *Health Education and Behavior, 26*(6), 774-787.

Page, R. M. and Hammermeister, J. (1997). Weapon-carrying and youth violence. *Adolescence, 32*, 505-513.

Sheley, J. F. (1994a). Drug activity and firearms possession and use by juveniles. *The Journal of Drug Issues, 24*(3), 363-382.

Sheley, J. F. (1994b). Drugs and guns among inner city high school students. *Journal of Drug Education, 24*(4), 303-321.

Sheley, J. F. (2000). Controlling violence: What schools are doing. In National Institute of Justice Report, *Preventing school violence* (pp. 37-57). Washington, DC: National Institute of Justice Report (NCJ 180972).

Sheley, J. F. and Wright, J. D. (1995). *In the line of fire: Youth, guns, and violence in urban America*. New York: Aldine de Gruyter.

Simon, T. R. (1996). *Self-help and problem proneness as predictors of weapon carrying among adolescents*. Los Angeles, CA: University of Southern California Graduate School.

Simon, T. R., Crosby, A. E., and Dahlberg, L. L. (1999). Students who carry weapons to high school: Comparisons with other weapon-carriers. *Journal of Adolescent Health, 24,* 340-348.

Simon, T. R., Richardson, J. L., Dent, C. W., Chih-Ping, C., and Flay, B. R. (1998). Prospective psychosocial, interpersonal, and behavioral predictors of handgun carrying among adolescents. *American Journal of Public Health, 88*(6), 960-963.

"Students speak out: Why do some students carry weapons to school?" (1988). *The Washington Post,* December 1, p. M15.

Sutherland, E. H. (1947). *Principles of criminology* (Fourth edition). Chicago: J.B. Lippincott Company.

United States Department of Justice (2000). *National integrated firearms violence reduction strategy.* Washington, DC: Department of Justice.

United States Department of the Treasury and United States Department of Justice (1999). *Gun crime in the age group 18-20.* Washington, DC: Government Printing Office.

United States Secret Service and United States Department of Education (2002). *The final report and findings of the safe school initiative: Implications for the prevention of school attacks in the United States.* Washington, DC: United States Government Printing Office. Available online at <http://www.treas.gov/usss/ntac_ssi.shtml>.

Webster, D. W., Gainer, P. S., and Champion, H. R. (1993). Weapon carrying among inner-city junior high school students: Defensive behavior vs. aggressive delinquency. *American Journal of Public Health, 83*(11), 1604-1608.

Wilcox-Rountree, P. (2000). Weapons at school: Are the predictors generalizable across context? *Sociological Spectrum, 20,* 291-324.

Wilcox-Rountree, P. and Clayton, R. R. (2001). A multilevel analysis of school-based weapon possession. *Justice Quarterly, 18*(3), 509-541.

Williams, F. P. III and McShane, M. D. (1999). *Criminological theory* (Third edition). Upper Saddle River, NJ: Prentice-Hall.

Wright, J. D. and Rossi, P.H. (1986). *Armed and considered dangerous.* New York: Aldine de Gruyter.

PART III:
INTERVENTIONS IN CASES
OF SCHOOL VIOLENCE

On March 5, 2001, at approximately 9:22 a.m., a 15-year-old freshman at Santana High School opened fire from a rest room onto a busy quad while hundreds of students changed classes. Two students were killed. Eleven students were wounded. One student teacher and one campus supervisor were wounded. Based upon a survey conducted four days after the shooting, it is estimated that over 500 people were in harm's way and witnessed the shootings. From that moment on, the world changed for 1,774 students, 130 staff and faculty at Santana High School, and an entire community.

This account of the Santana High School shooting in San Diego, California, is the lead paragraph from Chapter 11 of this book. Even though educators, in collaboration with professionals in law enforcement and human service agencies, may work diligently to prevent school violence, some incidents are likely to occur. How to deal with and manage these incidents is a major challenge. These approaches to intervention will necessarily involve the domains of human functioning that Lazarus (1981) identified with the acronym BASIC ID: behavior, affect, sensation, imagery, cognition, interpersonal relations, and diet and physical functioning. Following is a cursory examination of how each domain helps to guide interventions in cases of school violence.

Behavior

When violence occurs at school, professionals must deal with the act or acts themselves to limit physical harm to individuals close to the event. Professionals must also deal with copycat violence sometimes associated with violent acts in schools. Professionals must also cope with and manage appropriately the behavior of media personnel who work to communicate circumstances surrounding significant acts of violence in schools. Most important, educators and law enforcement officials must learn from the violence and prevent similar acts in the future.

Affect

School violence creates a variety of emotional responses that demand both immediate and long-term attention. Significant violent acts that receive national and international attention, for instance, usually result in deep sadness, anger, and fear. Victims' family members and friends typically need access to counseling and spiritual guidance. Witnesses to the violent acts may need similar help. Entire communities, whether urban or rural, often experience emotional reactions that demand short-term or long-term care, depending on the intensity of the emotional reactions. Perpetrators of the violence also need extensive services, including legal and psychological help. In short, the emotional fallout from school violence, particularly from significant acts, demands complicated and thorough interventions.

Sensation and Imagery

The wide range of sensations and mental images associated with acts of school violence often demand serious interventions. Teachers, students, and parents sometimes experience nightmares and mental flashbacks from observing violent acts, particularly acts involving weapons and resulting in serious physical injury or death. Teachers and students often find it difficult to return to school facilities because of the images associated with significant violent acts. Counselors, social workers, and medical professionals are usually needed to help individuals recover from the sensations and images associated with serious acts of school violence.

Cognition

Violence seriously impairs the effectiveness of schools as places of learning and cognitive development. Violent acts mark schools as places of danger and insecurity, making it difficult for educators and students alike to think clearly and function effectively toward achieving the central mission of schools, namely academic learning. School administrators, in collaboration with teachers and other school staff members, need to take reasonably quick action to remedy security problems and to assure communities that a safe environment exists for academic activity to resume.

Interpersonal Relations

When violence occurs at school, educators need to find ways of rebuilding community spirit and make available adequate opportunities for students and adults in schools to be with one another to discuss and to learn from violence. Following violent acts at school, many students become suspicious of peers, especially peers who appear not to be part of the mainstream. On the other hand, acts of violence offer teachers and school administrators the opportunity to forge new bonds among students, and build communities that promote cooperation and closeness for safety. Furthermore, educators can use school violence as a means of breaking down cultural and racial barriers that may have existed prior to the acts of violence. Students are able to see safety as a common objective, crossing all boundaries that previously separated students.

Diet and Physical Functioning

The physical domain is at the core of school violence. When violence occurs, it often results in physical trauma observed by many in the school community. Following incidences of violence, school administrators and medical personnel need to demonstrate that physical safety is paramount to the mission of the school.

An Overview of Part III

Part III of the *Handbook of School Violence* evolved as the result of the emerging work of Shane Jimerson (University of California, Santa Barbara) and his colleagues Stephen Brock (California State University, Sacramento) and Robert McGlenn (practicing clinical psychologist in San Diego). They have provided a splendid foundation for understanding how to intervene when school violence occurs.

In Chapter 9, "Characteristics and Consequences of Crisis Events: A Primer for the School Psychologist," Brock and Jimerson identify situations that may require school crisis intervention. The chapter discusses various indicators of the need for crisis intervention. In Chapter 10, "School Crisis Interventions: Strategies for Addressing the Consequences of Crisis Events," Brock and Jimerson discuss interventions that are needed to (1) prevent and/or mitigate common stress reactions, (2) identify those who may develop psychopathology, (3) prevent and/or mitigate dangerous coping behaviors, and (4) provide appropriate referrals to mental health professionals. Finally, in Chapter 11, "Support Services Following a Shooting at School: Lessons Learned Regarding Response and Recovery," McGlenn and Jimerson note that "when responding to a shooting on campus, the capturing of the shooter, the bandaging of the wounded, and the uniting of the families is only the start of the road to recovery." This final chapter provides guidance for immediate crisis management as well as for both short-term and long-term mental health services to support those who are affected by a school shooting.

As the *Handbook of School Violence* Internet site evolves, practitioners, graduate students, and other scholars will be able to go online to critique and build on what is presented on how to intervene in cases of school violence. Individuals may follow the evolution of the handbook's Internet site at the following address: <http://genesislight. com/hsv%20files/>.

REFERENCE

Lazarus, A. A. (1981). *The practice of multimodal therapy.* New York: McGraw-Hill.

Chapter 9

Characteristics and Consequences of Crisis Events: A Primer for the School Psychologist

Stephen E. Brock
Shane R. Jimerson

The school psychologist's crisis-intervention roles and responsibilities have received increasing attention during the past decade (Brock, Lazarus, and Jimerson, 2002). For example, it has recently become a training, field placement, and credentialing standard (National Association of School Psychologists, 2000). Given this increased attention, it is important to ensure that a solid crisis intervention foundation is built for those who provide these services. This chapter attempts to help lay such a foundation by offering an overview of the characteristics and consequences of crisis events with special emphasis on their impact upon schools. First, this chapter addresses crisis event characteristics and identifies situations that may require school crisis intervention. Then it discusses indicators of the need for crisis intervention, including

1. common signs of distress,
2. crisis reactions and maladaptive coping strategies that indicate a need for immediate assistance from a mental health professional,
3. possible psychopathological outcomes related to crises, and finally,
4. consequences unique to crises that affect schools.

With this knowledge school crisis intervenors will be better able to recognize situations that require their services and the crisis consequences that are a focus of their interventions.

WHAT IS A CRISIS? SITUATIONS THAT MAY REQUIRE SCHOOL CRISIS INTERVENTION [1]

Students face many school problems that might be referred to as "crises." These events range from failing a test to a playground fight. Although stressful, and often labeled as "traumatic," most of these events do not require crisis intervention. Given this fact, it is important for school crisis intervenors to understand the characteristics of events that may require their services. By understanding these characteristics intervenors will be able to distinguish between potentially traumatic events and those that are simply "stressful." Without this knowledge, crisis response resources may be inappropriately allocated.

The diagnostic criteria for post-traumatic stress disorder (PTSD) describe the essential features of crisis events. According to the *Diagnostic and Statistical Manual of Mental Disorders,* Fourth Edition, Text Revision (American Psychiatric Association, 2000) extreme traumatic stressors from trauma include (1) having an experience, (2) being in a place to observe an incident, and/or (3) acquiring some knowledge about an incident that involves death or injury and/or the threat of death or injury. Obviously, these events are not a part of the usual range of school experience (Everly and Mitchell, 2000; Silverman and La Greca, 2002). In fact, they are so far from the ordinary that they overwhelm previously developed problem-solving or coping strategies (Everly and Mitchell, 2000; Herman, 1992; Young, 1998). In other words, they present students with problems that (at least initially) appear to be without any solution.

Brock (2002a) provides further discussion of the characteristics of crisis events. Based on both practical experiences and other sources (Carlson, 1997; Matsakis, 1994; Slaikeu, 1990), Brock suggested that crisis events are extremely negative, uncontrollable, depersonalizing, and sudden and unexpected. Box 9.1 provides a summary of each of these characteristics.

From the description of these crisis event characteristics and several other sources (Carlson, 1997; Green, 1993; Matsakis, 1994; Slai-

BOX 9.1. Crisis Event Characteristics

Extremely negative—The primary characteristic of a crisis event is that it is perceived as being extremely negative (American Psychiatric Association, 2000; Carlson, 1997). These events have the potential to generate extreme pain. Specifically, they may cause physical pain, emotional pain, or be viewed as having the potential to cause such pain.

Uncontrollable—A crisis event generates feelings of helplessness, powerlessness, and/or entrapment (American Psychiatric Association, 2000; Carlson, 1997; Matsakis, 1994). Crises make people feel that they have lost control over their lives.

Depersonalizing—Crisis events strip away individuality and humanity (Matsakis, 1994). At the moment of the crisis, an individual's self-worth and value have very little meaning. Although degree of impact will vary, these events typically result in some stress reaction in all persons regardless of their prior level of physical and mental health (Silverman and La Greca, 2002).

Unpredictable—Crisis events typically occur suddenly, unexpectedly, and without warning. A key factor that makes the event traumatic is the relative lack of time to adjust or adapt to crisis-generated problems (Carlson, 1997).

Note: Adapted from S. E. Brock (2002a), Crisis Theory: A Foundation for the Comprehensive School Crisis Response Team. In S. E. Brock, P. J. Lazarus, and S. R. Jimerson (Eds.), *Best Practices in School Crisis Prevention and Intervention* (pp. 5-17). Bethesda, MD: National Association of School Psychologists.

keu, 1990; Young, 1998), Brock, Sandoval, and Lewis (2001) offer six classifications of crisis events. These classifications are severe illness or injury, violent and/or unexpected death, threatened death and/or injury, acts of war and/or terrorism, natural disasters, and man-made/industrial disasters. Examples of specific events that fall into each of these categories are provided in Table 9.1. People who experience or witness one of these events, or learn about a significant other being exposed to such an event, are potential psychological trauma victims and *may* require support and assistance from crisis intervenors. These crisis types do not have equivalent traumatizing

TABLE 9.1. Crisis Event Classifications and Examples

Classification	Examples
Severe illness and/or Injury	Life-threatening illnesses; disfigurement and dismemberment; road, train, and maritime accidents; assaults; suicide attempts; fires/arson; explosions
Violent and/or unexpected death	Sudden fatal illnesses; fatal accidents; homicides; suicides; fires/arson; explosions
Threatened death and/or injury	Human aggression (e.g., robbery, mugging, or rape); domestic violence (e.g., child and spouse abuse); kidnappings
Acts of war and/or terrorism	Invasions; terrorist attacks; taking hostages; prisoners of war; torture; hijackings
Natural disasters	Hurricanes; floods; fires; earthquakes; tornadoes; avalanches/landslides; volcanic eruptions; lightning strikes; tsunami
Man-made/industrial disasters	Nuclear accidents; airline crashes; exposure to noxious agents/toxic waste; dam failures; electrical fires; construction/plant accidents

Source: Adapted from S. E. Brock, J. Sandoval, and S. Lewis (2001), *Preparing for Crises in the Schools: A Manual for Building School Crisis Response Teams* (Second Edition). New York: Wiley.

potential. Some carry greater risk for psychological trauma than do others. For example, with all other conditions being equal (i.e., similar physical impact), acts of war or assaultive violence are much more traumatic than natural disasters. In addition, each event presents unique problems, issues, and crisis-response concerns. For example, events that involve sudden and unexpected death will be complicated by grief reactions. For a further discussion of the traumatizing potential of specific crisis events refer to Brock (2002b).

THE EFFECTS OF CRISES: REASONS FOR PROVIDING SCHOOL CRISIS INTERVENTION

Although the occurrence of a crisis event should prompt *consideration* of the need to provide school crisis intervention, an event in and of itself is insufficient to justify *provision* of a school crisis intervention. Rather it is the effect of the crisis that provides the rationale for provision of services. The following section reviews the adverse effects of crisis events that may signal the need to provide one or more school crisis intervention services.

Common Signs of Distress

The majority of people exposed to a crisis event will be distressed (Litz et al., 2002), and common signs of these stress reactions are provided in Box 9.2. When considering this list remember that a given crisis event will not involve the same type and intensity of crisis experience for all survivors, and that all survivors bring a different personal history of trauma into the disaster. Recognize that the developmental age and history of individuals will impact reactions to a crisis event (Pfohl, Jimerson, and Lazarus, 2002). Thus, individuals exposed to the same crisis event will have their own unique experiences and crisis reactions (Young et al., 1998). In addition, not all students and staff members will require an immediate school crisis intervention to cope with or manage their stress reactions. In fact, a guiding principle of crisis intervention should be to expect individuals to recover from these reactions (National Institute of Mental Health, 2002). With these cautions in mind, providing assistance and support (as needed) to students and staff who display these reactions is an important function of school crisis intervention.

Crisis Reactions That Indicate the Need for a Mental Health Referral

For most people, the initial distress generated by a crisis event will gradually decrease over time (Foa et al., 2001). However, some individuals (typically a minority of those exposed to a crisis event) will have persistent psychological problems that will require psychotherapeutic intervention. In general, the diagnosis of acute stress disorder has been found to be a powerful predictor of later psychopathology (post-traumatic stress disorder in particular; see Litz et al., 2002). More specifically, crisis reactions that might signal the impending development of a psychopathology are provided in Box 9.3. Ensuring

BOX 9.2.
Common Signs of Distress
Following Exposure to a Crisis Event

Emotional Effects

Shock
Anger
Despair
Emotional numbing
Terror/fear
Guilt
Phobias

Depression or sadness
Grief
Irritability
Hypersensitivity
Helplessness/hopelessness
Loss of pleasure from activities
Dissociation[a]

Cognitive Effects

Impaired concentration
Impaired decision-making
    ability
Memory impairment
Disbelief
Confusion
Distortion

Decreased self-esteem
Decreased self-efficacy
Self-blame
Intrusive thoughts/memories[b]
Worry
Nightmares

Physical Effects

Fatigue
Insomnia
Sleep disturbance
Hyperarousal
Somatic complaints
Startle response

Impaired immune response
Headaches
Gastrointestinal problems
Decreased appetite
Decreased libido

Interpersonal/Behavioral Effects

Alienation
Social withdrawal/isolation
Increased relationship conflict
Vocational impairment
Refusal to go to school
School impairment
Avoiding reminders

Crying easily
Change in eating patterns
Tantrums
Regression in behavior
Risk taking
Aggression

Sources: B. H. Young et al. (1998), *Disaster Mental Health Services: A Guide for Clinicians and Administrators,* Palo Alto, CA: National Center for Post Traumatic Stress Disorder; and A. H. Speier (2000), *Psychosocial Issues for Children and Adolescents in Disasters* (Second Edition), Washington, DC: U.S. Department of Health and Human Services.

Notes: [a]Examples include perceptual experience, e.g., "dreamlike," "tunnel vision," "spacey," or on "automatic pilot"; [b]Reenactment play among children.

**BOX 9.3.
Crisis Reactions That Indicate the Need
for a Mental Health Referral**

Dissociation—depersonalization, derealization, numbing, reduced awareness of surroundings, amnesia

Intrusive reexperiencing[a]—flashbacks, terrifying memories or nightmares, repetitive automatic reenactment

Avoidance—agoraphobic-like social withdrawal, isolation

Hyperarousal—panic episodes, startle reactions, fighting or temper problems

Anxiety—debilitating worry, nervousness, vulnerability or powerlessness

Depression—anhedonia, worthlessness, loss of interest in most activities, awakening early, persistent fatigue, lack of motivation

Psychotic symptoms—delusions, hallucinations, bizarre thoughts or images, catatonia

Source: Adapted from B. H. Young et al. (1998), *Disaster Mental Health Services: A Guide for Clinicians and Administrators,* Palo Alto, CA: National Center for Post Traumatic Stress Disorder.

Note: [a]It is important to acknowledge that among younger children symptoms of reexperiencing the trauma may be primarily displayed through reenacting play (Almqvist and Brandell-Forsberg, 1997) and is considered pathological only when it appears to be repetitive and automatic (Vogel and Vernberg, 1993).

---

that referral for professional mental health assistance has been offered to those who display these reactions is also an important function of school crisis intervention.

In addition to the reactions previously described, maladaptive coping strategies that present acute risk of harm to self or others may also emerge as a consequence of exposure to crisis events (American Red Cross, 1991; Azarian and Skriptchenko-Gregorian, 1998; Berman et al., 1996; Matsakis, 1994; de Wilde and Kienhorst, 1998). The presence of maladaptive coping strategies, such as those presented in the following list, also signals the need for an immediate mental health referral.

- Extreme substance abuse
- Self-medication
- Suicidal ideation
- Homicidal ideation
- Inappropriate anger toward others
- Abuse of others

Possible Psychopathological Consequences of Crisis Event Exposure

Post-traumatic stress disorder (PTSD) is the most common psychopathology associated with exposure to a crisis event. However, it is not the only diagnosis linked with such exposure (Green, 1994). Following is a list of the psychopathologies that may afflict individuals following crises. Ensuring that ongoing psychotherapeutic assistance has been provided to those who have these conditions is another important function of school crisis intervention.

Anxiety disorders (e.g., acute and post-traumatic stress disorders, panic disorder)
Substance-related disorders (e.g., substance dependence)
Dissociative disorders (e.g., dissociative amnesia)
Mood disorders (e.g., major depressive episode/disorder)
Sleep disorders (e.g., insomnia, sleep terror disorder)
Adjustment disorders (e.g., adjustment disorder with depressed mood)

Although these psychopathological outcomes are typically found among only a minority of those exposed to the crisis event, the exact percentage of the population who will have such outcomes will vary. Some events are more traumatic than others (Brock, 2002b). All other factors being equal (e.g., threat perceptions, relationships with crisis victims, proximity to the crisis, etc.), man-made crisis events (especially those that involve assaultive violence) are associated with a higher rate of psychopathology than are natural disasters. Furthermore, the number of individuals who develop a psychopathology will depend upon a complex interaction between the nature of the crisis event and the survivor's unique crisis experiences and personal vulnerabilities (Brock, 2002c; Pfohl, Jimerson, and Lazarus, 2002).

Exposure to a crisis event is necessary to trigger postcrisis psycho-pathology; however, it is not sufficient to explain its onset (McFarlane, 1988).

Crisis Effects Unique to the School Setting

In addition to the effects already mentioned, other consequences of crisis events are relatively unique to the school setting. In fact, disruptive behavior at school may be the primary outcome of exposure to a crisis event. These unique crisis effects include school absenteeism (Azarian and Skriptchenko-Gregorian, 1998; Silverman and La Greca, 2002); school behavior problems, such as aggressive, delinquent, and/or criminal behavior (Azarian and Skriptchenko-Gregorian, 1998; Carlson, 1997; Monahon, 1993; Nader and Muni, 2002); academic failure (Nader, 1999; Nader and Muni, 2002; Silverman and La Greca, 2002; Vogel and Vernberg, 1993; Yule, 1998), and exacerbation of preexisting educational problems (Vogel and Vernberg, 1993). Preventing, mitigating, and/or providing assistance and support to students and staff who demonstrate these effects is an important function of school crisis intervention.

CONCLUDING COMMENTS

The possible effects of crisis events identified in this chapter are by no means exhaustive, however, the effects of exposure to crises are quite varied. Effects that may require school crisis intervention include common stress reactions, and possible psychopathology and maladaptive coping strategies. In addition, school crisis intervention should include strategies that address those crisis issues or problems that are relatively unique to the school setting. Thus, the school crisis response should be multifaceted and capable of addressing a variety of crisis problems.

NOTE

1. Adapted from S. E. Brock (2000a). Crisis theory: A foundation for the comprehensive school crisis response team. In S. E. Brock, P. J. Laxarus, and S. R. Jimerson (Eds.), *Best practices in school crisis prevention and intervention* (pp. 5-17). Bethesda, MD: National Association of School Psychologists.

REFERENCES

Almqvist, K. and Brandell-Forsberg, M. (1997). Refugee children in Sweden: Post-traumatic stress disorder in Iranian preschool children exposed to organized violence. *Child Abuse and Neglect, 21,* 351-366.

American Psychiatric Association (2000). *Diagnostic and statistical manual of mental disorders* (Fourth edition, Text revision). Washington, DC: American Psychiatric Association.

American Red Cross (1991). *Disaster services regulations and procedures* (ARC Document 3050M). Washington, DC: Author.

Azarian, A. and Skriptchenko-Gregorian, V. (1998). Traumatization and stress in child and adolescent victims of natural disasters. In T. W. Miller (Ed.), *Children of trauma: Stressful life events and their effects on children and adolescents* (pp. 77-118). Madison, CT: International Universities Press.

Berman, S. L., Kurtines, W. M., Silverman, W. K., and Serafini, L. T. (1996). The impact of exposure to crime and violence on urban youth. *American Journal of Orthopsychiatry, 66,* 329-336.

Brock, S. E. (2002a). Crisis theory: A foundation for the comprehensive school crisis response team. In S. E. Brock, P. J. Lazarus, and S. R. Jimerson (Eds.), *Best practices in school crisis prevention and intervention* (pp. 5-17). Bethesda, MD: National Association of School Psychologists.

Brock, S. E. (2002b). Estimating the appropriate crisis response. In S. E. Brock, P. J. Lazarus, and S. R. Jimerson, (Eds.), *Best practices in school crisis prevention and intervention* (pp. 355-366). Bethesda, MD: National Association of School Psychologists.

Brock, S. E. (2002c). Identifying individuals at risk for psychological trauma. In S. E. Brock, P. J. Lazarus, and S. R. Jimerson (Eds.), *Best practices in school crisis prevention and intervention* (pp. 367-384). Bethesda, MD: National Association of School Psychologists.

Brock, S. E., Lazarus, P. J., and Jimerson, S. R. (Eds.) (2002). *Best practices in school crisis prevention and intervention.* Bethesda, MD: National Association of School Psychologists.

Brock, S. E., Sandoval, J., and Lewis, S. (2001). *Preparing for crises in the schools: A manual for building school crisis response teams* (Second edition). New York: Wiley.

Carlson, E. B. (1997). *Trauma assessments: A clinician's guide.* New York: Guilford Press.

de Wilde, E. J., and Kienhorst, C. W. M. (1998). Life events and adolescent suicidal behavior. In T. W. Miller (Ed.), *Children of trauma: Stressful life events and their effects on children and adolescents* (pp. 161-178). Madison, CT: International Universities Press.

Everly, G. S. and Mitchell, J. T. (2000). The debriefing "controversy" and crisis intervention: A review of lexical and substantive issues. *International Journal of Emergency Mental Health, 2,* 211-225.

Foa, E. B., Hebree, E. A., Riggs, D., Rauch, S., and Franklin, M. (2001). Guidelines for mental health professionals' response to the recent tragic events in the U.S. Retrieved November 11, 2001, from <http://www.ncptsd.org/facts/disasters/ fs_ foa_advice.html>.

Green, B. L. (1993). Identifying survivors at risk: Trauma and stressors across events. In J. P. Wilson and B. Raphael (Eds.), *International handbook of traumatic stress syndromes* (pp. 135-144). New York: Plenum Press.

Green, B. L. (1994). Psychosocial research in traumatic stress: An update. *Journal of Traumatic Stress, 7,* 341-361.

Herman, J. (1992). *Trauma and recovery.* New York: Basic Books.

Litz, B. T., Gray, M. J., Bryant, R. A., and Adler, A. B. (2002). Early intervention for trauma: Current status and future directions. *Clinical Psychology: Science and Practice, 9,* 112-134.

Matsakis, A. (1994). *Post-traumatic stress disorder: A complete treatment guide.* Oakland, CA: New Harbinger.

McFarlane, A. C. (1988). The longitudinal course of posttraumatic morbidity: The range of outcomes and their predictors. *The Journal of Nervous and Mental Disease, 176,* 30-39.

Monahon, C. (1993). *Children and trauma: A guide for parents and professionals.* San Francisco: Jossey-Bass.

Nader, K. (1999). *Psychological first aid for trauma, grief, and traumatic grief* (Third edition). Austin, TX: Two Suns.

Nader, K. and Muni, P. (2002). Individual crisis intervention. In S. E. Brock and P. J. Lazarus (Eds.), *Best practices in school crisis prevention and intervention* (pp. 405-428). Bethesda, MD: National Association of School Psychologists.

National Association of School Psychologists (2000). *Domains of school psychology training and practice.* Bethesda, MD: Author.

National Institute of Mental Health (2002). *Mental health and mass violence: Evidence-based early psychological intervention for victims/survivors of mass violence. A workshop to reach consensus on best practices* [NIH Publication No. 02-5138]. Washington, DC: U.S. Government Printing Office.

Pfohl, W., Jimerson, S. R., and Lazarus, P. J. (2002). Developmental aspects of psychological trauma and grief. In S. E. Brock, P. J. Lazarus, and S. R. Jimerson (Eds.), *Best practices in school crisis prevention and intervention* (pp. 309-332). Bethesda, MD: National Association of School Psychologists.

Silverman, W. K. and La Greca, A. M. (2002). Children experiencing disasters: Definitions, reactions, and predictors of outcomes. In A. M. La Greca, W. K. Silverman, E. M. Vernberg, and M. C. Roberts (Eds.), *Helping children cope with disasters and terrorism* (pp. 11-33). Washington, DC: American Psychological Association.

Slaikeu, K. A. (1990). *Crisis intervention: A handbook for practice and research* (Second edition). Newton, MA: Allyn & Bacon.

Speier, A. H. (2000). *Psychosocial issues for children and adolescents in disasters* (Second edition). Washington, DC: U.S. Department of Health and Human Services.

Vogel, J. M. and Vernberg, E. M. (1993). Children's psychological responses to disasters. *Journal of Clinical Child Psychology, 22,* 464-484.

Young, B. H., Ford, J. D., Ruzek, J. I., Friedman, M., and Gusman, F. D. (1998). *Disaster mental health services: A guide for clinicians and administrators.* Palo Alto, CA: National Center for Post Traumatic Stress Disorder.

Young, M. A. (1998). *The community crisis response team training manual* (Second edition). Washington, DC: National Organization for Victim Assistance.

Yule, W. (1998). Posttraumatic Stress Disorder in children and its treatment. In T. W. Miller (Ed.), *Children of trauma: Stressful life events and their effects on children and adolescents* (pp. 219-244). Madison, CT: International Universities Press.

Chapter 10

School Crisis Interventions: Strategies for Addressing the Consequences of Crisis Events

Stephen E. Brock
Shane R. Jimerson

A number of adverse outcomes are potentially associated with exposure to a crisis event. Given this fact it is not surprising that a variety of school crisis interventions are required to meet school community needs following crises. Interventions will be needed to

1. prevent and/or mitigate common stress reactions,
2. identify those who may develop psychopathology (e.g., post-traumatic stress disorder, depression),
3. prevent and/or mitigate dangerous coping behaviors (e.g., suicidal and homicidal behaviors), and
4. provide appropriate referrals to mental health professionals.

In addition, *school* crisis interventions need to address problems that are relatively unique to the school setting. These include truancy, poor school adjustment (e.g., aggressive and/or delinquent behavior), academic failure, and the exacerbation of preexisting educational problems (Brock and Jimerson, 2004). School crisis interventions that are able to address these crises outcomes and problems would be considered successful (Brock, 2002c).

To facilitate the provision of school crisis interventions, this chapter provides a chronology of crisis intervention efforts, and discusses specific crisis intervention activities, related goals, and relevant research; and then concludes with a discussion of multicomponent crisis intervention. This information is intended to facilitate the training of educational professionals for crisis intervention work.

CHRONOLOGY OF CRISIS INTERVENTION

Recognizing that the form and content of school crisis interventions will change over time (National Institute of Mental Health, 2002; Vernberg, 2002), this discussion of school crisis intervention employs a chronological system that divides crisis events into five phases (Valent, 2000). These phases are as follows:

1. Preimpact (the period before the crisis)
2. Impact (when the crisis occurs)
3. Recoil (immediately after the crisis event)
4. Postimpact (days to weeks after the crisis event)
5. Recovery and reconstruction (months or years after the event)

Making use of this system, Figure 10.1 provides an illustration of when the different school crisis interventions occur. In the pages that follow each of these interventions will be discussed and the empirical supports for their provision will be identified. In addition, future research needs related to each of the school crisis interventions will be identified.

SPECIFIC CRISIS INTERVENTIONS

As illustrated in Figure 10.1, the specific school crisis interventions discussed in this chapter include (1) crisis preparedness, (2) immediate prevention, (3) medical intervention, (4) reestablishment of family and social support systems, (5) risk screening and referral, (6) psychological education, (7) psychological intervention, and (8) rituals and memorials. The following outline lists the various activities, goals, and subgoals associated with each of these interventions.

Preimpact (the period before the crisis)	Impact (when the crisis occurs)	Recoil (immediately after the crisis)	Postimpact (days to weeks after the crisis)	Recovery Reconstruction (months or years after the crisis)
			Rituals and memorials	
			Psychological interventions	
			Psychological education	
			Risk screening and referral	
			Reestablish support systems	
			Medical interventions	
	Immediate prevention			
Crisis preparedness				

FIGURE 10.1. School crisis interventions during the different phases of a crisis event

I. Crisis Preparedness
   A. Goal: Students and staff are prepared to adaptively respond to crises.
      1. *Crisis education:* Students gain knowledge needed to respond to crises in a way that mitigates crisis-related dangers and traumatic stress.
      2. *Crisis drills:* Students practice behaviors needed to respond to crises in a way that mitigates dangers.
      3. *Crisis management planning:* Staff develops a crisis management protocol for responding to crises, and provides appropriate training and materials so that all school community members are familiar with the plan and procedures.
II. Immediate Prevention
   A. Goal: The physical and emotional harm generated by a crisis event is mitigated.
      1. *Protect from harm/danger:* Students are removed from harmful/dangerous situations.
      2. *Minimize crisis exposure:* Students are shielded from crisis images.
      3. *Ensure actual and perceived safety:* Security procedures are implemented in a way that reassures students of their safety.
III. Medical Interventions
   A. Goal: Medical crisis interventions are the primary interventions supported by all resources.
      1. *First aid:* Emergency medical needs are met.
      2. *Isolate medical triage:* Noninjured students are shielded from viewing injured students.
      3. *Meet preexisting medical needs:* Treatments for preexisting medical conditions are provided.
IV. Reestablish Support Systems
   A. Goal: Naturally occurring social supports are located and reunited with students following crises.
      1. *Reunite/locate primary caregivers:* Parents and other loved ones/caregivers are located and reunited with their children.

2. *Reunite with close friends and teachers:* Students are re-united with their close friends and teachers.

3. *Facilitate community communication:* The services/activities of community agencies and organizations are identified and/or made available to students/families.

4. *Return to school:* Students return to school.

V. Risk Screening and Referral

   A. Goal: Students who are at risk for and/or display adverse crisis effects are identified and referred.

      1. *Initial risk screening:* From crisis facts and knowledge of individual student vulnerabilities, students at greatest risk for adverse crisis outcomes are identified and referred for appropriate psychological intervention.

      2. *Individual risk screening:* From initial psychological interventions, students at risk for adverse crisis outcomes are identified and referred for appropriate psychological intervention.

      3. *Referral procedures:* Procedures are implemented that allow students, staff, and other caregivers to refer themselves and/or others for psychological intervention, including follow-up procedures to ensure that those referred receive appropriate support and assistance.

      4. *Schoolwide risk screening:* Questionnaires and/or rating scales are completed by all students and/or teachers to identify those at high risk for adverse crisis outcomes. High-risk students are referred for appropriate psychological intervention.

VI. Psychological Education

   A. Goal: Students, staff, and caregivers acquire knowledge that assists them in understanding, preparing for, and responding to the crisis, and the problems and reactions it generates.

      1. *Psychoeducational groups:* Students understand the crisis, are prepared for possible crisis reactions, acquire self-care strategies, and know how to obtain assistance.

      2. *Caregiver training:* Caregivers understand the crisis, are prepared for possible crisis reaction (both in themselves and among students), acquire strategies for supporting

students, and know how to make referrals for additional support.

3. *Disseminate informational handout:* Informational handouts are made available (through the school and/or the media) that facilitate understanding of the crisis and its possible effects, and identify available supports.

4. *Anniversary preparations:* Students, staff, and caregivers are made aware of the possible effects of crisis anniversaries.

VII. Psychological Interventions

    A. Goal: Students are able to adaptively cope with the problems and reactions generated by crises, and are able to achieve precrisis functioning levels.

        1. *Psychological first aid:* Psychological contact is made, crisis problems are identified, immediate coping is reestablished, and connections are made to appropriate helping resources.

        2. *Empowerment:* Students engage in crisis prevention and preparedness activities that involve some form of concrete action and, as a result, move them from the position of a victim to that of an actor.

        3. *Group crisis debriefing:* Crisis facts are understood, crisis experiences and reactions are shared/normalized, coping actions are taken (or at least planned), and the need for additional helping resources is identified.

        4. *Psychotherapy:* Ongoing professional mental health assistance is made available as needed.

        5. *Anniversary reaction support:* Making use of psychological first aid, students are able to cope with crisis reactions associated with significant anniversary dates and/or connections are made to appropriate helping resources.

VIII. Rituals and Memorials

    A. Goal: Students engage in activities that provide mutual support, opportunities to express shared grief and remembrance, and interpretation of crisis events and survivor actions. These activities also facilitate the process of bringing closure to the crisis event.

1. *Ritual participation:* Students are given the opportunity to participate in rituals that allow for public expressions of shared grief and mutual support, which summarizes and interprets the crisis, and begins the process of closure.
2. *Memorial development/implementation:* Students are able to develop and implement appropriate crisis-related memorials.

Crisis Preparedness

Crisis preparedness includes activities provided during the preimpact phase. The primary goal is to better ensure that students and staff are able to respond or react to crisis events in adaptive ways. Crisis preparedness includes crisis education and crisis drills. Crisis education programs help students to understand the dangers associated with crisis events (typically natural disasters) and the protective actions that can be taken (e.g., standing under a doorway and away from windows during an earthquake). Crisis education may also include instruction on how to manage crisis-related stress. Crisis drills include the traditional fire or natural disaster drill. The goal of these activities includes giving students an opportunity to practice the behaviors needed to mitigate the danger associated with crisis events. Recently, some schools have begun to employ crisis drills that require students, staff, and emergency response personnel to role-play the actions they will take in the event of assaultive violence (e.g., a school shooting).

Crisis preparedness also includes preimpact-phase planning activities. Applied at a school-system level, these activities are designed to facilitate school staff's response to the impact, recoil, postimpact, and recovery and reconstruction phases. Theoretically, these activities place schools in the best possible position to meet student and staff needs following a crisis event. For detailed discussions of these activities refer to Brock, Sandoval, and Lewis (2001), Brock (2002d), and Brock and Poland (2002). A written document emerging from these efforts should be a school crisis management plan, detailing policies and procedures related to crisis intervention (see Jimerson and Brock, 2002, for a sample crisis management plan).

Empirical Support

Clearly, in areas prone to certain types of recurrent natural disasters (e.g., earthquakes, floods, hurricanes, fires, tornadoes), crisis preparedness activities are easily justified (Vernberg, 2002). Theoretically, these activities should make certain types of crises appear more controllable and as a result less traumatic (Vernberg and Vogel, 1993). For example, one might expect that the student from California who had engaged in earthquake preparedness education would find such a crisis event less frightening than the child who has just moved to the area and never received such education. Despite the face validity of this hypothesis, however, the discussion that follows reveals only partial research-based support for crisis preparedness activities.

Research regarding the effects of crisis education, as it relates to natural and industrial disasters, appears positive. In a survey of 440 schoolchildren (ages five to thirteen years), Ronan et al. (2001) found that those who had participated in such programs had certain advantages over those who did not. Results suggested that hazard-educated children had more stable risk perceptions, reduced hazard-related fears, and a greater awareness of protective behaviors. Furthermore, children involved in two or more education programs had significantly greater awareness of these protective behaviors than children who participated in only one program.

Data that may be supportive of crisis-education activities designed to prepare students for crisis-related stress are found in research conducted by Kiselica et al. (1994); Deahl et al. (2000); and Holaday and Smith (1995). In the Kiselica et al. study the effect of a stress inoculation program was documented for a group of public high school students. This program included a discussion of stress, stressful events, anxiety and anxiety-related symptoms; instruction in relaxation techniques and how they can be used to manage anxiety-provoking situations; and cognitive restructuring. Results revealed greater declines in symptoms of stress and trait anxiety among the 24 program participants (as compared to students in a 24-student control group who were enrolled in traditional school guidance classes). However, this study's support for stress inoculation as a part of school crisis education is limited, as study participants did not experience what might be considered a "crisis event" during the study period. Thus, while the effect of this high school training program on "normal stress and anxiety" is documented by this research, its efficacy as a crisis education tool can only be partially supported by these data.

However, another study by Deahl et al. (2000) directly assessed the effects of crisis education on reactions to a traumatic situation. In this study, 106 British soldiers received an operational stress training package before being deployed for a six-month tour of duty in Bosnia. This half-day program included descriptions of stress and its physical, psychological, and behavioral consequences. In addition, it described anxiety reduction and relaxation techniques, and informed soldiers of the kind of situations they were likely to encounter. Despite the fact that during their tours of duty all soldiers were exposed to potentially traumatizing events, upon their return from Bosnia rates of psychopathology were approximately ten times less than figures reported in other military samples. However, generalizing from the results of this military research to school crisis intervention is clearly difficult. As a result, the ability of these data to support this form of crisis education in the schools is also limited.

In the Holaday and Smith (1995) study, in addition to providing a 35-minute coping skills training to 153 university students, this study also required participants to view a 31-minute videotape of disaster scenes. Approximately half of these participants ($n = 70$) viewed the video before the coping skills training (control group) and half ($n = 83$) viewed it after the training (experimental group). As they viewed the tape participants were asked to place themselves on the scene as helpers to disaster victims. Making use of a randomized, control-group posttest-only design, results obtained from a coping mechanisms questionnaire indicated that participants who had received coping skills training before viewing the disaster video used significantly more coping skills and felt more comfortable. Thus, this coping skills training (which emphasized social support, task-focused behaviors, emotional distancing, cognitive self-talk, and altruism) had promise as a tool for preparing individuals for disaster work. Although this finding has direct implications for the training of school staff members who are members of a school crisis intervention team, generalizing these data to schoolchildren is yet again problematic. This study's participants were young adults (mean male age 24, mean female age 27), not schoolchildren, and the focus was on preparing disaster workers for crisis work, not on helping students cope with a school crisis.

Regarding crisis drills, research by Hillman, Jones, and Farmer (1986) and Jones et al. (1989) highlights the effectiveness of fire drills for second- through fourth-grade students. The results of this research indicated that drills increase students' fire safety skills (when compared to an untrained control group). In addition, such drills were most effective when an explanation was given for the drill and when there was behavioral practice (versus verbal practice). When combined with data suggesting positive attitudinal responses to hazard education (Ronan et al., 2001), these data support the practice of preparing students for certain recurrent crises such as fires and natural disasters. However, this conclusion is specific only to certain types of disasters (e.g., fires and natural disasters). A PsycINFO database search (conducted July 2002) found no research that addressed the effect of crisis drills for less common events, such as school shootings.

Finally, a PsycINFO database search (conducted July 2002) found no research that documented the efficacy of school crisis response planning. Although the face validity of such procedures is strong and there are ample "how to" discussions of such planning (e.g., Brock, Sandoval, and Lewis, 2001; Petersen and Straub, 1992; Poland and McCormick, 1999), empirical data are lacking.

Future Research

Research examining the efficacy of crisis-preparedness activities needs to address four related questions, as they relate to different types of crisis events. Specifically, does crisis-preparedness result in

1. a reality-based understanding of crisis events (i.e., concern about the crisis event is consistent with the actual degree of danger);
2. improved preimpact knowledge of protective actions to be taken during crisis impact;
3. adaptive actions actually being taken during crisis impact, recoil, and postimpact phases (i.e., actions that mitigate crisis dangers and reactions); and
4. a reduction of adverse postimpact outcomes.

As was just discussed, student self-reports do suggest that some forms of crisis education develop positive attitudes toward, and knowledge of, certain types of natural and industrial disasters (Ronan et al., 2001). However, it has yet to be documented if in fact such education facilitates realistic views and helpful knowledge of other types of crises. For example, given the relatively low incidence of school-associated violent deaths (Anderson et al., 2001), it is possible that the emotional costs of holding "lockdown" drills and providing instruction in taking cover and avoiding attention during an attack, outweighs any potential benefit (Vernberg, 2002). Empirical study is needed to determine the degree to which this type of crisis preparedness either makes students feel more secure, or generates a climate of fear within which school violence is viewed as unrealistically likely. At present the role of these drills in contributing to school safety and crisis preparedness is not understood (Pagliocca, Nickerson, and Williams, 2002).

In addition, it has yet to be documented if in fact crisis education facilitates adaptive impact, recoil, and postimpact phase actions and adjustments among school-aged youths following exposure to a crisis event. For example, does crisis education translate into actions that make the situation less dangerous following a crisis? Does crisis education result in the use of adaptive coping strategies following such events? Regarding this latter question, future research might employ a design similar to Holaday and Smith (1995), but enlist school-aged youths (not college students) as participants.

Although the Deahl et al. (2000) study suggests that preparing soldiers for war-related stress does have certain benefits in terms of postimpact outcomes (i.e., lower-than-expected rates of psychopathology), the ability to generalize these findings to schools and schoolchildren's crisis preparedness is limited. Thus, it must be concluded that it has yet to be determined if school crisis preparedness translates to positive postimpact outcomes.

Finally, while the need for school staff to engage in crisis response planning appears to be self-apparent (schools that prepare for the crisis response should be better able to implement such a response), nevertheless a need exists to examine if in fact this planning is an effective use of resources. Do schools that engage in systemwide crisis planning respond to crisis events significantly better than schools that do not engage in these efforts? In other words, is crisis response planning worth the effort? Assuming that it is an effective use of resources, the question remains regarding the most important elements of crisis preparedness (Brock and Poland, 2002; Pagliocca, Nickerson, and Williams, 2002). In addition, are there certain crisis planning activities that have an effect on specific postimpact outcomes (e.g., do activities that are designed to develop psychological interventions translate to the identification of students with traumatic stress reactions?).

Immediate Prevention

Immediate prevention activities take place during the impact and recoil phases of a crisis and are designed to mitigate the physical and emotional harm generated by the event. Immediate prevention activities include protecting and/or shielding students from physical and emotional harm. This may be done by implementing crisis preparedness strategies (e.g., fire drill, lockdown, evacuation procedures, etc.). Immediate prevention also involves minimizing exposure to traumatic stimuli during the recoil phase. This can be done by directing children who are ambulatory away from the crisis site, and away from severely injured students (National Institute of Mental Health, 2001). Minimizing such exposure may also involve restricting television viewing of crisis events.

The need for these activities is documented by research that demonstrates the relationship between degree of exposure to a crisis event and subsequent stress reactions (Applied Research and Consulting et al., 2002; March et al., 1997; Pynoos et al., 1987). Regarding television exposure, research by Gurwitch and her colleagues (2002) has suggested it to be a risk factor for post-traumatic stress disorder (PTSD). They report that following the 1995 Oklahoma City bombing, children who were not physically or emotionally proximal to the bombing, but who reported having had extensive television viewing of the event, also reported having a higher number of traumatic stress symptoms than did other children who reported lower amounts of such television viewing. From these findings it is suggested that either direct exposure or simply being a passive observer of a traumatic event, even by viewing it on television, may place students at risk for traumatic stress reactions.

Finally, restoration of both actual and perceived safety during the recoil phase has been suggested to be a primary factor in promoting the natural adjustment to crisis events (Brewin, 2001; Gurwitch et al., 2002; Yule, 2001). It is not enough for students to *actually* be safe immediately following a crisis. For recovery to begin, students must *believe* that the potential for harm has passed and that they are no longer in any danger. Thus, schools should be certain that the steps taken to ensure student safety following crises are not only effective, but also concrete and visible (e.g., having a strong police presence on campus following acts of violence).

Psychological education and intervention activities (to be discussed later in this chapter) may also be important tools in facilitating perceptions of safety. Specifically, helping students to gain cognitive mastery over the event (i.e., understand the reality of the danger) may help them to feel safer. An example of how this might work is provided by Brock, Sandoval, and Lewis (2001) who reported that following a school shooting there was a persistent rumor that only one of two gunmen had been accounted for. In reality, the lone gunman had committed suicide after his assault. Interventions that dispelled this rumor were important to help students accurately understand that the danger of being shot had passed. This knowledge, combined with a strong police presence on school grounds for the first few days following the shooting, helped students to *believe* that they were safe.

Empirical Support

Clearly, protecting students from harm and danger, and minimizing exposure to the crisis, will reduce the degree of physical and psychological trauma. However, a PsycINFO database search (conducted July 2002), found no studies that investigated the effectiveness of specific immediate prevention activities designed to achieve these goals. In addition, no research could be located that investigated the effectiveness those immediate prevention activities designed to facilitate students' feelings of safety following a crisis event.

Future Research Needs

Crisis preparedness research should also address the future research needs in the area of immediate prevention. For example, it is important to identify those preparedness strategies that are most beneficial in preparing students and staff to engage in procedures that protect them from harm and/or minimize their exposure to the crisis event. In addition, future research should investigate the effects of restricting television viewing of crisis images on rates of traumatic stress. Is the relationship between amount of such viewing and degree of traumatic stress a casual relationship or is there a causal connection?

Interventions that are most helpful in ensuring students' subjective sense of safety and security following a crisis should be identified. For example, does a prominent police presence actually help students feel better, or does it create the impression that danger is still present? Are there interactions between such interventions and a student's developmental level? It is possible that police presence may be very reassuring for older students while very frightening for younger students. Finally, a related question is whether there are any specific actions associated with increases in subjective security following specific crisis events. For example, does a police presence increase feelings of safety following natural disasters as well as following school violence?

Medical Intervention

Although often not considered a "school crisis intervention" (as it is typically provided by professionals who are not school staff members), the primary importance of addressing medical needs during the impact and recoil phases argues for its inclusion in this discussion. With the exception of those crisis interventions that prevent injury in the first place, all other forms of crisis interventions are secondary in importance to medical treatment (e.g., triage and first aid). In addition, it is important to acknowledge the need for medical interventions that may guide crisis intervention. Specifically, some forms of crisis intervention (e.g., psychological debriefing) are contraindicated for those with acute physical injury (Everly and Mitchell, 2000).

Another medical treatment issue that is germane to this discussion is medical triage. Following a major disaster, the meeting of medical needs may require medical triage, which involves the screening and classification of the injured to determine priority needs for medical intervention (Thomas, 1993). When this procedure is used, psychological trauma (due to secondary exposure to crisis events) may be reduced by conducting triage in a location that cannot be directly viewed by noninjured students (Brock, Sandoval, and Lewis, 2001).

Finally, it is important for all crisis intervention teams to be aware of preexisting medical conditions and to make certain that the crisis event does not disrupt the treatment of these conditions (American Red Cross, 1991; National Institute of Mental Health, 2002). Clearly, failure to treat a preexisting condition following a crisis event will only make matters worse. For example, the failure to treat diabetes following a crisis event may turn a moderately stressful event into a critical medical emergency.

Empirical Support

A PsycINFO database search (conducted in June 2002) showed that there is no empirical research (at least in the psychological literature) that guides school crisis intervention practices associated with the meeting of medical needs in the school setting following crisis events. However, the importance of not exposing students to grotesque crisis scenes, such as medical triage, is supported by research suggesting increases in the probability of severe postcrisis reactions associated with such exposure (Vogel and Vernberg, 1993).

Although the empirical literature may not offer guidance on how the school crisis intervention can effectively support the meeting of medical needs, studies exist that can be interpreted as supporting the primary importance of medical treatment and the contraindication of some crisis interventions for those with acute injury. Specifically, Bisson et al. (1997) and Mayou, Ehlers, and Hobbs (2000) report that psychological debriefing, when provided as an individual and isolated crisis intervention temporally proximal to acute burn trauma or road traffic accident, may have had adverse long-term outcome (as documented by traumatic stress reactions).

Future Research Needs

Evaluation of school crisis intervention strategies for supporting and working with medical personnel during the recoil and postimpact phases of a crisis is needed. Documentation of specific crisis intervention strategies that both facilitate medical treatment and also minimize student exposure to those students who have been severely injured would be helpful.

Reestablish Support Systems

Individuals with strong familial and social support systems are better able to cope with life stressors than those without such supports (Cohen and Willis, 1985). Given this, it is not surprising that the reestablishment and use of naturally occurring supports is a frequently recommended crisis intervention (American Red Cross, 1991; Brewin, 2001; Foa et al., 2001; Gurwitch et al., 2002; Litz et al., 2002; National Institute of Mental Health, 2002; Norris et al., 2001). During the recoil phase this crisis intervention initially involves reuniting students with (or at least locating and determining the status of) parents, and other caregivers and loved ones. Priority is typically given to reuniting younger students with their parents (Brock, Sandoval, and Lewis, 2001). Later, typically during the recoil and/or postimpact phase, this intervention would include reuniting students with their close friends, teachers, and classmates. Facilitating communication among families, students, and community agencies and organizations may also facilitate natural support systems that are available in communities (Gist and Lubin, 1999). In addition, because the resumption of familiar roles and routines as soon as possible following crises reduces the intensity and duration of crisis reactions (Omer and Alon, 1994; Prinstein et al., 1996; Vernberg and Vogel, 1993), returning students to school as soon as possible is an important intervention (Vernberg, 2002).

The importance of facilitating family and social supports has been documented for both adults and children following several different traumatic stressors. For example, among adults, specifically Vietnam War veterans, studies show that dysfunctional and low-quality social supports are associated with psychiatric disorders (Boscarino, 1995; King et al., 1998). Furthermore, among those veterans with post-traumatic stress disorder, their social support had systematically declined over time relative to comparison groups (Keane et al., 1985). Among elementary school students who survived a hurricane it was found that higher levels of social support were associated with lower levels of traumatic stress reactions (La Greca et al., 1996; Vernberg et al.,

1996), and it was suggested that multiple sources of such support were important to meeting different support needs (La Greca et al., 1996). Interestingly, however, among Kuwaiti children exposed to the traumatic stressors of the Gulf War, social support buffered the effect of trauma on girls but not on boys (Llabre and Hadi, 1997). This may point to culturally specific reactions to social support and/or the differential effects of this particular stressor on boys and girls.

Psychological education (which will be discussed in greater detail later) is also important to the reestablishment of social supports. Specifically, it involves encouraging students (and staff) to access their existing social supports and educating caregivers about how to most effectively provide such support.

Empirical Support

A PsycINFO database search (conducted July 2002) showed only one study of a specific intervention to facilitate social support. Specifically, Hansell et al. (1998) report that healthy caregivers of children with HIV benefited from a "social support boosting" intervention as documented by increased social support levels. This individual intervention involved working with caregivers to identify stressful problems and the social supports available to help deal with the stressors. However, among caregivers who were themselves ill this intervention did not improve social support. This suggests that caregivers who are themselves significantly impaired (e.g., those who are suffering from a trauma-related psychopathology), may be limited in their ability to provide social support. This finding illustrates that social support systems have certain limitations and may not be able to meet the needs of all crisis victims.

Although there is a lack of research specifically investigating interventions designed to promote social support systems, several studies document the importance of other crisis intervention practices in this area. For example, the importance of ensuring the reunification of students with their parents as soon as possible is supported by research suggesting that parents and family are judged by children to be their primary sources of support following crises (Klingman, 2001; Leffler and Dembert, 1998; Vernberg et al., 1996). Prinstein et al.

(1996) document that after a hurricane elementary-aged children reported receiving the most coping assistance from their parents.

Support for the practice of making reunification between younger children and parents a priority is found in reports that preschool- and kindergarten-aged children show the strongest reactions (when compared to older students) when separated form parents during stressful events. Following an earthquake, preschool children showed more behavior problems if they had been separated from their parents during the quake (Vogel and Vernberg, 1993).

After parents and family, close friends and teachers are also reported to be important social supports (Klingman, 2001; Vernberg et al., 1996). For example, Prinstein et al. (1996) documented that children reported friends as primary providers of emotional processing coping. In addition, among soldiers, support from military leaders was found to moderate the relationship between this population's accumulated exposure to traumatic events and measures of health (Martin et al., 2000). This finding may point to the importance of school administrator leadership and support in helping school staff members cope with crisis events.

Data that may support a quick return to school following a crisis is offered in a study of elementary school children following a hurricane. Prinstein et al. (1996) found children's self-reports to yield an association between more severe traumatic stress symptoms and low levels of a return to predisaster roles and routines. In addition, it is obvious that a failure to return to precrisis settings will minimize opportunities for ongoing social support, the effects of which have been documented by Milne (1977). Results of this study revealed significantly higher disaster-related fear and school problems among children who were evacuated and unable to return to their community (as compared to those were either not evacuated or who were evacuated but had returned to the community).

The importance of encouraging students to make use of their social support systems has been documented by Jeney-Gammon et al. (1993) who found that following a natural disaster, the levels of depression among third, fourth, and fifth graders were lower among those students who had sought out social support (versus those who did not seek such support). With adults, Pennebaker and O'Heeron (1984) documented that among the spouses of suicide and accident fatalities, fewer health problems were associated with the ability to discuss these deaths with friends. It was speculated that not confiding in others increased physiological activity and had a cumulative stress on the body, with the long-term consequence being an increased probability of stress-related disease.

Future Research Needs

Crisis intervention research needs to systematically examine the effectiveness of programs designed to reestablish social support systems following crisis events. Essential questions include whether specific actions should be undertaken by schools to most effectively facilitate the reestablishment of familial and social support. In addition, are there specific strategies (such as parent meetings) that schools can employ to ensure that the potential of these support systems is realized?

It would also be helpful if future research were to give school crisis intervention guidance regarding which specific social supports are most important for specific age groups and populations. For example, is it most important to reunite younger children with parents and relatively more important to reunite adolescents with their close friends? Are there specific crisis events that make reestablishment of particular social supports more or less important?

Although naturally occurring social support systems provide important protections against adverse crisis outcomes, these very systems are themselves vulnerable to crises and as a result may decline or deteriorate in strength (as was documented by Hansell et al., 1998). In addition, naturally occurring social support systems may not be powerful enough to overcome the effects of severe crisis events (e.g., school shootings), which points to the importance of having more direct services (such as the psychological interventions discussed later in this chapter) be a component of school crisis intervention (Norris et al., 2001). Given this observation it would be helpful if future research were to examine the relationship between the power of social support systems, and the nature and impact of certain types of crisis events.

Risk Screening and Referral

Risk screening and referral (also known as psychological triage) is a dynamic process that includes activities provided during the recoil, postimpact, and recovery and reconstruction phases. Recognizing the fact that not all individuals will be equally affected by a crisis event (Stallard, 2000), and that different individuals will likely benefit from different interventions (Turner, 2000), the primary goals of this process are to identify students (and staff) who are at risk for, and/or display adverse crisis outcomes, and to make appropriate referrals. These interventions help school crisis intervention teams identify those individuals who *do* and *do not* need their services. The need to identify and assist students who are in need of support is readily apparent, however, less obvious is the need for crisis intervention teams to identify students who may not require assistance and to allow them to manage crisis reactions and problems independently. Providing crisis intervention assistance to students who do not need such support may unintentionally send the message that they are not capable of coping with the crisis independently. It may also stigmatize students and generate self-fulfilling prophecies (Litz et al., 2002).

During the recoil phase, an initial screening based on known crisis facts and prior knowledge of individual student vulnerabilities is conducted. From these data students at greatest risk for adverse crisis outcomes (e.g., those who were physically and/or emotionally proximal to the crisis event, have preexisting psychopathology, lack social resources, etc.) are identified and psychological first aid is made available (Brock, 2002b; Brock, Sandoval, and Lewis, 2001).

During the postimpact phase, risk screening involves individual screenings conducted as a part of the initial psychological interventions (e. g., psychological first aid and group crisis debriefings), implementation of referral procedures (i.e., mechanisms that allow students, staff, and parents to refer to the crisis intervention those who need crisis intervention support), and schoolwide screenings (i.e., questionnaires and rating scales completed by all students that further identify those in need of support). Because virtually anyone with sufficient exposure to a traumatic stressor will display initial crisis reactions (they are normal reactions to abnormal situations), initial referrals are typically directed toward psychological first aid resources (not to professional mental health resources) and are designed to flag those individuals who *may* require mental health intervention because they are statistically more likely to develop psychopathology (Litz et al., 2002). However, if dangerous coping strategies are displayed (e.g., substance abuse, suicidal/homicidal ideation, inappropriate expressions of anger) then immediate psychotherapeutic referrals to mental health professionals would be appropriate. Otherwise, screening for psychiatric disturbances (e.g., post-traumatic stress disorder) due to traumatic event exposure would typically not begin until a week or more after the crisis event (Brewin, 2001; Litz et al., 2002).

Although the intensity of traumatic memories and crisis reactions typically fade over time, memories of a traumatic event never completely go away, and a variety of life events can retrigger intense reactions to the trauma (Young et al., 1998). As a result, it is important to continue to conduct individual screenings during the recovery and reconstruction phase and provide both psychological first aid and psychotherapeutic interventions as indicated. For further discussions of risk screening and referral refer to Brock, Sandoval, and Lewis (2001), and Brock (2002b).

Empirical Research

Arguably, the most important outcome that would support the effectiveness of any risk screening and referral protocol would be a low incidence of failure to identify and refer students who have significant mental health problems secondary to crisis exposure. Based upon a PsycINFO database search (conducted July 2002), there is no research that assesses the effectiveness of any school-based risk screening and referral protocol. However, substantial data exist that can be used to validate the inclusion of specific risk factors in risk screening. These factors include physical proximity and duration of exposure to the crisis, emotional proximity to the crisis (i.e., having significant relationships with crisis victims and threat perceptions), the severity and type of crisis reactions (e.g., the diagnosis of an acute stress disorder is a powerful predictor of later PTSD), and a host of external and internal resources (Brock, 2002b; Litz et al., 2002). However, the individual development of psychopathology will depend upon a complex interaction between the nature of the crisis event, the survivor's unique crisis experiences, and his or her personal vulnerabilities. To date these interactions have not been studied (Silverman and La Greca, 2002) and are poorly understood.

Additional data indicate that specific symptoms are especially significant and suggestive of the need for psychotherapeutic referral. Specifically, research conducted by McFarlane and Yehuda (1996) revealed that individuals who displayed dissociative or panic reactions during a crisis event were more vulnerable to posttraumatic reactions. They also reported that "enduring exaggerated startle response, hypervigilance, increased irritability, sleep disturbed memory, and concentration" (p. 172) differentiated crisis survivors who developed PTSD from those who did not. Conversely, they suggested that distressing and intrusive memories, in the initial days after the crisis event, were common indicators of normal reappraisal. Thus, a psychotherapeutic referral might be particularly appropriate to consider for the individual who panics or dissociates during the trauma and who has ongoing difficulty regulating his or her arousal levels (Brock, 2002b), and/or has been diagnosed with an acute stress disorder.

Future Research Needs

The primary research need is to establish the efficacy of existing risk screening protocols (e.g., Brock, Sandoval, and Lewis, 2001; Brock 2002b). This would include establishing the effectiveness of initial risk screenings, psychological first aid, group crisis debriefings, and schoolwide screenings in risk assessment. The outcome variable of interest to such research would be the degree to which interventions are able to identify individuals in need of assistance (in particular psychotherapeutic assistance). To the extent that individuals in need of such assistance are not identified and offered appropriate referrals, these interventions could be judged ineffective. For example, the fact that two-thirds of New York City public schoolchildren who have reported symptoms of traumatic stress have not obtained any treatment (Applied Research and Consulting et al., 2002) might signal an ineffective risk screening and referral procedure. In addition, the importance of identifying low-risk individuals and giving them opportunities to independently cope with crisis events needs to be assessed. The question of whether it is counterproductive to provide psychological intervention assistance (e.g., psychological first aid, group crisis debriefings) to those who would be able to recover without it needs to be explored.

In addition, questions regarding the possible interactions between specific crisis events, unique crisis experiences, and personal resiliency and vulnerability needs further study. Such research would inform decisions regarding appropriate psychotherapeutic referrals.

Finally, the question of when to begin screening for psychotherapeutic referrals requires future research (Yule, 2001). This is a difficult question as the optimal time for beginning such treatment is not easily identified and has been the subject of some debate (Vernberg and Vogel, 1993). This question has, however, been addressed to a certain extent by diagnostic criteria. For example, the American Psychiatric Association's (2000) diagnostic criteria for post-traumatic stress disorder suggests that traumatic stress symptoms must be present for at least four weeks before this diagnosis can be made. Thus, following a crisis event it would appear inappropriate to immediately begin to conduct psychotherapeutic treatment screening.

Psychological Education

Psychological education includes a variety of activities provided primarily during the recoil and postimpact phases. However, they also continue to be important during the recovery and reconstruction phase (Vernberg, 2002). The primary goal of these activities is to provide students, staff, and caregivers with knowledge that assists in understanding, preparing for, and responding to the crisis, and resulting problems and reactions. During the recovery and reconstruction phase, activities are designed to predict and prepare the school community for anniversary reactions. Bisson, McFarlane, and Rose (2000) and McFarlane (2000) suggest such procedures should help to contain distress and facilitate coping. Advantages of these activities include their ability to present an array of intervention options to individuals (Litz et al., 2002). Specific activities include psychoeducational groups, caregiver trainings, and informational bulletins or handouts.

Supporting the need for psychological education following crisis events is found in research conducted by Allen et al. (1999). These researchers studied over 6,000 elementary schoolchildren in Oklahoma City following the bombing of the Alfred P. Murrah Building and found that younger children need to be provided with crisis facts. These children were the least likely to understand what was going on, were the most likely to be confused, and had the highest number of facts wrong. In addition, this same study highlights the need to provide students (particularly younger students) with adaptive coping strategies, as this group was most likely to use avoidance as a coping mechanism.

Psychoeducational groups (also referred to as crisis management briefings, Everly, 2000) may include small group discussions, classroom meetings, or schoolwide assemblies. These gatherings are highly directive and involve the dissemination of important information that will aid in coping with crisis problems and reactions. Specifically, these groups hope to achieve the following goals:

- Crisis facts are understood and rumors are dispelled. Students gain a degree of cognitive mastery over the event.
- Common crisis reactions are normalized. Students are prepared for common crisis reactions that might be seen in themselves or among their peers.
- Stress management strategies are identified and/or taught. Students develop their own plan for coping with crisis reactions.
- Problematic (psychopathological) crisis reactions and coping strategies are discussed and referral procedures identified. Students are able to identify psychopathological reactions and coping strategies, and know how to make referrals for professional assistance.[1]

Caregiver training is very similar to the psychoeducational group, however, its focus is on caregiver knowledge. These gatherings are also typically very directive and involve the dissemination of information that will help parents, teachers, and other caregivers to effectively support their children. The importance of this type of psychoeducation is documented by research conducted by Harvey et al. (1991). They found that among adult sexual assault survivors, "empathic reactions" occurring early after the assault were associated with more successful coping than were "nonempathic reactions." Thus, it would appear that at least among some groups of trauma victims, there are certain types of caregiving reactions that are helpful and certain types that are not.

Specifically, the psychoeducation offered to caregivers hopes to achieve the following goals:

- Crisis facts are understood and rumors are dispelled. Caregivers have the facts needed to help children understand the crisis event.
- Common crisis reactions are normalized. Caregivers are prepared for common crisis reactions that might be seen in their children and/or among themselves.
- Stress management strategies are identified and/or taught. Caregivers are given tools that can be used to help their children cope with crisis reactions and/or problems.
- Specific helpful reactions (i.e., empathic reactions) to children's traumatic stress are identified. Caregivers are instructed on how to best respond to their children. This includes educating them about the importance of their own crisis reactions in shaping their child's perceptions of the crisis event.[2]
- Problematic crisis reactions and coping strategies are discussed and referral procedures identified. Caregivers are able to identify psychopathological reactions and coping strategies, and know how to make referrals for professional assistance.[3]

Box 10.1 provides a list of suggestions for parents and teachers that might be used during a caregiver training.

Informational handouts parallel the information disseminated through psychoeducational groups and caregiver trainings. They are designed to facilitate understanding of the crisis event, predict possible crisis consequences, and identify available supports. Litz et al. (2002) have suggested that these documents be routinely made available. They can be used as complements to other psychological education activities. Everly (2000), for example, suggests that each psychoeducational group participant should be provided with a reference sheet that describes common crisis reactions, stress management techniques, and local professional resources. Alternatively, they can be disseminated via mail and/or media outlets. Brock (2001a,b,c), provides examples of such flyers.

Anniversary preparations may employ group discussion and/or informational handouts. The primary goal of the recovery and reconstruction phase activity is to ensure that students, staff, and caregivers are prepared for the possible effects of crisis anniversaries and other significant dates. Brock and Jimerson (2002) offer an example of a handout used for this purpose.

BOX 10.1. Suggestions for Caregivers

- Give yourself a bit of time to come to terms with the event before you attempt to reassure children.

- Take care of yourself so that you can take care of children.

- Explain the episode of violence or disaster. Replace crisis rumors with crisis facts. At the same time, however, do not give children un-asked-for details that might increase their threat perceptions.

- Encourage children to express their feelings and listen without passing judgment.

- Let children know that it is normal to feel upset.

- Allow time for children to experience and talk about their feelings.

- Do not try to rush back to ordinary routines too soon. However, a gradual return to routine can be reassuring.

- If children are fearful, reassure them that you will take care of them.

- Stay together as much as possible.

- If behavior at bedtime is a problem, give children extra time and re-assurance. Let them sleep with a light on or in your room for a limited time if necessary.

- Reassure children that the traumatic event was not their fault.

- Do not criticize regressive behavior or shame children with words such as "babyish."

- Do your best to let children know that you understand their perception of the crisis event. Try to put yourself in their shoes.

- Although it is important to understand children's crisis event perceptions, it is also important to correct misperceptions.

- Allow children to cry or be sad.

- Encourage children to feel in control. Let them make some decisions about meals, what to wear, etc.

- Encourage children to develop coping and problem-solving skills and age-appropriate methods for managing anxiety.

Source: Adapted from National Institute of Mental Health (2001).

Empirical Research

Three studies were identified that may document the effectiveness of psychological education activities following crisis events. Unfortunately, each of these studies examined the degree to which these activities benefited adults, not children. The first study, conducted by Chemtob et al. (1997) assessed the effectiveness of a combination of group psychological debriefing and two hours of lecture. The lectures described reactions to disaster, phases of recovery, and what to expect. Results revealed substantial reductions in hurricane distress relative to controls. However, given that psychological education was combined with group debriefing, it is not known which results were due to psychological debriefing or education.

A second study by Rose et al. (1999) assessed the effect of three different individual treatment conditions (control group, education-only group, and debriefing plus education group) on traumatic stress reaction among victims of violent crime. The education intervention lasted an average 30 minutes and involved providing information on normal reactions to traumatic stress and when there was a need to find help. No statistically significant differences were found in posttraumatic stress reactions among the three groups. All three demonstrated declines in stress reactions (as measured by a posttraumatic stress scale) over time. This led to the conclusion that there was no evidence for the effectiveness of brief, one-session educational intervention (or debriefing plus education) for the victims of violent crime. However, the largest declines in traumatic stress scores from baseline were found among education group participants. This observation combined with the fact that the intervention lasted an average only 30 minutes (versus Chemtob et al., 1997, two hours of lecture), and did not provide information on coping strategies, gives reason to question this finding as an indication that psychological education is ineffective.

The final study by Herman, Kaplan, and LeMelle (2002) examined the effect of an intervention for governmental and nonprofit agency workers following the events of September 11, 2001. The 90- to 120-minute interventions gave information about emotional responses (both normal and pathological), how to help children, and practical coping strategies. Two hundred three individuals participated in 12 different groups sessions. Of this number 129 (64 percent) responded to the survey designed to assess participant perceptions of the intervention. Results revealed that the vast majority (82 percent) found the sessions to be helpful. Ten percent reported that it did not help, and 3 percent ($n = 4$) reported that the intervention had been harmful (8 percent had no opinion). Seventy-three percent reported that the sessions assisted them in talking to their children about crisis events. Within the respondent subgroup who were "high exposure" (i.e., had lost someone in the disaster), 92 percent reported the intervention to have been helpful. Within the respondent subgroup that reported having crisis symptoms, 97 percent reported the intervention to have been helpful. This research, however, does not document the actual effects of the intervention on individual crisis outcome. Rather, it simply provided treatment acceptability data. In addition, the data on the four participants who reported the intervention to have been harmful clearly show a need for additional research in this area.

Future Research

Although the available data is suggestive, it is far from conclusive. Thus, a continued need exists for controlled research of psychological education interventions (Bisson et al., 2000; Everly, 2000). Regarding the current understanding of psychological education practices, Vernberg (2002) states:

> To date, little research has been conducted on the usefulness of postimpact-phase distribution of information related to children's psychological reactions. Common sense, as well as the continuity principle, argues that well conceived, factually accurate information should be made available as widely as possible. At the same time, it would be helpful to evaluate the scientific basis of information disseminated following disasters and to study how parents, teachers, and children interpret and use that information. (p. 63)

Especially relevant to school crisis intervention is a need to document the effect of these interventions on children and adolescents. Additional research questions should ask whether different types of interventions are more effective than others. For example, are programs that teach coping strategies more helpful than those that simply predict crisis reactions? Are group interventions more effective than individual educational sessions? Does the amount of education provided affect outcome? Also, the question remains of whether an interaction is evident between psychological education and specific types of trauma. For example, do individuals who have experienced a natural disaster benefit more from a certain type of psychological education than victims of violent crime? In addition, some have raised questions regarding how much information about a crisis event should be given to students. Gurwitch et al. (2002) have suggested that being given "too much" information about the more frightening consequences of a crisis may sensitize individuals to the crisis instead of alleviating distress. This suggests the question: How much is too much? Finally, the common school crisis intervention practice of disseminating informational handouts has yet to be empirically evaluated. Research on the efficacy of these materials is also needed (Vernberg and Vogel, 1993).

Psychological Intervention

Psychological interventions include a variety of activities provided during the recoil, postimpact, and recovery and reconstruction phases. The primary goal of these activities is to directly facilitate coping with crisis problems and reactions in a way that allows for a return to precrisis functioning levels. Psychological interventions include psychological first aid, empowerment, group crisis debriefings, psychotherapy, and anniversary reaction support.

Psychological first aid is the immediate helping response offered to students affected by crisis events, and typically occurs during the recoil and early postimpact phases. It requires the school crisis intervenor to make psychological contact with the person in crisis, identify crisis problems, examine possible solutions, help the person to take concrete problem-solving action, and, when necessary, ensure connections to appropriate helping resources. Its primary goal is to reestablish immediate coping. In doing so it places students in a position to resolve crisis problems (Slaikeu, 1990).

Empowerment activities elicit student involvement in the process of identifying (and as appropriate implementing) strategies designed to prevent and/or mitigate the future occurrences of the crisis event (e.g., crisis prevention and preparedness). The primary goal is to encourage students to engage in activities that involve some form of concrete action and, as a result, move them from the position of a victim to that of an actor. Doing this makes the crisis appear more controllable and thereby less traumatic. Although these activities are often a part of other psychological interventions (e.g., group crisis debriefing may include empowerment activities), they are also used as discrete interventions and thus are treated separately in this discussion.

Group crisis debriefings are typically provided during the postimpact phase. The activities that are typically part of debriefings are very similar to psychoeducational groups. In fact, psychoeducational groups are sometimes referred to as a debriefing. However, unlike psychoeducational groups, group crisis debriefings actively explore and process individual crisis experiences and share individual crisis reactions. In so doing, these interventions help students feel less alone and more connected to their classmates by virtue of their common experiences and reactions. They also help to normalize these experiences and reactions (Brock, 2002a).

Psychotherapeutic interventions are typically provided during the latter part of the postimpact and in the recovery and reconstruction phases. These are professional mental health interventions that are not typically provided by school personnel. However, given the possibility that a substantial minority of students exposed to a crisis event may have crisis outcomes that require this intervention, consideration of these activities needs to be a part of school crisis intervention. Although school-based personnel may not deliver this intervention, ensuring that such services are at least made available to all who need them is definitely a school crisis intervention responsibility.

The final psychological intervention involves providing psychological first-aid assistance during significant dates and anniversaries that occur during the recovery and reconstruction phase. As was mentioned earlier, it is not unusual to find a reawakening of crisis reactions during periods temporally proximal to significant dates and crisis anniversaries. The goals of these interventions are to normalize the reawakening of crisis reactions, offer assistance coping with these reactions, and making connections to additional helping resources as needed.

Empirical Support

Very little research exists regarding the efficacy of psychological interventions following crisis events. A PsycINFO search (conducted July 2002) found no research examining psychological first aid or empowerment within the school setting. However, given that these interventions facilitate coping strategies (i.e., they help students to take concrete problem-solving actions), and coping is associated with lower rates of mental illness (Seiffge-Krenke et al., 2001), and avoidant coping strategies are predictive of posttraumatic stress (McFarlane, 1988), these interventions may have some support.

The study of psychological debriefings, in particular group crisis debriefings, has recently been the subject of empirical investigations. The appendix provides a summary of the peer-reviewed group comparison investigations considered. Because none of these studies focused on children, it is at best difficult and at worst dangerous to generalize these findings to school crisis intervention. Furthermore, generalization is difficult, because of the unique effects of different types of exposure to different types of crisis events. Although some have suggested that the available data do not support the continued use of psychological debriefing following crisis events (Litz et al., 2002; Rose, Wessely, and Bisson, 1998), it is premature to make such a broad conclusion. Rather, more specific and relatively limited conclusions regarding this form of psychological intervention should be drawn from the available literature. These conclusions are offered in Box 10.2. From the information provided in the appendix and in Box 10.2, it is suggested that group crisis intervention is contraindicated as a brief (less than 60 minutes), stand-alone, individual (one-to-one) intervention for adult acute physical trauma victims. On the other hand, it might have some promise when used as a more involved (more than 60 minutes and/or combined with other interventions) group intervention for adults who have experienced a crisis but were not physically injured.

Although there is limited research examining the immediate crisis response, the literature regarding the psychotherapeutic (or professional mental health response) is much more substantial. In particular, cognitive-behavioral treatments have been found to be effective treatments for psychological trauma (Foa and Meadows, 1997, 1998). These treatments included exposure-based therapies, anxiety man-

BOX 10.2. Conclusions About Psychological Debriefing

- Among adults who experience property damage due to a natural disaster, the sharing and subsequent normalization of crisis experiences and reactions, combined with psychological education offered several months after the crisis event, appears to facilitate reductions in the impact of the crisis event (Chemtob et al., 1997).

- Among civilian employees who are robbery victims (but who were not physically injured nor threatened by a gun), immediate debriefing (offered less than ten hours after the crisis) appears to result in more rapid reductions of traumatic stress symptoms than does delayed debriefing (offered more than forty-eight hours after the event) (Campfield and Hills, 2001).

- Among soldiers exposed to war, debriefing offered immediately upon return from a war zone does not appear to add to the benefits of precrisis education when it comes to reducing traumatic stress. However, it would appear to reduce the rate of maladaptive coping strategies (e.g., alcohol misuse) (Deahl et al., 2000).

- Among adults and adolescents who were acute trauma victims (i.e., suffered a physical injury requiring hospitalization and/or were the victims of a violent crime), individual debriefings are not sufficient to prevent psychopathology (Bisson et al., 1997; Hobbs et al., 1996; Mayou, Ehlers, and Hobbs, 2000) and do not appear to promote a more rapid rate of recovery than would occur without intervention (Rose et al., 1999).

- Among adults who suffer an acute physical injury requiring hospitalization (such as a burn), individual debriefings may cause harm when offered in close temporal proximity to the injury (Bisson et al., 1997).

- Among adolescents and adults who suffered an acute physical injury requiring hospitalization (following a traffic accident) an individual one-hour intervention (that includes a review of the traumatic event, expression of emotions and education about stress reactions, the value of talking about the crisis, and time importance of returning to normal travel) may make those who were most psychologically traumatized worse (Mayou, Ehlers, and Hobbs, 2000).

(continued)

(continued)

- Among adolescents and adults who suffered a minor physical injury not requiring hospitalization (following a traffic accident) an individual 30-minute intervention (that includes expression of emotional and cognitive reactions and education about traumatic stress symptoms and coping strategies) does not appear to promote a more rapid rate of recovery than would have occurred without intervention (Conlon, Fahy, and Conroy, 1999).

- Natural disaster worker self-reports of having been "debriefed" are not associated with a more rapid rate of recovery (as compared to those who did not report having been debriefed) (Kenardy et al., 1996).

- Among bank employees who were victims of armed robberies (but who were not injured, shot at, or taken hostage) a combination of precrisis education, debriefing, and individual support is associated with lower rates of psychological trauma than is debriefing as a stand-alone intervention (Richards, 2001).

agement, and cognitive therapy. Of these treatments, exposure-based therapies are the most effective. Based upon basic principles of human learning (i.e., classical and operant conditioning), these treatments involve asking psychological trauma victims to systematically confront their fears.

From their review of the empirical literature, Foa and Meadows (1997, 1998) suggest that prolonged exposure is the most efficacious treatment approach for traumatic stress reactions. Their description of this treatment indicates that it has the following five components:

1. information gathering,
2. breathing retraining,
3. psychoeducation,
4. imaginal exposure (i.e., mentally reliving the traumatic event), and
5. in vivo exposure (i.e., directly confronting reminders of the trauma).

The last component involves instructing the traumatized individual to begin to visualize the traumatic event. The visualization is narrated in the present tense and the individual is instructed to provide as much detail as possible (including related thoughts, perceptions, and feelings). At the end of this visualization period, the individual is asked to use previously taught relaxation skills. The power of this treatment approach is thought to rest in the pairing of a sense of physical calm (resulting from use of relaxation techniques) with the traumatic stress.

Finally, from a PsycINFO database search (conducted July 2002) no research was found that addresses interventions designed to support individuals who experience a reawakening of their symptoms associated with significant dates or crisis anniversaries.

Future Research Needs

When considering future research needs it is critical to acknowledge the complexity of psychological interventions following crisis events. The negative outcomes that these interventions address are the result of complex interactions among specific types of crises (different events generate different effects); the environments within which crises occur (some environments are better able to respond to crises); the individual's precrisis history (some individuals are more vulnerable to crises than others); and the individual's unique crisis experiences (some individuals will judge a crisis as more threatening than will others). As a result, future research will not be able to give absolute answers to questions about the efficacy of psychological interventions following school crisis events. Rather, for now such data must be considered guides that will influence, but not dictate, our actions. With this caution in mind, the following offers some ideas for future research in this area.

Perhaps most important, future research should study the efficacy of psychological interventions when used with children. As was previously stated, much of the existing research examines the effects of these interventions with adults. Generalizing such research to work with children is very difficult if not dangerous. It would be especially helpful if this research was conducted in the school setting.

Future research should examine the efficacy of psychological interventions following crises by using outcome variables other than traumatic stress. Specifically, it will be important to use the prevention or mitigation of other psychopathologies and maladaptive coping, and the impact on crisis effects unique to the school setting (e.g., school avoidance, academic failure, behavior problems) as measures of the success (or failure) of school crisis intervention. In addition, it would be important to identify if these interventions increase treatment alliances and acceptability (as has been suggested by Bisson, McFarlane, and Rose, 2000). Finding that early psychological interventions make it more likely for individuals to seek mental health assistance would be especially exciting given that individuals with traumatic stress symptoms often do not seek treatment (Applied Research and Consulting et al., 2002).

Methodological problems abound in the literature. The failure to clearly standardize the independent variable is arguably the most problematic. Thus, future research should clearly operationalize interventions and, whenever possible, a well-developed, standardized protocol should be employed. School crisis intervenors should continue to develop and document their practices.

Finally, future research must begin the long process of helping crisis intervenors understand the complex interrelationship between specific crisis events, specific crisis event settings, and specific individuals or populations. What works best for whom and under what circumstances will provide important guidance to school crisis intervention. Timing also requires further investigation as the optimal time to begin psychological interventions remains unclear.

Rituals and Memorials

Rituals and memorials occur during the postimpact and recovery and reconstruction phases. The primary goal is to engage students in activities that provide mutual support, security, and reduce feelings of isolation and vulnerability, as well as opportunities to express shared grief and remembrance, and provide interpretations of the crisis event. This begins the process of closure; the crisis event is placed in the past as survivors begin to move on with their lives. Rituals include religious services and memorials. They may involve relatively simple activities such as listing the attributes of lost friends or loved ones; developing memory books; planting a flower or a tree; saying a prayer; and writing a poem, story, or song about the person(s) who died (Brock and Jimerson, 2002; Vernberg and Vogel, 1993).

Empirical Support

A PsycINFO database search (conducted June 2002) found no research addressing the efficacy of rituals and/or memorials. However, given the timelessness of such activities across all cultures, it can be strongly argued that these activities have at the very least a strong appeal, if not an adaptive function (Vernberg and Vogel, 1993).

Future Research Needs

Although the universal and timeless appeal of rituals and memorials speaks for itself, future research would nevertheless benefit the practice of school crisis intervention. Knowing what type of memorial or ritual is most appropriate for given groups and individuals following specific types of crisis events would be helpful. Some people benefit from certain types of memorials, under certain types of circumstances, and other individuals may find them to be counterproductive. Ethnic, cultural, and/or religious factors may play a significant role in determining whether a given memorial activity will be of benefit.

MULTICOMPONENT CRISIS INTERVENTION

As highlighted in the discussion of various intervention strategies, no single activity will provide resolution for all in the aftermath of crisis events. When it comes to crisis intervention, it is clear that one size does not fit all. Considering the complexity inherent in the multitude of individual and contextual factors influencing responses following a crisis and recognizing changes that are likely across time, systematic, and multifaceted crisis intervention approaches are encouraged. Making use of a chronological framework, the intervention strategies previously discussed address unique considerations of crises impacting children in the school context. Insights based on research, practical experience, and theory should be incorporated into school crisis management plans aimed at facilitating the coping and adjustment of students in the wake of crises. School crisis management plans should include strategies to

1. prevent and/or mitigate common stress reactions,
2. identify those who may develop psychopathology (e.g., posttraumatic stress disorder, depression),
3. prevent and/or mitigate dangerous coping behaviors (e.g., suicidal and homicidal behaviors),
4. provide appropriate referrals to mental health professionals, and
5. address unique school-related issues (e.g., truancy, achievement, behavior problems, learning problems).

APPENDIX:
SUMMARIES OF "DEBRIEFING" RESEARCH STUDIES

Authors:	Bison, Jenkins, Alexander, and Bannister (1997)
Interventions:	45-minute Mitchell Model of Debriefing (adapted for use with individuals and couples)
Participants:	65 adults (consecutive admissions to a hospital burn unit)
Stressor:	Acute physical trauma (burn)
Groups/timing:	Random assignment of individuals to debriefing and control (no intervention) groups. Intervention offered 2 to 19 days (mean 6.3) after the burn trauma.
Results:	At 13-month follow-up, interview and questionnaire data suggested the debriefing group to have significantly worse symptoms of depression, anxiety, and traumatic stress than the control group. In addition, among debriefed individuals, the closer the temporal relationship of the trauma to the debriefing, the worse the outcome.

Authors:	Campfield and Hills (2001)
Interventions:	60- to 120-minute Mitchell Model of Debriefing
Participants:	77 civilian employees
Stressor:	Robbery (no physical injuries, gun not used)
Groups/timing:	Random assignment of individuals to two groups. Immediate group: debriefing provided less than ten hours posttrauma. Delayed group: debriefing provided more than forty-eight hours posttrauma.
Results:	The number and severity of PTSD symptoms were no different at the time of debriefing but were lower for the immediate (compared to the delayed group) at two-day, four-day, and two-week follow-up.

Authors:	Chemtob, Tomas, Law, and Cremniter (1997)
Interventions:	300-minute group sharing and normalization of crisis experiences and reactions combined with lecture
Participants:	43 adults (Group 1: FEMA counseling project staff; Group 2: local mental health staff)
Stressor:	Hurricane exposure (Average exposure: homes damaged, but inhabitable). Intact groups assigned to one of two groups. Group 1: intervention offered six months postdisaster. Group 2: intervention offered nine months postdisaster.
Results:	At 90-day follow-up, both groups showed significant reductions of Impact of Events Scale scores. No group dif-

ferences were observed, suggesting that stress reductions were not simply a matter of time.

Authors:	Conlon, Fahy, and Conroy (1999)
Interventions:	30-minute psychological debriefing (individual, expression of emotion/cognitive effects and psychoeducation)
Participants:	40 consecutive trauma clinic attenders (16 to 65 years of age)
Stressor:	Road traffic accident victims (minor injuries, no hospitalization)
Groups/timing:	Random assignment (coin flip) of individuals to two groups: Intervention group ($n = 18$) or Monitoring group ($n = 22$).
Results:	Three-month follow-up interview and self-report questionnaires did not reveal any significant differences between groups. Four monitoring group and two intervention group members developed PTSD. This distribution was not significant.

Authors:	Deahl et al. (2000)
Interventions:	Half-day predeployment crisis education combined with 120-minute Mitchell Model Debriefing
Participants:	106 British soldiers
Stressor:	War (six months in Bosnia)
Groups/timing:	All participants were provided predeployment crisis education. Immediately following return from Bosnia, random assignment of individuals to two groups: Debriefed and Nondebriefed.
Results:	At three-, six-, and twelve-month follow-ups, both groups showed lower than expected rates of PTSD. The debriefed group showed lower rates of alcohol misuse than was found in the nondebriefed group.

Authors:	Hobbs, Mayou, Harrison, and Warlock (1996)
Interventions:	60-minute psychological debriefing (individual review of the accident, expression of emotions, and psychoeducation)
Participants:	106 adults (consecutive admissions to a hospital following traffic accident)
Stressor:	Acute physical trauma (hospitalization following a traffic accident)
Groups/timing:	Random assignment of individuals to an intervention group ($n = 54$) and to a control group ($n = 52$). Intervention offered 24-48 hours after the accident in most cases.

Results:	Four-month follow-up interview and self-report questionnaire did not find either group to demonstrate a significant reduction in posttraumatic symptoms, mood disorder, anxiety, intrusive thoughts, travel anxiety, PTSD, or phobic anxiety.

Authors:	Kenardy et al. (1996)
Interventions:	Group stress debriefing (no information provided regarding the models that may have been used)
Participants:	195 emergency response and disaster personnel
Stressor:	Earthquake
Groups/timing:	Participant self-reports regarding whether or not they had participated in a group stress debriefing session was used to create intervention groups. No information available regarding the form or timing of the "debriefing."
Results:	At an average follow-up of 27, 50, 86, and 114 weeks postdisaster, questionnaire results did not suggest any differences between groups. Self-reports of having been "debriefed" did not yield lower scores on measures of event impact, general health, or level of stress.

Authors:	Mayou, Ehlers, and Hobbs (2000)
Interventions:	60-minute debriefing (individual review of the accident, expression of emotions, and psychoeducation)
Participants:	61 adolescents and adults (consecutive admission to a hospital following traffic accident)
Stressor:	Acute physical trauma (hospitalization following a traffic accident)
Groups/timing:	Random assignment of individuals to an intervention group and to a nonintervention group. Intervention offered within 24 hours after hospital admission or as soon as the individual was physically able to be debriefed.
Results:	Three-year follow-up questionnaire data suggested the intervention group did not appear to benefit from debriefing. They had worse physical and functional outcomes than the control group. Of those with high initial traumatic stress, individuals in the intervention group had a worse outcome than those in the nonintervention group.

Author:	Richards (2001)
Interventions:	90- to 120-minute Mitchell Model of Debriefing or pretrauma training, debriefing, and individual support
Participants:	524 bank employees

Stressor: Armed robbery (no physical injuries, gunshots, or hostage taking)

Groups/timing: Intact groups of robbery victims were initially offered debriefing as a stand-alone intervention. Subsequently, different groups of victims were offered the services of an integrated stress management system that included pretrauma education and individual support.

Results: At three- to twelve-month follow-up, groups who had received support from an integrated stress management system scored lower on measures of psychological trauma and had fewer clinically significant cases than did groups who were offered debriefing as a stand-alone intervention.

Authors: Rose, Brewin, Andrews, and Kirk (1999)

Interventions: 30-minute psychoeducation and/or 60-minute Mitchell Model of Debriefing (adapted for use with individuals and couples)

Participants: 157 adults (victims of violent crime; 2,161 solicited, 243 replied, 157 eligible)

Stressor: Actual or attempted physical or sexual assault, or purse snatching

Groups/timing: Random assignment of individuals to assessment only, education only, and education plus debriefing groups. Intervention offered within one month after the crime (mean 21 days).

Results: At 11-month follow-up rating scales suggested all groups to improve over time. No significant differences between groups were found. However, the assessment-only group had the lowest baseline and the highest posttraumatic stress scale scores at follow-up.

NOTES

1. The importance of providing information about self-referral is emphasized by reports that two-thirds of students with PTSD subsequent to the events of September 11, 2001, have not sought any treatment (Applied Research and Consulting et al., 2002).

2. Green et al. (1991) and McFarlane (1987) highlight the importance of educating parents about how their own reactions influence the reactions of their children. Specifically, these researchers found that parental reactions to disaster (a dam disaster and an Australian bushfire) were better predictors of child posttraumatic stress reactions, than was direct exposure to the disaster.

3. Handford et al. (1986) highlight the importance of educating caregivers about possible crisis reaction among their children. This study found that children reported much stronger and more symptomatic responses to the Three Mile Island nuclear accident than their parents reported having observed.

REFERENCES

Allen, S. F., Dlugokinski, E. L., Cohen, L. A., and Walker, J. L. (1999). Assessing the impact of a traumatic community event on children and assisting with their healing. *Psychiatric Annals, 29,* 93-98.

American Psychiatric Association (2000). *Diagnostic and statistical manual of mental disorders* (Fourth edition, Text revision). Washington, DC: American Psychiatric Association.

American Psychological Association (2002). PsycINFO. Available: <http://www.apa.org/psycinfo/>.

American Red Cross (1991). *Disaster services regulations and procedures* (ARC Document 3050M). Washington, DC: Author.

Anderson, M., Kaufman, J., Simon, T. R., Barrios, L., Paulozzi, L., Ryan, G., Hammond, R., Modzeleski, W., Feucht, T., Potter, L., and the School-Associated Violent Deaths Study Group (2001). School associated violent deaths in the United States, 1994-1999. *Journal of the American Medical Association, 286*(21), 2695-2702.

Applied Research and Consulting, Columbia University Mailman School of Public Health, and New York State Psychiatric Institute (2002). Effects of the World Trade Center Attack on NYC public school students: Initial report to the New York City Board of Education. New York: New York City Board of Education. Retrieved July 8, 2002, from <http://www.nycenet.edu/offices/spss/wtc/_needs/firstrep.pdf>.

Bisson, J. I., Jenkins, P. L., Alexander, J., and Bannister, C. (1997). Randomized controlled trial of psychological debriefing for victims of acute burn trauma. *British Journal of Psychiatry, 171,* 78-81.

Bisson, J. I., McFarlane, A. C., and Rose, S. (2000). Psychological debriefing. In E. B. Foa, T. M. Keane, and M. J. Friedman (Eds.). *Effective treatments for*

PTSD: Practice guidelines from the International Society for Traumatic Stress Studies (pp. 39-59, 317-319). New York: Guilford Press.

Boscarino, J. A. (1995). Post-traumatic stress and associated disorders among Vietnam veterans: The significance of combat exposure and social support. *Journal of Traumatic Stress, 8,* 317-336.

Brewin, C. R. (2001). Cognitive and emotional reactions to traumatic events: Implications for short-term interventions. *Advances in Mind-Body Medicine, 17,* 160-196.

Brock, S. E. (2001a). America under attack: What to tell children. CASP guidelines on how to discuss the national tragedy with children and students. Sacramento, CA: California Association of School Psychologists. Retrieved September 13, 2001, from <http://www.casponline.org/whattodo.htm>.

Brock, S. E. (2001b). Identifying seriously traumatized children: Tips for parents and educators. *Communiqué: National Association of School Psychologists, 30*(2), Insert, October.

Brock, S. E. (2001c). Our national tragedy: What to tell children. *CASP Today: Quarterly Newsletter of the California Association of School Psychologists, 50*(4), 14.

Brock, S. E. (2002a). Group crisis intervention. In S. E. Brock, P. J. Lazarus, and S. R. Jimerson (Eds.), *Best practices in school crisis prevention and intervention* (pp. 385-403). Bethesda, MD: National Association of School Psychologists.

Brock, S. E. (2002b). Identifying psychological trauma victims. In S. E. Brock, P. J. Lazarus, and S. R. Jimerson (Eds.), *Best practices in school crisis prevention and intervention* (pp. 367-383). Bethesda, MD: National Association of School Psychologists.

Brock, S. E. (2002c). The nature and consequence of crisis events: A primer for the school psychologist. Unpublished manuscript. California State University, Sacramento.

Brock, S. E. (2002d). Preparing for the school crisis response. In J. Sandoval (Ed.), *Handbook of crisis counseling, intervention and prevention in the schools* (Second edition) (pp. 25-38). Hillsdale, NJ: Erlbaum.

Brock, S. E. and Jimerson, S. R. (2002). One year later. Remembering September 11, 2001: Suggestions for professional educators and other caregivers. Bethesda, MD: National Association of School Psychologists. Retrieved June 23, 2002, from <http://www.nasponline.org/NEAT/oneyearlater.htm/#ftnl>.

Brock, S. E. and Jimerson, S. R. (2004). Characteristics and consequences of crisis events: A primer for the school psychologist. In E. R. Gerler (Ed.), *Handbook of school violence* (pp. 273-284). Binghamton, NY: The Haworth Press.

Brock, S. E. and Poland, S. (2002). School crisis preparedness. In S. E. Brock, P. J. Lazarus, and S. R. Jimerson (Eds.), *Best practices in school crisis prevention and intervention* (pp. 274-288). Bethesda, MD: National Association of School Psychologists.

Brock, S. E., Sandoval, J., and Lewis, S. (2001). *Preparing for crises in the schools: A manual for building school crisis response teams* (Second edition). New York: Wiley.

Campfield, K. M. and Hills, A. M. (2001). Effect of timing of critical incident stress debriefing (CISD) on posttraumatic symptoms. *Journal of Traumatic Stress, 14,* 327-339.

Chemtob, C., Tomas, S., Law, W., and Cremniter, D. (1997). Postdisaster psychosocial interventions: A field study of the impact of debriefing on psychological distress. *American Journal of Psychiatry, 154,* 415-417.

Cohen, S. and Willis, T. A. (1985). Stress, social support, and the buffering hypothesis. *Psychological Bulletin, 98,* 310-355.

Conlon, L., Fahy, T. J., and Conroy, R. (1999). PTSK in ambulant RTA victims: A randomized controlled trial of debriefing. *Journal of Psychosomatic Research, 46,* 37-44.

Deahl, M., Srinivsan, M., Jones, N., Thomas, J., Neblett, D., and Jolly, A. (2000). Preventing psychological trauma in soldiers: The role of operational stress training and psychological debriefing. *British Journal of Medical Psychology, 73,* 77-85.

Everly, G. S. (2000). Crisis management briefings (CMB): Large group crisis intervention in response to terrorism, disasters, and violence. *International Journal of Emergency Mental Health, 2,* 53-57.

Everly, G. S. and Mitchell, J. T. (2000). The debriefing "controversy" and crisis intervention: A review of lexical and substantive issues. *International Journal of Emergency Mental Health, 2,* 211-225.

Foa, E. B., Hebree, E. A., Riggs, D., Rauch, S., and Franklin, M. (2001), Guidelines for mental health professionals' response to the recent tragic events in the U.S. Retrieved November 11, 2001, from <http://www.ncptsd.org/facts/disasters/fs_foa_advice.html>.

Foa, E. B. and Meadows, E. A. (1997). Psychosocial treatments for posttraumatic stress disorder: A critical review. *Annual Review of Psychology, 48,* 449-480.

Foa, E. B. and Meadows, E. A. (1998). Psychosocial treatments for posttraumatic stress disorder. In R. Yehuda (Ed.), *Psychological trauma* (pp. 179-204). Washington, DC: American Psychiatric Press.

Gist, R. and Lubin, B. (Eds.) (1999). *Response to disaster: Psychosocial, community, and ecological approaches.* Philadelphia, PA: Brunner-Mazel.

Green, B. L., Korol, M., Grace, M. C., Vary, M. G., Leonard, A., Gleser, G. C., and Smitson-Cohen, S. (1991). Children and disaster: Age, gender, and parental effects on PTSD symptoms. *Journal of the American Academy of Child and Adolescent Psychiatry, 30,* 945-951.

Gurwitch, R. H., Sitterle, K. A., Young, B. H., and Pfefferbaum, B. (2002). The aftermath of terrorism. In A. M. La Greca, W. K. Silverman, E. M. Vernberg, and M. C. Roberts (Eds.), *Helping children cope with disasters and terrorism* (pp. 327-357). Washington, DC: American Psychological Association.

Handford, H. A., Mayes, S. D., Mattison, R. E., Humphrey, F. J., Bagnato, S., Bixler, E. O., and Kales, J. D. (1986). Child and parent reactions to the Three Mile Island nuclear accident. *Journal of the American Academy of Child Psychiatry, 25,* 346-356.

Hansell, P. S., Hughes, C. B., Caliandro, G., Russo, P., Budin, W. C., Hartman, B., and Hernandes, O. C. (1998). The effect of a social support boosting intervention on stress, coping, and social support in caregivers of children with HIV/AIDS. *Nursing Research, 47,* 79-86.

Harvey, J. H., Orbuch, T. L., Chwalisz, K. D., and Garwood, G. (1991). Coping with sexual assault: The roles of account-making and confiding. *Journal of Traumatic Stress, 4,* 515-531.

Herman, R., Kaplan, M., and LeMelle, S. (2002). Psychoeducational debriefings after the September 11 disaster. *Psychiatric Services, 53,* 479.

Hillman, H. S., Jones, R. T., and Farmer, L. (1986). The acquisition and maintenance of fire emergency skills: Effects of rationale and behavioral practice. *Journal of Pediatric Psychology, 11,* 247-258.

Hobbs, M., Mayou, R., Harrison, B., and Warlock, P. (1996). A randomized trial of psychological debriefing for victims of road traffic accidents. *British Medical Journal, 313,* 1438-1439.

Holaday, M. and Smith, A. (1995). Coping skills training: Evaluating a training model. *Journal of Mental Health Counseling, 17,* 360-346.

Jeney-Gammon, P., Daugherty, T. K., Finch, A. J., Belter, R. W., and Foster, K. Y. (1993). Children's coping styles and report of depressive symptoms following a natural disaster. *Journal of Genetic Psychology, 154,* 259-267.

Jimerson, S. R. and Brock, S. E. (2002). *School crisis management plan: An exemplar.* Sacramento, CA: California Association of School Psychologists.

Jones, R. T., Ollendick, T. H., McLaughlin, K. J., and Williams, C. E. (1989). Elaborative and behavioral rehearsal in the acquisition of fire emergency skills and the reduction of fire fear. *Behavior Therapy, 20,* 93-101.

Keane, T. M., Scott, W. O., Chavoya, G. A., Lamparski, D. M., and Fairbank, J. A. (1985). Social support in Vietnam veterans with post-traumatic stress disorder: A comparative analysis. *Journal of Consulting and Clinical Psychology, 53,* 95-102.

Kenardy, J. A., Webster, R. A., Lewin, T. J., Carr, V. J., Hazell, P. L., and Carter, G. L. (1996). Stress debriefing and patterns of recovery following a natural disaster. *Journal of Traumatic Stress, 9,* 37-49.

King, L. A., King, D. W., Fairbank, J. A., Keane, T. M., and Adams, G. A. (1998). Resilience-recovery factors in post-traumatic stress disorder among female and male Vietnam veterans: Hardiness, postwar social support, and additional stressful life events. *Journal of Personality and Social Psychology, 74,* 420-434.

Kiselica, M. S., Baker, S. B., Thomas, R. N., and Reedy, S. (1994). Effects of stress inoculation training on anxiety, stress, and academic performance among adolescents. *Journal of Counseling Psychology, 41,* 335-342.

Klingman, A. (2001). Stress responses and adaptation of Israeli school-age children evacuated from homes during massive missile attacks. *Anxiety, Stress, and Coping, 14,* 149-172.

La Greca, A. M., Silverman, W. K., Vernberg, E. M., and Prinstein, M. J. (1996). Symptoms of posttraumatic stress after Hurricane Andrew: A prospective study. *Journal of Consulting and Clinical Psychology, 64,* 712-723.

Leffler, C. T. and Dembert, M. L. (1998). Posttraumatic stress symptoms among U.S. Navy divers recovering TWA flight 800. *Journal of Nervous and Mental Disease, 186,* 574-577.

Litz, B. T., Gray, M. J., Bryant, R. A., and Adler, A. B. (2002). Early intervention for trauma: Current status and future directions. *Clinical Psychology: Science and Practice, 9,* 112-134.

Llabre, M. M. and Hadi, F. (1997). Social support and psychological distress in Kuwaiti boys and girls exposed to the Gulf crisis. *Journal of Consulting and Clinical Psychology, 26,* 247-255.

March, J. S., Amaya-Jackson, L., Terry, R., and Costanzo, P. (1997). Posttraumatic symptomatology in children and adolescents after an industrial fire. *Journal of the American Academy of Child and Adolescent Psychiatry, 36,* 1080-1088.

Martin, L., Rosen, L. N., Durand, D. B., Knudson, K. H., and Stretch, R. H. (2000). Psychological and physical health effects of sexual assaults and nonsexual traumas among male and female United States Army soldiers. *Behavioral Medicine, 26,* 23-33.

Mayou, R. A., Ehlers, A., and Hobbs, M. (2000). Psychological debriefing for road traffic accident victims: Three-year follow-up of a randomized controlled trial. *British Journal of Psychiatry, 176,* 589-593.

McFarlane, A. C. (1987). Posttraumatic functioning in a longitudinal study of children following a natural disaster. *Journal of the American Academy of Child and Adolescent Psychiatry, 26,* 764-769.

McFarlane, A. (1988). The longitudinal course of post-traumatic morbidity: The range of outcomes and their predictors. *Journal of Nervous and Mental Disease, 176,* 30-39.

McFarlane, A. (2000). Can debriefing work? Critical appraisal of theories of interventions and outcomes, with directions for future research. In B. Raphael and J. P. Wilson (Eds.), *Psychological debriefing: Theory, practice and evidence* (pp. 327-336). New York: Cambridge University Press.

McFarlane, A. C. and Yehuda, R. (1996). Resilience, vulnerability, and the course of posttraumatic reactions. In B. A. van der Kolk, A. C. McFarlane, and L. Weisaeth (Eds.), *Traumatic stress: The effects of overwhelming experience on mind, body, and society* (pp. 155-181). New York: Guilford Press.

Milne, G. (1977). Cyclone Tracy: II. The effects on Darwin children. *Australian Psychologist, 12,* 55-62.

National Institute of Mental Health (2001). *Helping children and adolescents cope with violence and disasters.* Retrieved June 17, 2002, from <http://www.nimh.nih.gov/anxietymenu.cfm>.

National Institute of Mental Health (2002). *Mental health and mass violence: Evidence-based early psychological intervention for victims/survivors of mass violence. A workshop to reach consensus on best practices* [NIH Publication No. 02-5138]. Washington, DC: U.S. Government Printing Office.

Norris, F. H., Byrne, C. M., Diaz, E., and Kaniasty, K. (2001). Psychosocial resources in the aftermath of natural and human-caused disasters: A review of the empirical literature, with implications for intervention. Retrieved June 13, 2002, from <http://www.ncpstd.org/fact/disasters/fs_resources.html>.

Omer, H. and Alon, N. (1994). The continuity principle: A unified approach to disaster and trauma. *American Journal of Community Psychology, 22,* 273-287.

Pagliocca, P. M., Nickerson, A. B., and Williams, S. H. (2002). Research and evaluation directions in crisis intervention. In S. E. Brock and P. J. Lazarus (Eds.), *Best practices in school crisis intervention and prevention* (pp. 771-790). Bethesda, MD: National Association of School Psychologists.

Pennebaker, J. W. and O'Heeron, R. C. (1984). Confiding in others and illness rate among spouses of suicide and accident-death victims. *Journal of Abnormal Psychology, 93,* 473-476.

Petersen, S. and Straub, R. L. (1992). *School crisis survival guide: Management techniques and materials for counselors and administrators.* West Nyack, NY: Center for Applied Research in Education.

Poland, S. and McCormick, J. S. (1999). *Coping with crisis: Lessons learned.* Longmont, CO: Sopris West.

Prinstein, M. J., La Greca, A. M., Vernberg, E. M., and Silverman, W. K. (1996). Children's coping assistance: How parents, teachers, and friends help children cope after a natural disaster. *Journal of Clinical and Child Psychology, 25,* 463-475.

Pynoos, R. S., Frederick, C., Nader, K., Steinberg, A., Eth, S., Nune, F., and Fairbanks, L. (1987). Life threat and posttraumatic stress in school-age children. *Archives of General Psychiatry, 44,* 1057-1063.

Richards, D. (2001). A filed study of critical incident stress debriefing versus critical incident stress management. *Journal of Mental Health, 10,* 351-362.

Ronan, K. R., Johnston, D. M., Daly, M., and Fairley, R. (2001). Schoolchildren's risk perceptions and preparedness: A hazards education survey. *The Australasian Journal of Disaster and Trauma Studies, 5*(1), NP.

Rose, S., Brewin, C. R., Andrews, B., and Kirk, M. (1999). A randomized controlled trial of individual psychological debriefing for victims of violent crime. *Psychological Medicine, 29,* 793-799.

Rose, S., Wessely, W., and Bisson, J. (1998). Brief psychological interventions ("debriefing") for trauma-related symptoms and prevention of posttraumatic stress disorder (Cochrane Review). In *The Cochrane Library, 2.* Oxford: Update Software.

Seiffge-Krenke, I., Weidemann, S., Fentner, S., Aegenheister, N., and Poeblau, M. (2001). Coping with school-related stress and family stress in healthy and clinically referred adolescents. *European Psychologist, 6,* 123-132.

Silverman, W. K. and La Greca, A. M. (2002). Children experiencing disasters: Definitions, reactions, and predictors of outcomes. In A. M. La Greca, W. K. Silverman, E. M. Vernberg, and M. C. Roberts (Eds.), *Helping children cope with disasters and terrorism* (pp. 11-33). Washington, DC: American Psychological Association.

Slaikeu, K. (1990). *Crisis intervention: A handbook for practice and research* (Second edition). Newton, MA: Allyn & Bacon.

Stallard, P. (2000). Debriefing adolescents after critical life events. In B. Raphael and J. P. Wilson (Eds.), *Psychological debriefing: Theory, practice and evidence* (pp. 213-224). New York: Cambridge University Press.

Thomas, C. L. (Ed.) (1993). *Taber's encyclopedic medical dictionary* (Seventh edition). Philadelphia: F. A. Davis.

Turner, A. L. (2000). Group treatment of trauma survivors following a fatal bus accident: Integrating theory and practice. *Group Dynamics: Theory, Research, and Practice, 4,* 139-149.

Valent, P. (2000). Disaster syndrome. In G. Fink (Ed.), *Encyclopedia of stress,* Volume 1 (pp. 706-709). San Diego, CA: Academic Press.

Vernberg, E. M. (2002). Intervention approaches following disasters. In A. M. La Greca, W. K. Silverman, E. M. Vernberg, and M. C. Roberts (Eds.), *Helping children cope with disasters and terrorism* (pp. 55-72). Washington, DC: American Psychological Association.

Vernberg, E. M., La Greca, A. M., Silverman, W. K., and Prinstein, M. J. (1996). Predictors of children's post-disaster functioning following Hurricane Andrew. *Journal of Abnormal Psychology, 105,* 237-248.

Vernberg, E. M. and Vogel, J. (1993). Interventions with children following disasters. *Journal of Clinical Child Psychology, 22,* 485-498.

Vogel, J. M. and Vernberg, E. M. (1993). Children's psychological responses to disasters. *Journal of Clinical Child Psychology, 22,* 464-484.

Young, B. H., Ford, J. D., Ruzek, J. I., Friedman, M., and Gusman, F. D. (1998). *Disaster mental health services: A guide for clinicians and administrators.* Palo Alto, CA: National Center for Post Traumatic Stress Disorder.

Yule, W. (2001). When disaster strikes—the need to be "wise before the event": Crisis intervention with children and adults. *Advances in Mind-Body Research, 17,* 191-196.

Chapter 11

Support Services
Following a Shooting at School:
Lessons Learned Regarding Response
and Recovery

Robert L. McGlenn
Shane R. Jimerson

On March 5, 2001, at approximately 9:22 a.m., a 15-year-old freshman at Santana High School (Santee, California) opened fire from a rest room onto a busy quad while hundreds of students changed classes. Two students were killed. Eleven students were wounded. One student teacher and one campus supervisor were wounded. Based upon a survey conducted four days after the shooting, it is estimated that over 500 people were in harm's way and witnessed the shootings (see Table 11.1 for a summary of survey results). From that moment on, the world changed for 1,774 students, 130 staff and faculty at Santana High School, and an entire community.

When responding to a shooting on campus, the capturing of the shooter, the bandaging of the wounded, and the uniting of the families is only the start on the road to recovery. The visions of that day continue for days, weeks, months, and for some even years. Although limited research specifically addresses school crisis response and intervention efforts, many lessons are learned from those who have been involved with response and intervention efforts in the aftermath of school shootings (Brock, Lazarus, and Jimerson, 2002). The response efforts include immediate crisis management and long-term mental health and counseling services to support students. While acknowledging contextual and individual variation, the experiences following the shootings at Santana High School warrant consideration by

TABLE 11.1. Summary of School Survey Results Four Days After the Shooting (*n* = 871 students and staff)

Item	Number Affirming	Percentage of Respondents
Injured during the shooting	5	1
Believed you were shot at	94	11
Were fearful that you could have been shot at	480	55
Witnessed other(s) being shot	298	34
Cared for someone wounded	327	38
Had a close relationship with the deceased	136	16
Have close relationship with a shooting victim	249	29
Have close relationship with the shooter	62	7

other professionals preparing school crisis management plans. This chapter provides an overview and lessons learned regarding the immediate response, aftershocks, and student support services. This information is offered as a contribution to emerging knowledge addressing student support services following a crisis on campus (e.g., Brock, Lazarus, and Jimerson, 2002).

THE IMMEDIATE RESPONSE

As an off-duty policeman and two deputies stormed the rest room a little over six minutes had passed since the initial sounds of "firecrackers" resonated from the rest room. By then the streets and skies were filled with emergency personnel and media responding to the crisis. SWAT team members stormed the school carefully searching each classroom for wounded individuals or possible accomplices. The wounded were ushered to the front of the school where paramedics triaged the casualties and evacuated them to area hospitals. The other students were evacuated to a small mall across the street where they were reunited with their parents amidst a frenzy of media. Because the school immediately became a crime scene and under control of law enforcement, the principal and administrative staff united at the fast-food restaurant that became the impromptu crisis command center. Their initial tasks focused on accounting for all staff and students. Administrators, psychologists, and counselors from across the district were joined by mental health volunteers in comforting students, staff, and parents. Once all of the students were accounted for, the staff was briefed and assistance was given to get the students home.

The structured response to the communities' need for information and support went into effect immediately. A phone bank was established in the district office to provide the latest official information. A church near the school was designated the location for the next three days where individuals and families could come for information and counseling. Care was taken to ensure all information provided to the media came directly from the superintendent or his designate. On the night of the first day students returned to school, a meeting occurred in the school's gym in which the superintendent, principal, sheriff, district attorney, and a psychologist spoke directly to parents. They were told what was being done, what they could expect to happen, and explained the procedure to access victim/witness resources. Information was prepared to be sent home in the coming weeks that described expected emotional occurrences in the coming months and possible referral sources for mental health support.

During the days immediately following the shooting, emphasis was placed on debriefing, confirming the normalcy of the broad range of emotions that had been stimulated from this abnormal situation, and identifying those individuals who needed immediate or individual support services. A group debriefing utilizing the Sanford model was conducted the morning following the shooting for the entire Santana staff. The staff was divided into groups of equal size. Each group leader presented four questions. Each person had two minutes to respond to the question and then it was the next person's turn. The questions were:

> The Fact Question—"Could you please introduce yourself, including your name and job responsibilities, and tell us where you were when the shooting occurred?"
> The Thought Question—"What was your first thought when you had realized what had happened?"

The Feeling Question—"What was your worst feeling?"
The Assessment Question—"What would help you to feel safer right now?"

While this process occurred in unison for all of the groups, mental health professionals were present to give individual support when needed. Once the staff had completed this debriefing, they were told they were released until later in the afternoon when they would be allowed back on campus to collect personal items and organize their classroom. It was explained to them that by that time the campus would be released as a crime scene and it would have been cleaned of all effects of the shooting. They were also informed that the following day the faculty and students would return to the school, which would begin in the midmorning period.

The first day back at school was devoted to giving support and processing the students' experiences. Before the start of school 250 mental health volunteers met in the gymnasium to be prepared to implement the Sanford model of group debriefing. Two mental health professionals were assigned to each classroom to lead the class in the debriefing. They stayed with the teacher and his or her classes upon the discretion of the teacher. The other volunteers were assigned throughout the campus in the halls, in the office, and at the makeshift monuments that had emerged. Volunteer mental health professionals were also available in the three safe rooms that had been established for students, staff, and parents to receive counseling. During the first day the students also received a letter from the principal sharing her thoughts and asking them to write to her regarding their experiences and feelings.

Direct individual and group support services and counseling continued on campus for the coming weeks. To monitor the outcome of those contacts, the mental health professionals wrote a brief assessment each time a student or staff member was counseled. This information, along with the responses to the principal's letter and a survey that was completed four days after the shooting, was compiled to create a hierarchy of risk assessment. Those students and staff who were closest to the shooting or who knew the victims or the shooter well were considered to have the highest priority. The results of the initial surveys demonstrated that many students and staff were involved in various ways, through their experiences and relationships (see Table

11.1). High-risk students and staff were monitored and met frequently with the mental health volunteers (see Jimerson and Brock, 2001, for a review of immediate crisis response activities from the perspective of the California National Emergency Assistance Team through collaborative efforts of the U.S. Department of Education, the National Association of School Psychologists, and the California Association of School Psychologists).

AFTERSHOCKS

As with an earthquake, those who are closest to the epicenter during a school crisis are usually the most traumatized (Pfohl, Jimerson, and Lazarus, 2002). The model of an earthquake continues to apply in that events after the initial shooting may stimulate an increase in PTSD symptoms and may possibly retraumatize victims. The first such aftershock occurred on the second day after school reopened, when an e-mail to campus computers threatened to finish the job the next day. The entire school was quickly ushered into the gym and a rally was held to take back the school and not let someone interfere with education. The next day over 90 percent of the student body attended school and were supported by 18 members of the San Diego Chargers professional football team who signed autographs where and at the time that the shooting had taken place.

The next aftershock to the school came 16 days later on March 22, when a shooting occurred at Granite Hills High School, a school five miles away and in the same district. This resulted in a need for increased services at Santana and other schools in the district. Other events outside the school that created anxiety included the terrorist attacks on September 11 and news programs related to the shooting. Normal campus occurrences such as a fire drill or a fight between students resulted in anxiety attacks for some people. The anniversary date was anticipated with trepidation by many and required extensive planning to reduce fears and encourage attendance. As a result of these efforts and despite the emotions it elicited, 94 percent of the students attended that day. For some, the day was an affirmation of their experience while for others it unleashed repressed feelings and fears.

THE SHORT-TERM TREATMENT PLAN

In designing a treatment system certain factors were taken into consideration including (1) the large number of traumatized, (2) the accessibility of services, (3) the wide range of responses possible in terms of onset and nature, and (4) the reluctance of adolescents to willingly admit to needing help. When faced with similar criteria other locations such as the Oklahoma City bombing (Pfefferbaum, Call, and Sconzo, 1999), Columbine High School shootings (Weintraub, Hall, and Pynoos, 2001), Northridge, California, earthquakes (Pynoos, Goenjian, and Steinberg, 1998), and community violence (Saltzman et al., in press) found school-based treatment services an essential part of a successful recovery program. After reviewing the literature and consulting with Dr. Robert Pynoos, Director of the Trauma Psychiatry Services at UCLA Neuropsychiatric Institute and the local district and school officials, a school-based trauma unit was established at Santana High School.

The mission of the Santana Recovery Project was to

1. serve as an information and referral agency to the campus and the community and to serve as a clearinghouse for other agencies that provided services,
2. provide direct mental health services to those traumatized by the shooting, and
3. help develop and participate in campus activities which promoted healing.

The project was housed in a large trailer that was added to the campus, and services were provided by four licensed mental health professionals. The therapists included one psychologist, one licensed clinical social worker, one marriage/family therapist/registered nurse, and the project coordinator who held licenses as a clinical psychologist, marriage/family therapist, and a school psychologist. All four professionals had extensive experience working with victims of trauma. The project was principally funded by grants from the U.S. Department of Education's Safe and Drug-Free Schools Program (Project SERV [School Emergency Response to Violence]), San Diego County Health and Human Services, and monies from the Grossmont Union High School District.

The integration of a school-based mental health treatment unit on a school campus necessitated adjustments to be made by all parties. The protocol-driven, decision-making model of the health services professions with its clear-cut formulas of right or wrong are contrary to the principle-driven, decision-making model of schools which focus on situational variables, resources and options, strategic priorities, and cultural and political climate (Johnson, 2000). Educating district and school officials as to what to expect in the aftermath of the shooting and how to treat it was the first crucial step in establishing the clinic component of the project. In turn, the project staff had to learn to adjust to the mores, culture, and procedures of the school in order to be accepted by the administration and staff. Consequently the project maintained a balance between being part of yet separate from the campus. Free-flowing communication about students occurred between the school's counseling staff and the therapists. This allowed for collaboration in helping students in all areas of need. Limited exchange of information occurred between the project and the school's administration in regard to school staff in treatment. This allowed staff to feel safe to contact the project for therapy.

The philosophy of the Santana Recovery Project was to seek out those in need rather than wait for them to step forward. This occurred with the staff through education and personal contact. By assigning one particular therapist to the staff, a sense of exclusivity and trust developed between the staff and the therapist thus contributing to a greater sense of confidentiality. The students were sought out more directly by administration of a survey which measured levels of PTSD, depression, anxiety, and existence of previous loss or grief.

In late May and early June, 268 of the soon-to-graduate seniors completed the Santana Recovery Project Survey that was designed by the UCLA Trauma Psychiatry program specifically for Santana. From this survey students were identified who had higher levels of PTSD, many of whom had not previously recognized or acknowledged their symptoms. When interviewed, many of them better understood feelings they were experiencing and agreed to participate in private support services or those offered through the project. A similar survey with some variations was administered in November and December to all of the 2001-2002 tenth, eleventh, and twelfth graders. As was done in the previous survey, an implied consent permission form was sent home to the parents. Twenty-two parents refused to have their child surveyed. During the administration of the survey 52 students refused to complete the form. Twenty of the surveys completed were determined to be invalid or incomplete. Of the 1,160 valid surveys, 95 had scored significantly high on a combination of the scales to warrant further investigation and an immediate interview. Other students were interviewed based on their responses to certain sections or questions. For example, in response to the question "I feel like hurting myself . . ." 16 checked "most of the time." These students, along with the 47 that checked "sometimes," were immediately interviewed and interventions were initiated when necessary.

In addition to individual and group therapy conducted at the project trailer, other therapeutic interventions were provided in collaboration with the school. Through the project, Scripps Hospital donated, designed, and implemented a project titled "Reflections of Hope." All seniors and staff members were given disposable cameras to take pictures of things that brought them hope, joy, or inspiration. Each participant selected one photo that was enlarged and displayed at graduation. On another occasion the artwork of the staff was displayed at Scripps Mercy Hospital under the title "The Art of Healing." The anniversary date posed a potential trigger for PTSD symptoms for many in the school. To counterbalance fears and to address emotions, a day consisting of classes, a brief ceremony, and a barbecue was designed, preceded by extensive communication with parents, students, and the media. The weekend prior to the anniversary date a 5K run/walk titled "Safe Schools Tribute" attracted 1,001 entrants and an even larger crowd of supporters in a positive affirmation of life and moving forward.

OBSERVATIONS AND LESSONS LEARNED

Given an almost overwhelming request for services, it is clear that a school shooting such as the one at Santana High School can have a major impact on the emotional state of a large number of people. Clearly, when services are provided in a convenient and timely fashion, victims of such a tragedy can improve quickly. By the end of the 2002 school year, 16 months after the shooting, the project practitioners had officially treated over 500 students and over 75 staff. Of the 130 staff that worked at Santana at the time of the shooting, nine took a leave of absence of four weeks or more at some time during the first year and then returned to work. One employee retired as a result of suffering a heart attack during the shooting and another went out on disability and eventually transferred to another school after the anniversary. Although anecdotal data suggested an increase in reckless behavior and substance abuse among the students, no hard data confirmed this. No reported deaths or serious accidents occurred to any students or staff 16 months after the shooting.

Some life-altering changes did occur for some of the students and staff. A few students who had enlisted in the armed services were discharged due to flashbacks. Others had difficulty concentrating in college and found college more difficult than expected. At least one young lady, who previously had no history of drug abuse, was treated for addiction and selling cocaine. In addition, there are the "silent sufferers" who never sought treatment, yet continue to have difficulty sleeping, concentrating, and lack motivation.

Some changed their lives for the better. Several students reported that after the shooting they had stopped abusing substances and focused more on graduating. Some students and staff made significant progress in confronting old traumas and as a result felt free and at peace for the first time. Many dedicated themselves to achieving more in their lives.

The following observations emerged from the response and intervention services following the tragic shooting at Santana High School:

- Victims respond to and recover from a school shooting in different ways and at different rates.
- A school-based treatment facility is an effective way to provide services to large numbers of trauma victims.
- Surveying students is an effective way to identify those who are experiencing posttraumatic stress and related mental health difficulties.
- A significant number of individuals identified through the survey who were experiencing symptoms of posttraumatic stress had not sought assistance, even ten months after the shooting.
- The trauma of the shooting ignited, and made worse, in many individuals, previous traumas and mental health issues.

- The institution experiences and responds to trauma in a similar fashion, as does an individual.
- Events on campus, such as anonymous threats of more shootings, student fights, and fire drills as well as off-campus events, such as the shooting at Granite Hills and the September 11 terrorist attacks, served as aftershocks which retraumatized many individuals.

Although the trauma from a school shooting can be extensive, through the use of immediate, convenient, and proactive mental health interventions, the damage may be addressed and recovery can be achieved. Tragic crisis events such as school shootings affect children, families, educational professionals, schools, and communities in innumerable ways, thus, schools and communities should prepare for such events (Jimerson and Huff, 2002). Ongoing preparation and training of educational and mental health professionals will help to address the relevant issues by acquiring knowledge of the issues and methods for supportive intervention in both the classroom and a group setting.

Comprehensive school crisis management plans and advanced preparation are important in preparing to respond to a crisis event at school (Dwyer and Jimerson, 2002). Such plans must include professional mental health resources that can assist in providing appropriate support services for diverse students, families, faculty, and staff. "Because it is not a matter of 'if,' but rather 'when,' an event will occur" (Jimerson and Huff, 2002, p. 466), educational professionals are encouraged to engage in professional development and prepare a comprehensive crisis management plan. The lessons learned regarding response and recovery following a school shooting may facilitate the efforts in preparing and providing support services following a crisis on campus.

REFERENCES

Brock, S. E., Lazarus, P. J., and Jimerson, S. R. (Eds.) (2002). *Best Practices in School Crisis Prevention and Intervention.* Bethesda, MD: National Association of School Psychologists.

Dwyer, K. and Jimerson, S. (2002). Enabling prevention through planning. In S. E. Brock, P. J. Lazarus, and S. R. Jimerson (Eds.), *Best Practices in School Crisis*

Prevention and Intervention (pp. 23-46). Bethesda, MD: National Association of School Psychologists.

Jimerson, S. R. and Brock, S. E. (2001). NASP/CASP response following shootings on school campuses. *National Association of School Psychologists—National Association of School Psychologists Communiqúe, 29*(6), 7.

Jimerson, S. and Huff, L. (2002). Responding to a sudden, unexpected death at school: Chance favors the prepared professional. In S. E. Brock, P. J. Lazarus, and S. R. Jimerson (Eds.), *Best Practices in School Crisis Prevention and Intervention* (pp. 451-488). Bethesda, MD: National Association of School Psychologists.

Johnson, K. (2000). Crisis response to schools. *International Journal of Emergency Mental Health, 2*(3), 173-180.

Pfefferbaum, B., Call, J. A., and Sconzo, G. M. (1999). Mental health services for children in the first two years after the 1995 Oklahoma City terrorist bombing. *Psychiatric Services, 50*(7), 956-958.

Pfohl, W., Jimerson, S. R., and Lazarus, P. J. (2002). Developmental aspects of trauma and grief. In S. E. Brock, P. J. Lazarus, and S. R. Jimerson (Eds.), *Best Practices in School Crisis Prevention and Intervention* (pp. 311-334). Bethesda, MD: National Association of School Psychologists.

Pynoos, R. S., Goenjian, A. K., and Steinberg, A. M. (1998). A public mental health approach to the postdisaster treatment of children and adolescents. *Child and Adolescent Psychiatric Clinics of North America, 7,* 195-210.

Saltzman, W. R., Pynoos, R. S., Layne, C. M., Steinberg, A., and Aisenberg, E. (in press). School-Based Trauma/Grief Group Psychotherapy Program for Youth Exposed to Community Violence, UCLA Psychotherapy Modules.

Weintraub, P., Hall, H. L., and Pynoos, R. S. (2001). Columbine High School shootings: Community response. In M. Shafii and S. L. Shafii (Eds.), *School Violence: Assessment, Management, Prevention* (pp. 129-161). Washington, DC, American Psychiatric Publishing.

Index